Brain-Wise

Patricia Smith Churchland

Brain-Wise

Studies in Neurophilosophy

A Bradford Book
The MIT Press
Cambridge, Massachusetts
London, England

This book was set in Times New Roman on 3B2 by Asco Typesetters, Hong Kong, and was printed and bound in the United States of America.

Library of Congress Cataloging-in-Publication Data

Churchland, Patricia Smith.
  Brain-Wise : studies in neurophilosophy / Patricia Smith Churchland.
       p.   cm.
  Includes bibliographical references and index.
  ISBN 0-262-03301-1 (hc : alk. paper) — ISBN 0-262-53200-X (pbk : alk. paper)
  1. Neurosciences—Philosophy. 2. Cognitive science—Philosophy. I. Title: Studies in neurophilosophy. II. Title.
  [DNLM: 1. Neuropsychology. 2. Knowledge. Metaphysics. 4. Neurology.
5. Philosophy. 6. Religion and Psychology.   WL 103.5 C563b 2002]
  RC343 .C486   2002
  153′.01—dc21   2002066024

10 9 8 7 6 5 4 3 2 1

Contents

Preface

A lot of water has passed over the dam since I published *Neurophilosophy* in 1986. Groundbreaking advances have been made in computational methods, in neuroscientific techniques, and in cross-field connections. Fruitful interactions have developed, for example, between molecular biology and neuroscience, and between experimental psychology and neuroscience. Philosophers, initially wary (to put it politely) of the idea that neuroscience might have some relevance to the problems they call their own, have slowly warmed to the idea of neurophilosophy. Two decades ago, proposing an undergraduate course in neurophilosophy was more or less a bad joke. Now such courses are beginning to spring up even in departments that had been proudly "antibrain." Students not only in philosophy but also in the sciences are signing up and eagerly attacking philosophy's Big Problems—such as the nature of consciousness, free will, and the self—in full recognition that neuroscientific data are indispensable to making progress. Alert to the change in philosophical winds, various people began to needle me concerning the absence of an introductory, single-authored neurophilosophy text. This book is the response to that needling.

I have assumed that an introductory text should provide a basic framework for how the brain sciences—the neurosciences and cognitive science—can interface with traditional topics in philosophy. Insofar as it is *elementary*, such a text should be as compact and uncluttered as is consistent with being pedagogically serviceable. Of necessity, this means keeping in-text references to an almost indecent minimum; it means slimming the number of suggested readings. It means making incendiary choices about which research best illustrates a point and which debates are worth recounting. Although selectivity serves the goal of presenting a fairly clean picture of how I see things, it carries a price, not least of which is the undying wrath of colleagues who feel stiffed by the trade-off between spare functionality and congested citation. The chips will have to as fall they may, however, since my primary goal is that the book be *useful* to those who want a panoramic view of philosophical problems as they appear from the vantage point of the brain sciences. I could not reasonably aim to make this book encyclopedic; I could aim to make it coherent and compact.

To be useful as an introduction, a book ought not to presuppose very much background knowledge of the subject. I have tried to abide by that rule. What I have presupposed is that readers totally unacquainted with neuroscience or with cognitive science will choose a good text to have handy in case of need. To assist in that choice, I make some general suggestions in the reading list of the introductory chapter, and topic-specific suggestions in subsequent chapters. There are excellent journals, websites, and encyclopedias to augment a beginner's background, and I have also listed a subset of those journals that contain good review papers or that are widely considered indispensable to keeping abreast of the developments in the brain sciences.

The book contains more neurobiological detail than one would typically find in a philosophy text. The rationale derives from the need to illustrate—and not merely preach—that understanding the neuroscientific detail is no mere frill if you intend to do more than play at philosophical problems, such as the nature of consciousness or learning. A continuing difficulty for philosophers is to be sufficiently versed in basic neuroscience to be able to tell whether the results of a reported experiment mean anything, and if so, what. Though I cannot solve this difficulty, I might reduce its size by conveying the need to understand the experimental design, the nature of the controls, possible flaws of interpretation, and so forth by discussing detail from selected experiments.

Though experimental detail is crucial, it is also important not to smother one's cognitive operations. They need time and space to mull. As philosopher and computer scientist Brian Smith once mused, some things that brains do *very* well, they do *very* slowly, over long stretches of time, and in a chewing-on-the-cud sort of way. These are typically the problem-solving and creative things that existing computers cannot do at all. In the same vein, Francis Crick observes that if you are too busy, you are probably wasting your time. With this thought in mind, I have reigned in my impulse to recommend readings ad infinitum. Since those readings I do recommend reflect my particular prejudices, curious readers will want to go afield for other points of view.

Again and again I have found the history of science invaluable in getting my bearings. The fact is, neuroscience is still an immature science, in the sense that it is still groping for the fundamental explanatory principles governing brain function. In this respect, it contrasts with molecular biology, for example, where the basic principles of the chemical structure of genes, how genes get turned on and off, and how proteins get made are essentially in place. Because neuroscience is still wet behind the ears, we probably have only the vaguest glimmerings of what remains to be discovered and no idea how the discoveries will change our heartfelt convictions about the nature of the mind. Heartfelt convictions, unavoidable though they may be, can be an intellectual nuisance. They have a way of posing as *nonnegotiable certainties*, as *verities*, and as *metaphysical truths*. Despite their convincing pose, they in fact are just bits of *conventional* wisdom. The history of science provides bracing tales of conventional wisdom as obstructing progress, as failure of imagination, and as dogma. History also shows both that *sometimes* the crackpots turn out to be right, but that being a crackpot is *no* guarantee of being right.

In hopes that the history might be likewise useful for others, I found myself telling science stories where they provide a helpful slant on current problems. These are tales about scientific error and scientific discovery, about scientific tenacity and humility, as well as about scientific arrogance and scientific oblivion. Many are stories of conventional wisdom turned arse over teakettle. Their particular relevance pertains to the search for knowledge in the broadest sense, irrespective of the topic. By putting some distance between us and our heartfelt convictions, these stories give us room to think. Oddly, the history of science is seldom taught to science students, yet it is this history that helps generate a sense of how to ask the right questions and how progress on the tough problems can be made.

Not surprisingly, I have also found the history of *philosophy* invaluable in putting current philosophical orthodoxy at arm's length. This is not because I subscribe to the goofy theory according to which the historical giants knew more because they knew less. I emphatically do not. Rather, it is because some of the greats were just a whole lot broader in their interests and a whole lot more curious about nature in general than are many of today's mainstream philosophers. This is manifestly true of those oldies for whom I have enduring fondness: Aristotle, Hume, and Peirce. My fondness is also explained by the get-on-with-it reason that they are clear and sensible, logical and bold. While these are not virtues for cult figures, they are virtues if one is trying to understand the nature of things.

In my opinion, much of what is considered *not quite mainstream* philosophy is where the exciting action is now to be found in academic philosophy. This work is enthusiastically cross-disciplinary. It leaves the borders between academic disciplines looking like the mere administrative conveniences they should be. Philosophy students are plugging into congenial labs, while students in neuroscience, cognitive science, and computer science are coming to realize that philosophical questions about the mind are at bottom just broad questions about the mind, and they can be addressed through experimental techniques. They are also learning that philosophy is often useful in showing where the logical minefields lie. This trend is putting blood back into philosophy, making it much more akin to the vigorous and expansive discipline it has been through most of its very long history. This trend is also heartening to those students who were lured into neuroscience by the big questions but found themselves endlessly tagging proteins.

Over the years so many people have taught me about the brain and about how to do science that I cannot begin properly to thank them all. Let me start, however, with Francis Crick, who has been a constant fount of ideas, not only of predictably ingenious ones but also, occasionally at least, of reassuringly flawed ones. His relentlessness in addressing a problem, accompanied by warnings to avoid falling in love with one's own theory, gave me the pluck to try things I might otherwise have shied away from. Additionally, Francis has been a consistently fair-minded critic of both my enduring enthusiasms and my ranch-hand skepticism. His knowledge of the history of science, and especially his personal and detailed knowledge of the history of molecular biology, has given me a perspective on neuroscience *as a science* that I could not have had in any other way.

Antonio and Hannah Damasio have patiently taught me how to think about systems-level neuroscience, and have generously shared their insights gleaned from clinical studies. They also firmly but kindly hoisted me out of a rut into which I had comfortably settled. In particular, they caused me to begin looking at consciousness from the perspective of the brain's fundamental "coherencing" functions, as well as from its perceptual functions. In turn, this led me to follow them to consider subcortical brain structures, especially brainstem structures, as the anchor for coherent behavior, and hence for self-representational capacities.

Brain-Wise also turned out to be every inch a family endeavor. Paul Churchland, as always, shared all his hunches and insights with me, laughed at my mistakes, and gave me broad shoulders to stand on. He also drafted many of the illustrations. Mark Churchland and Anne Churchland, steeped in philosophy as a matter of household routine and in neuroscience as a matter of professional training, took earlier versions of the manuscript to the woodshed. Free of any need to be polite, they repeatedly sent me back for wholesale, and badly needed, rethinking and rewriting. Marian Churchland did me the honor of letting loose her cartoonist's whimsy to compose the cover, and Carolyn Churchland gave me sensible advice for the chapter on religion. I am profoundly grateful.

I the world at large, Roderick Corriveau taught me about neural development, and added depth to chapters on representations and knowledge. My UCSD colleague Rick Grush has been a collaborator on several projects, and his ideas about emulators have been a central element in my thinking about how nervous systems self-represent. I must especially thank my friend and colleague Clark Glymour, who, with his mixture of intellectual rigor and take-no-prisoners honesty, taught me a lot about causation and gave me the spine to say what I really think. David Molfese went over the manuscript page by page and consistently suggested very smart improvements, both substantive and editorial. Save for the methodical determination of David, this book would have been forever in progress. Ilya Farber was also wonderfully helpful, both critically and in his perspective on the integration of scientific domains. Steve Quartz gave me ideas about brain evolution that helped reorient my thinking about modules and brain organization generally. Michael Stack, my long-time philosophical chum, helped me tighten up many arguments and spotted sections that sounded pompous. Terry Sejnowski kindly read some of the manuscript and gave me advice and ideas, especially about learning and memory, and spatial representation. My editor at the MIT Press, Alan Thwaits, gave me the kind of invaluable advice one gets from a top-notch editor. I owe him a large debt of thanks.

Others who read the manuscript and commented, browbeat, or encouraged me into improvements are Bill Casebeer, Carmen Carrillo, Lou Goble, Mitch Gunzler, Andrew Hamilton, John Jacobson, Don Krueger, Ed McAmis, and Clarissa Waites. The Sejnowski lab at the Salk Institute is my second home, where I can learn about the latest developments and try out ideas. I am grateful to all those in the lab who have taken the time to bring me up to speed on their experiments and share their speculations, doubts, and wild ideas. I have taken the liberty of testing the manuscript on two undergraduate classes at UCSD, and their feedback has provoked many revisions, especially in the choice of topics to emphasize. Too numerous to mention, these students have my gratitude for their comments and complaints. Pippin "Bubbles" Schupbach gave me cheerful assistance in a vast range of chores.

UCSD has been the most exciting place in the world for me during the eighteen years it has been my home, and I am deeply grateful to many colleagues for having the kindness to teach me what they know. This is especially true of Liz Bates, Gilles Fauconnier, "Rama" Ramachandran, Marty Sereno, and Larry Squire. Finally, I am particularly pleased to note that when he was chancellor at UCSD, Dick Atkinson was uncommonly encouraging, even in the early days when my work was dismissed by mainstream philosophers as not real philosophy. As president of the University of California, he continues to keep abreast of what "his" faculty are thinking and doing, and gives us feedback. He is a visionary, and I have much to thank him for.

La Jolla, California, 2002

Brain-Wise

1   Introduction

The goal of science is not to open the door to everlasting wisdom, but to set a limit on everlasting error.
Galileo, in *Galileo*, by Bertolt Brecht

1   Core Questions

Bit by experimental bit, neuroscience is morphing our conception of what we are. The weight of evidence now implies that it is the *brain*, rather than some nonphysical stuff, that feels, thinks, and decides. That means there is no soul to fall in love. We do still fall in love, certainly, and passion is as real as it ever was. The difference is that now we understand those important feelings to be events happening in the physical brain. It means that there is no soul to spend its postmortem eternity blissful in Heaven or miserable in Hell. Stranger yet, it means that the introspective *inside*—one's own subjectivity—is *itself* a brain-dependent way of making sense of neural events. In addition, it means that the brain's *knowledge* that this is so is likewise brain-based business.

Given what is known about the brain, it also appears highly doubtful that there is a special nonphysical module, the *will*, operating in a causal vacuum to create voluntary choices—choices to be courageous in the face of danger, or to run away and fight another day. In all probability, one's decisions and plans, one's self-restraint and self-indulgences, as well as one's unique individual character traits, moods, and temperaments, are all features of the brain's general causal organization. The self-control one thinks one has is anchored by neural pathways and neurochemicals. The mind that we are assured can dominate over matter is in fact certain brain patterns interacting with and interpreted by other brain patterns. Moreover, one's *self*, as apprehended introspectively and represented incessantly, is a brain-dependent construct, susceptible to change as the brain changes, and is gone when the brain is gone.

Consciousness, almost certainly, is not a semimagical glow emanating from the soul or permeating spooky stuff. It is, very probably, a coordinated pattern of neuronal activity serving various biological functions. This does not mean that consciousness is not real. Rather, it means that its reality is rooted in its neurobiology. That a brain can come to know such things as these, and in particular, that it can do the science of itself, is one of the truly stunning capacities of the human brain.

This list catalogues but a few of the scientific developments that are revolutionizing our understanding of ourselves, and one would have to be naive to suppose that things have "gone about as far as they can go." In general terms, the mind-body problem has ceased to be the reliably tangled conundrum it once was. During the last three decades, the pace of discovery in neuroscience has been breathtaking. At every level, from neurochemicals to cells, and onwards to the circuit and systems levels, brain research has produced results bearing on the nature of the mind (figures 1.1 and 1.2). Coevolving with neuroscience, cognitive science has probed the scope of large-scale functions such as attention, memory, perception, and reasoning both in the adult and in the developing infant. Additionally, computational ideas for linking large-scale *cognitive* phenomena with small-scale *neural* phenomena have opened the door to an *integration* of neuroscience, cognitive science, and philosophy in a comprehensive theoretical framework.

There remain problems galore, and the solution to some of these problems will surely require conceptual and theoretical innovation of a magnitude that will surprise the pants off us. Most assuredly, having achieved significant progress does *not* imply that only mopping-up operations remain. But it does mean that the heyday of unfettered and heavy-handed philosophical speculation on the mind has gone the way of the divine right of kings, a passing that has stirred some grumbling among those wearing the mantle of philosopher-king. It does mean that know-nothing philosophy is losing ground to empirically constrained theorizing and inventive experimentation.

If the aforementioned changes have emerged from discoveries in the various neurosciences—including neuroanatomy, neurophysiology, neuropharmacology, and cognitive science—wherefore *philosophy*? What is *neurophilosophy*, and what is *its* role? Part of the answer is that the nature of the mind (including the nature of memory and learning, consciousness, and free will) have traditionally been subjects within the purview of philosophy. Philosophers, by tradition,

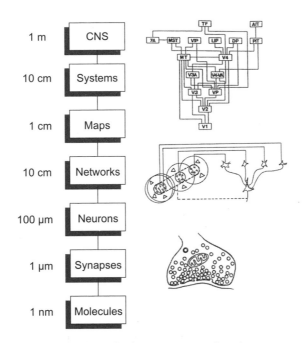

1 m — CNS

10 cm — Systems

1 cm — Maps

10 cm — Networks

100 μm — Neurons

1 μm — Synapses

1 nm — Molecules

Figure 1.1 Organized structures are found at many spatial scales in nervous systems. Functional levels may be even more fine-grained. Thus dendrites are a smaller computational unit than neurons, and networks may come in many sizes, including local networks and long-range networks. Networks may also be classed according to distinct dynamical properties. Icons on the right depict distinct areas in the visual system (top), a network (middle), and a synapse (bottom). (Based on Churchland and Sejnowski 1988.)

have wrestled with these topics, and the work continues. Neurophilosophy arises out of the recognition that at long last, the brain sciences and their adjunct technology are sufficiently advanced that real progress can be made in understanding the mind-brain. More brashly, it predicts that philosophy of mind conducted with no understanding of neurons and the brain is likely to be sterile. Neurophilosophy, as a result, focuses on problems at the intersection of a greening neuroscience and a graying philosophy.

Another part, perhaps the better part, of the answer is that philosophy, traditionally and currently, is quintessentially the place for synthesizing results and integrating theories across disciplinary domains. It is panoramic in its scope and all-encompassing in its embrace. It unabashedly bites off much more than it can chew. *Any* hypothesis, be it ever so revered or ever so scorned, is considered fair game for criticism. Philosophy deems it acceptable to kick the

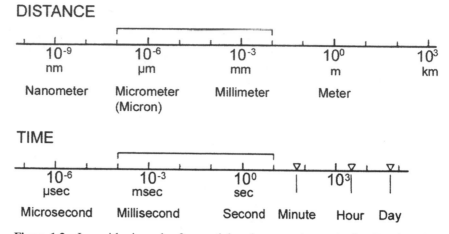

Figure 1.2 Logarithmic scales for spatial and temporal magnitudes. Brackets indicate the scales especially relevant to synaptic processing. (Based on Shepherd 1979.)

tires of every governing paradigm, examine every sacred cow, and peer behind the curtains of every magic show.

Under *this* description, we are all philosophers from time to time. Certainly, scientists have their philosophical hours, when they push back from the bench and stew on the broad questions, or when they beat on the conventional wisdom and strike a blow for originality. Such philosophical hours prepare the ground for the germination of new ideas and new experimental techniques.

Politely, we can consider philosophy the theoretical companion to experimental science; less politely, we can consider it merely woolgathering and freelancing. Certainly, some philosophy *is* just horsing around. Yet that is no bad thing, especially when a science is in its nascent stages. Neuroscience *is* a nascent science, and theoretical innovation is needed in every subfield of that broad über-field. Most theoretical ideas are bound to be losers, of course, but unless we are courageous enough to nurture lots and lots of new ideas, the rightful winners will never see the light of day.

This description highlights the positive side of philosophizing, but as with anything else, there is a seamier side. This is the side revealed when one is lulled into taking one's untested theoretical fancies as fact, or equating theory *beautiful* with theory *true*, or rejecting unorthodox ideas as heresy *because* they are unorthodox, or supposing that some chummy circle has the corner on clever ideas. If this applies to philosophy, it applies just as well to science, government, finance, and war.

This book is about neurophilosophy. It aims to take stock of various philosophical problems concerning the nature of the mind, given the recent bonanza of developments in neuroscience and cognitive science. In finding a path through the thicket of relevant neuroscientific studies and discoveries, I found material assembling itself into two classical categories: metaphysics and epistemology. Ethics gets a brief look in my discussion of free will and responsibility, but is mainly undiscussed on this occasion. Religion is the subject of the closing chapter, and has both a metaphysical and an epistemological dimension.

Before plunging on, we shall limber up with a few brief historical points and a short discussion on *reductionism*, a pivotal concept whose clarity is no luxury as we begin to assay the integration of hitherto separated domains.[1]

2 Natural Philosophy

Greek thought in the period 600 B.C. to 200 A.D. was the fountainhead for Western philosophy generally, as well as for modern science. In those days, *philosophy* literally meant "love of wisdom," and for the ancient Greeks, philosophy targeted a vast range of questions, such as, What is the nature of change such that water can freeze or wood burn? What is the nature of the moon and stars, and where did Earth come from? Are there fundamental particles of which all objects are composed? How do living things reproduce? In addition, of course, they raised questions about themselves—about what it is to be human, to think and perceive, to reason and feel, to plan and decide, to live a good life, to organize a harmonious and productive political state.

Theories about the *natural* world were considered part of *natural philosophy*. By contrast, theories of ethics and politics and practical life were part of *moral* philosophy. To a first approximation, this classification separates questions about *how things are* from questions about *what we should do*. Though distinct, these two domains share concepts and theories. In particular, sometimes questions about the mind will have one foot in each of these areas.

When did philosophy come to be considered a separate discipline? By the end of the nineteenth century, advances in some domains of natural philosophy had developed so extensively that separate subfields—physics, chemistry, astronomy and biology—branched off as distinct sciences. With progress and specialization, the expression "natural *science*" gained currency, while the more old-fashioned term, "natural *philosophy*" faded from use, now being essentially archaic. Nonetheless, this broad title can still be found on science buildings and doorways in older universities such as Cambridge in England and St. Andrews in Scotland. Until the middle of this century, St. Andrews's degrees in physics were officially degrees in Natural Philosophy. The title Ph.D. (*Philosophae Doctor*, or "teacher of philosophy") is awarded not only to philosophers, but to scientists of all sorts. It is a vestige of the older classification, which embraces all of science as a part of natural philosophy.

If the stars, the heart, and the basic constituents of matter became understood well enough to justify a separate science, what about the mind? Ancient thinkers, such as the physician Hippocrates (460–377 B.C.), were convinced that thoughts, feelings, and perceptions were activities of the brain. He believed that events such as sudden paralysis or creeping dementia had their originating causes in brain damage. And this implied, in his view, that normal movement and normal speech had *their* originating causes in the *well-tempered* brain. On the other hand, philosophers favoring a nonnatural framework—Plato (427–347 B.C.), and especially later Christian thinkers such as St. Thomas Aquinas (1225–1274) and St. Augustine (354–430)—believed the soul to be distinct from the body and divine in origin. Plato, in perhaps the first systematic theorizing on the soul, hypothesized it to have a sensible part (which determines perceptions), an emotional part (by virtue of which we feel honor, fear, and courage), and a rational part. This last was considered unique to humans and allowed us to reason, think, and figure things out. Theologically minded philosophers concluded that the mind (or, one might say, *the soul*) was a subject for study by means other than those available to natural science. If supernaturalism was true of the soul, then the nature of the soul could not be revealed by natural science, though perhaps other methods—such as meditation, introspection, and reason—might be useful.

Descartes (1595–1650) articulated the modern version and systematic defense of the idea that the mind is a *nonphysical* thing. This dual-substance view is known as *dualism*. Reason and judgment, in Descartes's view, are functions inhering in the mental, *immaterial* mind. He surmised that the mind and the body connect at *only* two points: sensory input and output to the muscles. Apart from these two functions, Cartesian dualism assumes that the mind's operations in thought, language, memory retrieval, reflection and conscious awareness proceed *independently* of the brain. When clinical studies on brain-damaged patients showed clear dependencies between brains and *all* these ostensibly brain-independent functions, classical dualism had to be reconfigured to allow that brain-soul interactions were not limited to sensory and motor functions. Achieving this correction without rendering the soul explanatorily redundant has been the bane of post-Cartesian dualism.

What about dualism appealed to Descartes? First, he was particularly impressed by the human capacity for reasoning and language, and the degree to which language use seems to be governed by reasons rather than causes. More exactly, he confessed that he was completely unable to imagine how a mechanical device could be designed so as to reason and use language appropriately and creatively.

What sort of mechanical devices were available to propel Descartes's imagination? Only clockwork machines, pumps, and fountains. Though some of these were remarkably clever, even the most elaborate clockwork devices of the seventeenth century were just *mechanical*. Well beyond the seventeenth-century imagination are modern computers that can guide the path of a cruise missile or regulate the activities of a spacecraft on Mars. In an obvious way, Descartes's imagination was limited by the science and technology he knew about. Had he been able to contemplate the achievements of computers, had he had even an inkling of electronics, his imagination might have taken wing. On the other hand, the core of Descartes's argument was revived in the 1970s by Chomsky[2] and Fodor[3] to defend their conviction that nothing we will ever understand about the brain will help us very much to understand the nature of language production and use.

The second reason dualism appealed is closely connected to the first. Descartes was convinced that exercise of free will was inconsistent with causality. He was also sure that humans did indeed have free will, and that physical events were all caused. So even if the body was a just a mechanical device, the mind could not be. Minds, he believed, must enjoy *uncaused* choice. We can undertake an action for a reason, but the relations between reasons and choices are not causal. Animals, by contrast, he believed to be mere automata, without the capacity for reason or for free choice. In its core, if not in its details, this argument too is alive and well even now, and it will be readdressed in greater detail in chapter 5 in the context of the general topic of free will.

Third, Descartes was impressed by the fact that one seems to know one's own conscious experiences simply by *having* them and *attending* to them. By contrast, to know about *your* experiences, I must draw inferences from your behavior. Whereas I know I have a pain simply by having it, I must draw an inference to know that my body has a wound. I cannot be wrong that *I* am conscious, but I can be wrong that *you* are conscious. I can even be wrong that you exist, since "you" might be nothing but *my* hallucination. According to Descartes's argument, differences in *how* we know imply that the thing that has knowledge—the mind—is fundamentally different from the body. The mind, he concluded, is essentially immaterial and can exist after the disintegration of the body. Like the other two arguments for dualism, this argument has remained powerful over the centuries. It has been touched up, put in modern dress, and in general reworked to look as good as new, but Descartes's insights regarding knowledge of mental states constitute the core of virtually all recent work on the nonreducibility of consciousness.[4] Because it continues to be persuasive, this argument will be readdressed and analyzed in detail when we discuss self-knowledge and consciousness. (See especially chapter 3, but also chapters 4 and 6.)

How, in Descartes's view, is the body able causally to affect the mind so that I feel pain when touching a hot stove? How can the mind affect the body so that when I decide to scratch my head, my body does what I intend it should do? Although Descartes envisioned interaction as limited to sensory input and motor output, notice that the business of interaction—*any* interaction—turns out to be a vexing problem for dualism, no matter how restricted or rich the interactions are believed to be. The interaction problem was, moreover, recognized as trouble right from the beginning. How could there be any causal interaction *at all*, was the question posed by other philosophers, including his contemporary, Princess Elizabeth of Holland, who put her objection bluntly in a letter of 10/20 June 1643: "And I admit that it would be easier for me to concede matter and extension to the soul than to concede the capacity to move a body and be moved by it to an immaterial thing" (*Oeuvres de Descartes*, ed. C. Adam and P. Tannery, vol. III, p. 685). As Princess Elizabeth realized, the mind, as a mental substance, allegedly has *no* physical properties; the brain, as a physical substance, allegedly has *no* mental properties. Slightly updated, her question for Descartes is this: how can the two radically different substances interact? The mind allegedly has no extension, no mass, no force fields—*no physical properties at all*. It does not even have spatial boundaries or locations. How could a nonphysical thing *cause a change* in a physical thing, and vice versa? What could be the causal basis for an interaction? Somewhat later, Leibniz (1646–1716) described the problem as intractable:[5] "When I began to meditate about the union of soul and body, I felt as if I were thrown again into the open sea. For I could not find any way of explaining how the body makes anything happen in the soul, or vice versa, or how one substance can communicate with another created substance. Descartes had given up the game at this point, as far as we can determine from his writings" (from *A New System of Nature*, translated by R. Ariew and Daniel Garber, p. 142).

Descartes almost certainly did recognize that mind-body interaction was a devastating difficulty, and indeed it has remained a stone in the shoe of dualism ever since. (For additional discussion, see chapter 2.)

The difficulty of giving a positive account provoked some philosophers, Leibniz being the first, to assert that events in a nonphysical mind are simply separate phenomena running in parallel to events in the brain. The mind causes nothing in the brain, and the brain causes nothing in the mind. Known as psychophysical parallelism, the idea was that the parallel occurrence of mental and brain events gives the illusion of causal interaction, though in fact no such causation ever actually occurs. What keeps the two streams in register? Some parallelists, such as Malebranche, thought this was a job God regularly and tirelessly performs for every conscious subject every waking hour. Leibniz, who preferred the idea that God kicked off the two streams and then let them alone, disparaged "occasionalists" such as Malebranche: "[Descartes's] disciples ... judged that we sense the qualities of bodies because God causes thoughts to arise in the soul on the occasion of motions of matter, and that when our soul, in turn, wishes to move the body, it is God who moves the body for it" (p. 143).

Descartes's best attempt to explain the interaction between mind and body was the suggestion that some unobserved but very, *very* fine material—*material* —in the pineal gland of the brain brokered the interaction between nonphysical mind and physical brain. His critics, such as Leibniz, were not fooled.

Perhaps Descartes was not fooled either. Some historians argue that Descartes's defense of a fundamental difference between mind and body was actually motivated by political rather than intellectual considerations.[7] Descartes was unquestionably a brilliant scientist and mathematician. This is, after all, the Descartes of the Cartesian coordinate system, a stunning mathematical innovation for which he is rightly given credit. He also understood well the bitter opposition of the Church to developments in science, and had left France to live in Holland to avoid political trouble. It is possible that he feared that developments in astronomy, physics, and biology would be cut off at the knees unless the Church was reassured that the "soul" was its unassailable proprietary domain. Such a division of subject matter might permit science at least to have the body as *its* domain. Whether this interpretation does justice to the truth remains controversial.

Certainly some of Descartes's arguments, both for the existence of God as well as for the mind/body split, are sufficiently flawed to suggest that they are ostentatiously flawed. On this hypothesis, the genius Descartes knew the logic full well and planted the flaws as clues for the discerning reader. And certainly Descartes had good reason to fear the Church's power to thwart scientific inquiry and to punish the scientist. Burning, torturing, and exiling those who inquired beyond official Church doctrine was not uncommon. Galileo, for example, was "shown the instruments of torture" to force him to retract his claim that Earth revolved around the Sun, a claim based on observation and reasoning. Recant he did, rather than submitting to the rack and iron maiden, but even so, he spent the rest of his life under house arrest by Church authorities. By vigorously postulating the mind/body division, perhaps contrary to his own best scientific judgment, Descartes may have done us all a huge, if temporary, favor in permitting the rest of science to go forward.

And go forward it did. By the end of the nineteenth century, physics, chemistry, astronomy, geology, and physiology were established, advanced scientific disciplines. The science of nervous systems, however, was a much slower affair. Though some brilliant *anatomical* work had been done on nervous systems, particularly by Camillo Golgi (1843–1926) and Santiago Ramón y Cajal (1852–1934), even at the end of the nineteenth century, little was known about the brain's functional organization, and almost nothing was understood concerning how neurons worked. That neurons signaled one another was a likely hypothesis, but how and to what purpose was a riddle.

Why did progress in neuroscience lag so far behind progress in astronomy or physics or chemistry? Why is the blossoming of neuroscience really a late-twentieth-century phenomenon? This question is especially poignant since, as noted, Hippocrates some four hundred years B.C. had realized that the brain was the organ of thought, emotion, perception, and choice.

The crux of the problem is that brains are exceedingly difficult to study. Imagine Hippocrates observing a dying gladiator with a sword wound to the head. The warrior had lost fluent speech following his injury, but remained conscious up to the end. At autopsy, what theoretical resources did Hippocrates possess to make sense of something so complex as the relation between the loss of fluent speech and a wound in the pinkish tissue found under the skull? Remember, in 400 B.C. nothing was understood about the nature of the cells that make up the body, let alone of the special nature of cells that make up the brain. That *cells* are the basic building blocks of the body was not really appreciated until the seventeenth century, and neurons were not seen until 1837, when Purkyně, using a microscope, first saw cell bodies in a section of brain tissue (figure 1.3).[8] Techniques for isolating neurons—brain cells—to

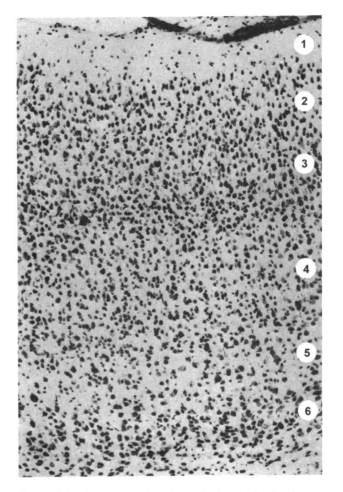

Figure 1.3 A cross-section through the mink visual cortex, with cresyl violet used to stain all cell bodies. Cortical layers are numbered at the right. (Courtesy of S. McConnell and S. LeVay.)

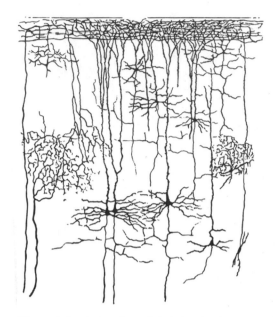

Figure 1.4   A drawing of Golgi-stained neurons in the rat cortex. About a dozen pyramidal neurons are stained, a tiny fraction of the neurons packed into the section. The height of the section depicted is about 1 mm. (Based on Eccles 1953.)

reveal their long tails and bushy arbors were not available until the second half of the nineteenth century, when stains that filled the cell were invented by Deiters (carmine stain) and then Golgi (silver nitrate stain) (figure 1.4). Neurons are *very* small, and unlike a muscle cell, each neuron has long branches—its axon and dendrites. There are about a 10^5 neurons per cubic *millimeter* of cortical tissue, for example, and about 10^9 synapses. (A handy rule of thumb is about 1 synapse/μm^3.) Techniques for isolating living neurons to explore their function did not appear until well into the twentieth century.[9]

By contrast, Copernicus (1473–1543), Galileo (1564–1642), and Newton (1643–1727) were able to make profound discoveries in astronomy without highly sophisticated technology. Through a clever reinterpretation of traditional astronomical measurements, Copernicus was able to figure out that Earth was not the center of the universe, thus challenging geocentrism. With a low-tech telescope, Galileo was able to see for the first time the moons of Jupiter and the craters of our own moon, thus undermining the conventional wisdom concerning the absolute perfection of the Heavens and the uniqueness of Earth.

Figuring out how neurons do what they do requires *very* high-level technology. And *that*, needless to say, depends on an immense scientific infrastructure: cell biology, advanced physics, twentieth-century chemistry, and post-1953 molecular biology. It requires sophisticated modern notions like molecule and protein, and modern tools like the light microscope and the electron microscope, and the latter was not invented until the 1950s. Many of the basic ideas can be grasped quite easily now, but discovering those ideas required reaching up from the platform of highly developed science.

To have a prayer of understanding nervous system, it is essential to understand how neurons work, and that was a great challenge technically. The most important *conceptual* tool for making early progress on nervous systems was the theory of electricity. What makes brain cells special is their capacity to signal one another by causing fast microchanges in each others' *electrical* states. Movement of ions, such as Na^+, across the cell membrane is the key factor in neuronal signaling, and hence in neuronal function. Living as we do in an electrical world, it is sobering to recall that as late as 1800, electricity was typically considered deeply mysterious and quite possibly occult. Only after discoveries by Ampere (1775–1836) and Faraday (1791–1867) at the dawn of the nineteenth century was electricity clearly understood to be a *physical* phenomenon, behaving according to well-defined laws and capable of being harnessed for practical purposes. As for neuronal membranes and ions and their role in signaling, understanding these took much longer (figures 1.5 and 1.6).

Once basic progress was made on how neurons signal, it could be asked *what* they signal; that is, what do the signals mean. This question too has been extremely hard to address, though the progress in the 1960s correlating the response of a visual-system neuron to a specific stimulus type, such as a moving spot of light, opened the door to the neurophysiological investigation of sensory and motor systems,[10] and to the discovery of specialized, mapped areas.

Beginning in the 1950s, progress had been made in addressing learning and memory at the systems level, and by the late 1970s, intriguing data on neuronal changes mediating system plasticity permitted the physiology of learning and memory to really take off. Meanwhile the role of specific neurochemicals in signaling and modulating neuronal function was beginning to be unraveled, and associated with large-scale effects such as changes from being awake to being asleep, to memory performance, to pain regulation, and to pathological conditions such as Parkinson's disease and obsessive-compulsive disorder. By the 1980s, attention functions came within the ambit of neuroscience, and changes at the neuronal level could be correlated with shifts in attention.

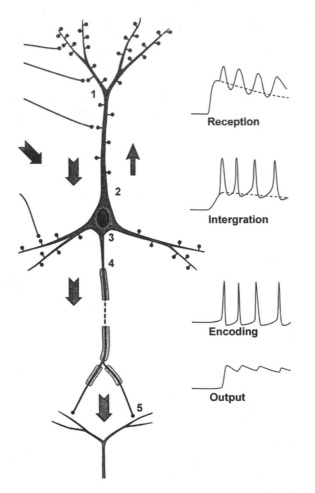

Figure 1.5 Neurons have four main structural regions and five main electrophysiological functions. The dendrites (2) have little spines (1) projecting from them, which are the major sites of in-coming signals from other neurons. The soma (3) contains the cell nucleus and other organelles involved in cell respiration and polypeptide production. Integration of signals takes place along the dendrites and soma. If signal integration results in a sufficiently strong depolarization across the cell membrane, a spike will be generated on the membrane where the axon emerges and will be propagated down the axon (4). Spikes may also be propagated back along dendritic membrane. When a spike reaches the axon terminal, neurotransmitter may be released into the synaptic cleft (5). The transmitter molecules diffuse across the cleft and some bind to receptor sites on the receiving neuron. (Adapted from Zigmond et al. 1999.)

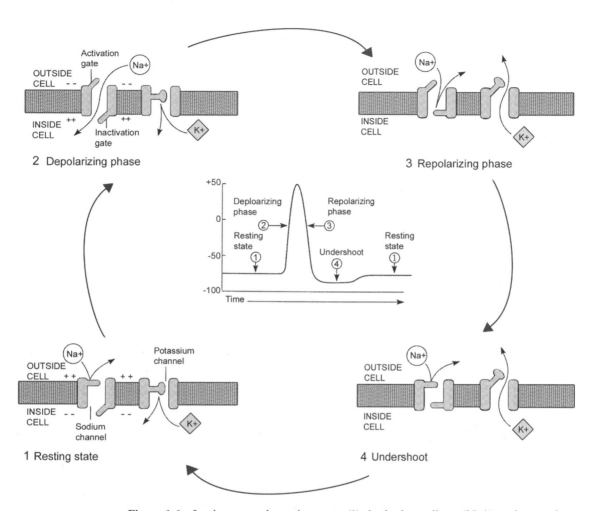

Figure 1.6   In the neuron's resting state (1), both the sodium (Na$^+$) and potassium (K$^+$) channels are closed, and the outside of the cell membrane is positively charged with respect to the inside. Hence there is a voltage drop across the membrane. If the membrane is depolarized (2), sodium ions enter the cell until the cell's polarity is reversed; that is, the inside of the cell is positively charged with respect to the outside. In the repolarization phase (3), the potassium channel then opens to allow efflux of potassium ions, the sodium gate closes, and sodium ions are actively pumped out of the cell. All of these activities help bring the membrane back to its resting potential. Because the potassium gate does not close as soon as the resting potential is reached (4), the voltage drop across the membrane briefly drops a little below the resting voltage. Equilibrium is reached once the resting potential is restored. (Based on Campbell 1996.)

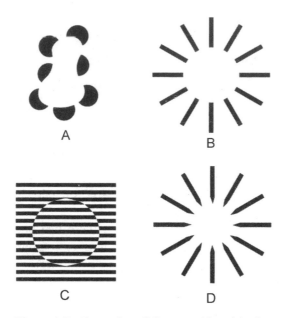

Figure 1.7 Examples of figures with subjective contours. Each of (A) through (C) seems to have a border (luminance contrast) where none exists. The borders are induced by line terminations that are consistent with the existence of an occluding figure. Thus the tapered ends in (D) do not give rise to a subjective contour. (From Palmer 1999.)

Progress on all these cognitive functions required adapting human psychophysical experiments, such as detection of illusory contours, to animals such as monkeys and cats (figure 1.7). In the animal studies, the responses of individual neurons under highly constrained conditions could be determined in order to test for sensitivity to a stimulus or a task (figure 1.8). And while cognitive functions at the network and neuronal level were being explored, details continued pour in to update the story of the ultrastructure of neurons—their synapses, dendrites, and gene expression within the nucleus—and how cognitive function was related to various ultrastructural operations.

Nevertheless, many fundamental questions about how the nervous system works remain wide open. In particular, bridging the gap between activity in individual neurons and activity in networks of neurons has been difficult. Macrolevel operations depend on the orchestrated activity of many neurons in a network, and presumably individual neurons make somewhat different contributions in order for the network to achieve a specific output, such as recog-

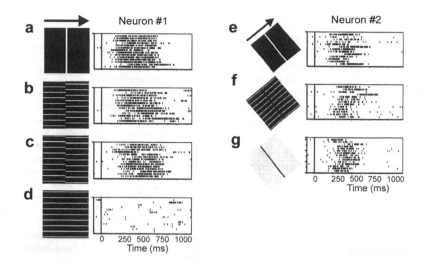

Figure 1.8 Neurons in owl visual forebrain areas (visual Wulst) respond to subjective contours about as well as to a real contour. The four contours (a) to (d) were randomly presented to the owl until each was viewed 15 times. The left column illustrates the stimuli; the right column shows the corresponding dot-raster displays for several presentations. Black dots represent the occurrences of spikes. Arrows indicate the direction of motion of the contours (motion onset at 0 ms). Notice that the neuron responds poorly in (d), where there is no subjective contour, but responds as well to (b) and (c) as to (a), the real contour. (Reprinted with permission from Nieder and Wagner 1999. Copyright by the American Association for the Advancement of Science.)

nition of visual motion or a command to move the eyes to a specific location. Moreover, understanding the dynamics of patterns of activity in neural networks and across many networks is undoubtedly essential to understanding how integration and coherence are achieved in brains. For example, there appear to be "competitions" between networks as the brain settles on a decision whether to fight or flee, and if to flee, whether to run in *this* direction or *that*, and so on. We are just beginning to feel our way toward concepts that might be helpful in thinking about the problems of coherencing.[11]

Until very recently, neuronal responses could be probed only one neuron at a time, but if we cannot access many neurons in a network, we have trouble figuring out how any given neuron contributes to various network functions, and hence we have trouble understanding exactly how networks operate. Significant technical progress has been made in recording simultaneously from more than one neuron, and the advent of powerful computers has made the problems of data analysis somewhat more tractable. Nevertheless, the search is on for technical breakthroughs that will really mesh microlevel experimentation with systems-level data. We are also uncertain how to identify what, among the billions of neurons, *constitutes one particular network*, especially since any given neuron undoubtedly has connections to many networks, and networks are likely to be distributed in space. To make matters yet more interesting, what constitutes a network may change over time, through development, and even on very short time scales, such as seconds, as a function of task demands. Obviously, these problems are partly technical, but they are also partly conceptual, in the sense that they require innovative concepts to edge them closer to something that can motivate the right technological invention for neurobiological experiments.

The advent of new safe techniques for measuring brain activity in humans has resulted in increasing numbers of fruitful collaborations between cognitive scientists and neuroscientists. When the results of techniques such as functional magnetic resonance imaging (fMRI)[12] and positron emission tomography (PET)[13] converge with results from basic neurobiology, we move closer to an integrated mind-brain science (figure 1.9). These techniques can show something about the changes in regional levels of activity over time, and if set up carefully, the changes can track changes in cognitive functions. It is important to understand that none of the imaging techniques measure neuronal activity directly. They track changes in blood flow (hemodynamics). Because the evidence suggests that localized increases in blood flow are a measure of local increases in neuronal activity (more active neurons need more oxygen and more glucose), they are believed to be an indirect indication of changes in levels of activity in the local neuronal population. Note also that the recorded changes are insensitive to what individual neurons in a region are doing. The best spatial resolution of PET is about 5 mm, and in fMRI it is about 2 mm, though these resolutions may improve. Since one mm^3 of cortex contains about 100,000 neurons, the spatial resolution of these techniques does not get us very close to single-neuron activity.[14]

If the images from scanning techniques reflect changes across time, one conceptual problem concerns how to interpret the changes, and that means figuring out what should count as the baseline activity in any given test. Suppose that a subject is awake and alert, and is given a task, for example, visually imaging moving his hand. How do we characterize the state before he is to begin the task? We ask the subject to just rest. But his brain does not rest. His brain will be doing *lots* of things, including making eye movements, monitoring

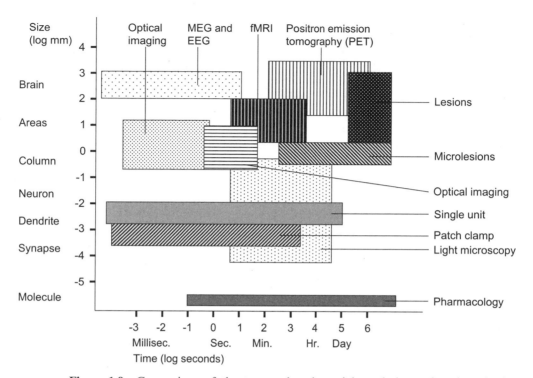

Figure 1.9 Comparison of the temporal and spatial resolutions of various brain-mapping techniques. MEG indicates magnetoencephalography; ERP, evoked response potential; EROS, event-related optical signal; MRI, magnetic resonance imaging; fMRI, functional MRI; PET, positron emission tomography; and 2-DG, 2-deoxyglucose. (Adapted from Churchland and Sejnowski 1988.)

glucose levels, perhaps thinking about missing breakfast, feeling an itch in his scalp, maintaining posture, and so forth. The subject cannot command the cessation of all cognitive functions, and certainly not all brain functions.

The problem of the baseline was recognized right from the beginning, and various strategies for reducing confounds have been developed, especially by Michael Posner and his colleagues.[15] These involve subtracting the level of activity in the "rest" condition from the level in the task condition, to reveal the difference made, presumably, by the task. There are other problems in getting meaningful interpretations of image data. For example, if a region shows increased activity during a cognitive task, does that mean it is *specialized* for that task? At most, it probably shows that the region has some role in executing the task, but this is a much weaker conclusion. Performance of the task may involve a fairly widely distributed network, and the noticed change may reflect a local blip in which one segment of the network happens to have a high density of neurons that contribute, though collectively other low-density regions may be more important to the execution of the function. Until we know more about brain organization at the neuronal and network levels, some of these problems in interpretation will persist.

These cautionary remarks regarding interpretation of image data should *not* be taken to imply that the new imaging techniques are too problematic to be useful. They are in fact *very* useful, but experiments do have to be carefully controlled so as to reduce confounds, and conclusions have to be carefully stated to avoid exaggerated claims. It is relatively easy to get image data, but very difficult to know whether the data reveal anything about brain function and organization. The main point is that the imaging techniques are indeed marvelous and are indeed useful, but not all imaging studies yield meaningful results. What we want to avoid is drawing strong conclusions about localization of function when only weak conclusions or no conclusions are warranted.

3   Reductions and Coevolution in Scientific Domains

The possibility that mental phenomena might be understood in a neuroscientific framework is associated with *reductive explanation* in science generally. An example where one phenomenon is successfully reduced to another is the reduction of heat to molecular kinetic energy. In this case, the prereductive science was dealing with two sets of phenomena (i.e., heat and energy of motion), and had a good deal of observational knowledge about each. It was not initially obvious that heat had anything at all to do with motion, which seemed a wholly separate and unrelated phenomenon. As it turned out, however, they have quite a lot to do with each other, initial appearances notwithstanding.

An understanding of mental phenomena—such as memory, pains, dreaming, and reasoning—in terms of neurobiological phenomena is a *candidate* case of reduction, inasmuch as it looks reasonable to expect that they are brain functions. Because the word "reduction" can be used in wildly different ways, ranging from an honorific to a term of abuse, I now outline what I do and do not mean by "reduction."[16]

The baseline characterization of scientific reduction is tied to real examples in the history of science. Most simply, a reduction has been achieved when the causal powers of the macrophenomenon are explained as a function of the physical structure and causal powers of the microphenomenon. That is, the macro-properties are discovered to be the entirely natural outcome of the nature of the elements at the microlevel, together with their dynamics and interactions. For example, *temperature* in a gas was reduced to *mean molecular kinetic energy.*[17]

Does a reduction of a macrotheory to a microtheory require that the key words of the macrotheory *mean* the same as the words referring to the micro-properties? Not at all. A common misunderstanding, especially among philosophers, is that if macrotheory about α is reduced to microtheory features β, γ, δ, then α must *mean the same* as β and γ and δ. Emphatically, this is not a requirement, and has never been a requirement, in science. In fact, meaning identity is rarely, if ever, preserved in scientific identifications. Temperature of a gas is *in fact* mean molecular kinetic energy, but the phrase "temperature of a gas" is not *synonymous* with "mean molecular kinetic energy." Most cooks are perfectly able to talk about the temperature of their ovens without knowing about anything about the movement of molecules. Second, it often happens that as the macrotheory and the microtheory coevolve, the meanings of the terms change to better mesh with the discovered facts. The word "atom" used to mean "indivisible fundamental particle." Now we know atoms are divisible, and "atom" means "the smallest existing part of an element consisting of a dense nucleus of protons and neutrons surrounded by moving electrons."[18] Usually, the meaning change is first adopted within the relevant scientific community and propagates more widely thereafter.

What does the history of science reveal about reductive explanations that might be helpful in understanding what a reduction of psychology to neuroscience will entail? A nagging question about the connection between cognition and the brain is this: can we ever get beyond mere *correlations* to actual identification and hence reduction? If so, how? Let us try to address this question by briefly discussing three cases. The first concerns the discovery that the identification of temperature of a gas with the mean kinetic energy of its constituent molecules permits thermal phenomena such as conduction, the relation of temperature and pressure, and the expansion of heated things to get a coherent, unified *explanation*. Correlations give you reasons for testing to evaluate the explanatory payoff from identification, but without *explanatory* dividends, correlations remain mere correlations. In the case of thermal phenomena, the first explanatory success with gases allowed the extension of the same explanatory framework to embrace liquids and solids, and eventually plasmas and even empty space. As a theory, statistical mechanics was far more successful than the caloric theory, the accepted theory of heat in the nineteenth century. Let us look at little more closely at how people came to realize that temperature was actually molecular motion.

It is very natural to think of heat as a kind of stuff that moves from hot things to cold things. As natural philosophers investigated the nature of changes in temperature, they gave the name "caloric" to the stuff that presumably made hot things hot. Caloric was thought to be a genuine fluid—a fundamental stuff of the universe, along with atoms, and existing in the spaces between atoms. When Dalton (1766–1844) proposed his atomic theory, his sketches of tiny atoms showed them as surrounded by tiny atmospheres of caloric fluid. Within this framework, a hot cannonball was understood to have more caloric than a cold cannonball; snow has less caloric than steam.

Given that caloric is a kind of fluid, this entails that a thing should weigh more when hot than when cold. Weighing a cannon ball before and after heating tested this theory. The results showed that no matter how hot the cannon ball became, its weight remained the same. Faced with a possible refutation of a very plausible theory (what *else* could heat be?), some scientists were tempted by the hypothesis that caloric fluid was *very* special in that it had no mass.

Heat created through friction was also a puzzle, because there was no evident fluid *source* of caloric. The conventional wisdom settled on the idea that rubbing released the caloric fluid that was normally sequestered in the spaces between atoms. Rubbing jostled the atoms, and the jostling allowed the caloric to escape. To test the solution to the friction puzzle, Count Rumford Benjamin Thompson (1753–1814) traveled from England to a factory in Bavaria that bored holes in iron cannons. The boring, of course, continuously produced a huge amount of heat through friction, and the cannons under construction were constantly cooled by water. Rumford reasoned that if caloric fluid was released by friction during boring, then the caloric should eventually run out. No additional heat should be produced by further boring or rubbing. Needless to say, he observed that heat never ceased to be produced as the holes down the cannon shaft were continuously bored. At no point did the caloric fluid in the iron show the slightest sign of depletion.

Either there was an *infinite* amount of this allegedly massless fluid in the iron, or something was fundamentally wrong with the whole idea of caloric. Rumford realized that the first option was not seriously believable. Were it true, even one's hands would have to contain an infinite amount of caloric, since you can keep rubbing them without decline in heat production. Rumford concluded that not only was caloric fluid not a *fundamental* kind of stuff, it was not a stuff of *any* kind. Heat required a different sort of explanation altogether. Heat, he proposed, just *is* micromechanical motion.[19]

Notice that a really determined calorist could persist in the face of Rumford's experiments, preferring to try to develop the option that every object really does contain an infinite amount of (massless) caloric fluid. And undoubtedly some believers did persist well after Rumford's presentation. The possibility of such persistence shows only that refutations of empirical theories are not as straightforward as refutations of mathematical conjectures. The caloric-fluid theory of heat was eventually rejected because its fit with other parts of science slowly became worse rather than better, *and* because, in the explanatory realm, it was vastly outclassed in explanatory and predictive power by the theory that heat is a matter of molecular motion. The fit of the newer theory with other parts of science, moreover, became *better* rather than worse. These developments also led to the distinction between heat (energy transfer as a result of difference in temperature) and temperature (movement of molecules).

The explanation of the nature of light can be seen as another successful example of scientific reduction. In this instance, visible light turned out to be electromagnetic radiation (EMR), as did radiant heat, x-rays, ultraviolet rays, radio waves, and so forth (see plate 1). Note also that in these examples, as in most others, further questions always remain to be answered, even after the reductive writing is on the wall. Hence, there is a sense in which the reduction is always incomplete. If the *core* mysteries are solved, however, that is usually sufficient for scientists to consider an explanation—and hence a reduction—to be well established and worthy of acceptance as the basis for further work.

Reductions can be very messy, in the sense that the mapping of properties from micro to macro can be *one-many* or even *many-many*, rather than the ideal *one-one*. While the case of light reducing to EMR is relatively clean, the case of phenotypic traits and genes is far less clean. Genes, as we now know, may not be single stretches of DNA, but may involve many distinct segments of DNA. The regulatory superstructure of noncoding DNA means that identification of a stretch of coding DNA as a "gene for ..." is a walloping simplification. Additionally, a given DNA segment may participate in different macroproperties as a function of such things as stage of development and extracellular milieu. Despite this complexity, molecular biologists typically see their explanatory framework as essentially reductive in character. This is mainly because a causal route from base-pair sequences in DNA to macrotraits, such as head/body segmentation, can be traced. The details, albeit messy,

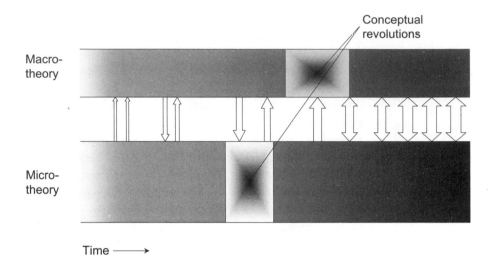

Conceptual
revolutions

Macro-
theory

Micro-
theory

Time ⟶

Figure 1.10   Macrolevel theories and microlevel theories coevolve through time. Initially, the connection between the macro- and microlevels may be tenuous and only suggestive, but their interactions may increase as experiments reveal correlations between macro- and microphenomena. As the experimental and theoretical interactions increase, the theories become increasingly interdigitated. The central concepts classifying macrophenomena and microphenomena are inevitably revised, and when the conceptual revision is very dramatic, this may be described in terms of a scientific revolution. Such revolutions are crudely indicated by a tunnel in the darkening pattern.

can be expected to fill out, at least in general terms, as experimental results come in.

This brings us to a second major point. Reductive explanations typically emerge in the later stages of a long and complicated courtship between higher-level and lower-level scientific domains. Earlier phases involve the *coevolution* of the scientific subfields, where each provides inspiration and experimental provocation for the cohort subfield, and where the results of each suggest modifications, revisions, and constraints for the other (figure 1.10). As theories coevolve, they gradually knit themselves into one another, as points of reductive contact are established and elaborated. Initially, contact between a high-level science and a lower-level science may be based merely on suggestive correlations in the occurrences of phenomena. Some such suggestive connections may prove to be genuine; some may turn out to be coincidental.

Reductive links begin to be forged when mechanisms at one level begin to explain and predict phenomena at another level. Not until there exist reasonably well-developed theories on both levels do the reductive explanations emerge. If you don't know beans about the macrolevel phenomenon of heat, you will not get very far trying to explain it in terms of some deeper and invisible property of matter. Sometimes the coevolution involves major revisions to the basic ideas defining the sciences, and the history of science reveals a wide spectrum of revisionary modifications. Caloric fluid, as we saw, got the boot as thermodynamics and statistical mechanics knit themselves together. Galileo and Newton rewrote the book on *momentum* and threw out the medieval conception of "impetus." Michael Faraday demonstrated, contrary to received opinion, that electricity is fundamentally the same phenomenon, whether it is produced by a battery, an electromagnetic generator, an electric eel, two hot metals brought into contact, or a hand rubbing against cat fur. In reality, the varieties of electrical phenomena are at bottom just one thing: electricity.

Reductive achievements sometimes fall short of the complete reduction of one theory to another because the available mathematics are insufficient to the task. Thus quantum mechanics has succeeded in explaining the macroproperties of the elements, such as the conductivity of copper or the melting point of lead, but not why a specific protein folds up precisely as it does. Whether more is forthcoming depends on developments in mathematics. In the case of quantum mechanisms, the mathematical limitations entail not that the macroproperties of complex molecules (e.g., serotonin) are emergent in some spooky sense, but only that we cannot now fully explain them.

It may come as a surprise that the great majority of philosophers working now are not reductionists, and are not remotely tempted by the hypothesis that understanding the brain is essential to understanding the mind. Such philosophers typically also see the details of neuroscience as *irrelevant* to understanding the nature of the mind.[20] The reason for their skepticism about the role of neuroscience is not rooted in substance dualism. Rather, the key idea is that the mind is analogous to software running on a computer. Like Adobe Photoshop, the cognitive program can be run on computers with very different hardware configurations. Consequently, although mind software can be run on the brain, it can also run on a device made of silicon chips or Jupiter goo. Hence, the argument goes, there is nothing much we can learn about cognition per se from looking at the brain.

Known as functionalism, this view asserts that the nature of a given type of cognitive operation is wholly a matter of the role it plays in the cognitive economy of the person.[21] Thus the draw operation of Adobe Photoshop is what it is solely and completely in virtue of its *role* in Adobe Photoshop. Its nature, so to speak, is exhausted by the description of its interactions when Photoshop is running. Obviously, therefore, understanding the draw operation in Photoshop will not be helped by understanding the capacitors and transistors and circuits of one's computer.[22] Likewise, understanding what it is for a person to want a banana or believe that cows can fly will not be helped by understanding neurons, circuits, or anything else about how the brain works.[23]

Considerations of this sort motivated Jerry Fodor to emphasize the importance of experimental psychology, but also to firmly reject the relevance of neuroscience. He defends a thesis he calls the *autonomy of psychology*. This is a methodological claim. Its label embodies his conviction that psychology, as a science, is independent in its concepts and generalizations, of the concepts and generalizations of neuroscience. Briefly, the crux of the claim is that cognition cannot be explained in neurobiological terms and will not be usefully explored by neuroscientific techniques. The claim supports investigating cognition using *behavioral* measures, such as reaction times, and developing theories by constructing models that reflect the cognitive organization supposedly revealed by behavioral and introspective experiments. Neuroscientific data allegedly have a bearing only on how the cognitive program can be implemented in a particular physical arrangement, but have very little bearing on the actual nature of the cognitive functions. Neuroscience, from this perspective, may be of clinical interest, but it has no major significance for cognitive science.

There are many well-known criticisms of the autonomy-of-psychology thesis.[24] One powerful objection, repeatedly raised but never answered by those who live by the software analogy, is that the conceptual distinction between hardware and software does not correspond to any real distinction in nervous systems.[25] There are many levels of brain organization, ranging from protein channels in membranes, to neurons, microcircuits, macrocircuits, subsystems, and systems (see again figures 1.1 and 1.2). At many brain levels there are operations fairly describable as computations, and *none* of these levels can be singled out as *the* hardware level. For example, computations are performed by parts of dendrites, as well as by whole neurons, as well as by networks of neurons. Learning and memory, for example, involve computational operations at many levels of structural organization.[26] (This will be discussed in more detail in chapter 8.) The fact is, in nervous systems there are no levels of brain organization identifiable as *the* software level or *the* hardware level. Consequently, the linchpin analogy (mind/brain = software/hardware) is about as accurate as saying that the mind is like a fire or the mind is like a rich tapestry. In a poetic context, the metaphors are perhaps charming enough, but they are far too unconnected to the real phenomena do very much to advance the scientific project of understanding cognition.

Another major concern is as practical as wearing boots in the snow. There is no point in turning your back on a vast range of data that might very well narrow your search space. To do so is perversely counterproductive. Keeping psychology pure from the taint of neuroscience seems strangely puritanical. Why not take advantage of every strategy, every technique, every well-controlled and well-run experiment? Why turn up your nose at some data when it might be useful?

Fodor, however, takes the software/hardware analogy to license assurance that neuroscientific data will not be useful. As noted, the analogy stipulates that neuroscientific data pertain to *implementation* rather than software. Unfortunately, and rather obviously, this response is untenable, because the analogy is untenable. By insisting that experimental psychology cut itself off from potentially useful neurobiological data, theory dualism is steering resolutely into the past instead of into the future. In a curious way, brain-averse functionalism is methodologically close to Cartesianism. In place of Descartes's *nonphysical mental substance*, functionalism substituted "*software.*" Otherwise, things are much the same: no interest in or search for mechanisms of cognitive functions, no credence given to the possibility that we might learn fundamental facts about the mind by understanding how the brain works.

Notwithstanding the strictures of functionalism, the fact is that neuroscience and cognitive science are coevolving, like it or not. This coevolution is motivated not by ideology, but by the scientific and explanatory rewards derived from the interactions. Increasingly, this trend means that data from neuroscience are having an impact on how we frame questions about the mind and how we rethink how best to characterize psychological phenomena themselves. Examples of these developments will be seen in later chapters, and they will make us wonder whether some folk-psychological "verities" are as much in need of revision as were the "verities" of geocentrism. Exactly how the cognitive sciences and the neurosciences will knit into one another and how coevolution will change *both* is not easily predicted.

Though we can expect in a general way that mental phenomena will reduce to neurobiological phenomena, in the qualified sense of "reduction" used here, that achievement is certainly not yet in hand and could well be thwarted by the reality of the brain. For all we can be sure of now, a loose, if revealing, integration of domains may be the best we can achieve. Detailed explanatory mechanisms may elude us, and we might have to settle for general explanatory principles that give us a story about mechanisms. Then again, maybe not. Science often surprises us with progress we thought impossible.[27]

There are still some very general worries about reduction to be addressed and allayed in advance of further progress, and I shall turn to three of those now.[28]

3.1   If We Get an Explanatory Reduction of Mental Life in Terms of Brain Activity, Should We Expect Our Mental Life to Go Away?

This worry is based on misinformation concerning what reductions in science do and do not entail. The short answer to the question, therefore, is "No." Pains will not cease to be real just because we understand the neurobiology of pain. That is, a reductive explanation of a macrophenomenon in terms of the dynamics of its microstructural features does not mean that the macrophenomenon is not real or is scientifically disreputable or is somehow explanatorily unworthy or redundant. Even after we achieved an explanation of light in terms of EMR, the classical theory of optics continues to be useful, even in discovering new things. Nobody thinks that light is not real, as result of Maxwell's explanatory equations. Rather, we think that we understand more about the real nature of light than we did before 1873. Light is real, no doubt about it. But we now see visible light as but one segment of a wider spectrum that includes x-rays, ultraviolet light, and radio waves (plate 1). We can now explain a whole lot at the macrolevel that we were unable to explain before, such as why light can be polarized and why light is refracted by a lens.

Sometimes, however, hitherto respectable properties and substances do turn out to be unreal. The caloric theory of heat, as we mentioned, did not survive the rigors of science, and caloric fluid thus turned out not to be real. As neuroscience proceeds, the fate of our current conception of consciousness, for example, will depend on the facts of the matter and the long-term integrity of current macrolevel concepts.[29]

3.2   Should We Expect a One-Step Integration of the Behavioral Domain with the Neuronal Domain?

Nervous systems appear to have many levels of organization, ranging in spatial scale from molecules such as serotonin, to dendritic spines, neurons, small networks, large networks, areas, and systems. Although it remains to be empirically determined what exactly are the functionally significant levels, it is unlikely that explanations of macroeffects such as perceiving motion will be explained directly in terms of the lowest microlevel. More likely, high-level network effects will be the outcome of interacting subnetworks; subnetwork effects the outcome of participating neurons and their interconnections; neuron effects the outcome of protein channels, neuromodulators, and neurotransmitters; and so forth. One misconception about the integrationist strategy sees it as seeking a *direct* explanatory bridge between the highest level and lowest levels. This idea of "explanation in a single bound" does stretch credulity, and neuroscientists are not remotely tempted by it. My approach predicts that integrative *explanations* will proceed stepwise from highest to lowest, and that the *research* should proceed at all levels simultaneously.[30]

3.3   How Can You Have Any Self-Esteem If You Think You Are Just a Piece of Meat?

The first part of the answer is that brains are not *just* pieces of meat. The human brain is what makes humans capable of painting the Sistine Chapel, designing airplanes and transistors, skating, reading, and playing Chopin. It is a truly astonishing and magnificent kind of "wonder-tissue," as the philosopher Dennett jokingly puts it.[31] Whatever self-esteem justly derives from our accomplishments does so *because* of the brain, not in spite of it.

Second, if we thought of ourselves as glorious creatures before we knew that the brain is responsible, why not continue to feel so after the discovery? Why does the knowledge not make us more interesting and remarkable, rather than less so? We can be thrilled by the spectacle of a volcano erupting or a calf being born or a bone healing before we understand what volcanoes are and how reproduction and healing work. Being the creatures we are, however, commonly we are even more thrilled in the embrace of the knowledge about volcanoes and birth and bones. Understanding why we sleep and dream or how we distinguish so many smells makes us so much more glorious, rather than less so. At the same time, understanding why someone is demented or gripped by a handwashing compulsion or tormented by a phantom arm after amputation helps replace superstition with sympathy and panic with calm reason.

Third, self-esteem, as we all know, depends on many complex factors, including things that happened or didn't happen during childhood and social recognition of a certain kind. None of this is altered one iota by realizing that one's feelings are caused by brain activity. When I step on a thorn, it still hurts in the same way, whether I know that the pain is really an activity in neurons or not. When a teacher sincerely compliments a student's essay as insightful, well-researched, and clearly written, he esteems the student's accomplishment. In consequence, she is entitled to self-esteem, and it would be utterly irrelevant to add, "Too bad, though, this paper is just a product of your brain" as a deflationary remark.

4   Concluding Remarks

Three hypotheses underpin this book:

Hypothesis 1   Mental activity *is* brain activity. It is susceptible to scientific methods of investigation.

Hypothesis 2   Neuroscience needs cognitive science to know *what* phenomena need to be explained. To understand the scope of the capacity you want to explain—such as sleep, temperature discrimination, or skill learning—it is insufficient to simply rely on folk wisdom and introspection. Psychophysics, and experimental psychology generally, are necessary accurately to characterize the organism's behavioral repertoire and to discover the composition, scope, and limits of the various mental capacities.

Hypothesis 3   It is necessary to understand the brain, and to understand it at many levels of organization, in order to understand the nature of the mind.

Hypothesis 1 is a front-and-center topic of the entire book. It will be continually dissected, tested, and defended when we address the nature of the self, consciousness, free will, and knowledge. Ultimately, its soundness will be settled by what actually happens as the mind/brain sciences continue to make progress. Conceivably, it will turn out that thinking, feeling, and so on, are in fact carried out by nonphysical soul stuff. At this stage of science, however, the Cartesian outcome looks improbable. As noted earlier, hypothesis 3 is hotly contested by those psychologists and philosophers who favor the "mind as software" approach.[32] Hypothesis 2, on the other hand, though it may be embraced *in principle* by neuroscientists, is sometimes ignored in practice. For example, molecular-level neuroscientists may be apt to scoff at systems-level neuroscientists who are groping for ways to test psychophysical hypotheses in monkeys.

The more serious problem, however, is that brain-averse philosophers and psychologists tend to assume that those who believe hypothesis 3 (e.g., neuroscientists) are bound and determined to *dis*believe hypothesis 2.[33] *No such conclusion follows*, of course. The important point is that psychology and neuroscience are coevolving and will continue to do so. The fields are not mutually incompatible, but *mutually dependent*. Temporarily focusing on one level of organization is often a practical experimental expedient, but that is very different from making it a principle of research strategy.

One further observation concerns our ideas about ourselves, including our philosophical ideas. The main business of our brains is to help us adapt to changing circumstances, to predict food sources and dangers, to recognize mates and shelter, in general, to allow us to survive and reproduce. The human brain, as a rather fancy defense against variability and disaster, also generates stories—call them *theories*—to explain *why* things happen and thus help predict what *will* happen.

Some theories are better than others. The theory that bubonic plague is God's punishment is not as successful as the theory that it is a rat-borne bacterial infection. The first suggests prayer as a preventative, the second predicts that hand washing, rat killing, and water boiling will be more effective. As indeed they are. The theory that Zeus makes thunder by hurling luminous bolts is not as successful as the theory that lightning causes a sudden heating of adjacent air and therewith a sudden expansion. And so forth.

What about theories concerning ourselves—*our* natures? Our ideas about why people do certain things, and indeed why one does something oneself, are part of a wider network of story structures, with some cultural variability and some commonality. We explain and predict one another's behavior by relying on stories about attitudes, will power, beliefs, desires, superegos, egos, and selves. For example, we explain a certain basketball player's demands for attention in terms of his big ego; we may describe a backsliding smoker as lacking will power, an actor as moody or as obsessed with popularity or as having a narcissistic personality disorder, and so on. Freud (1856–1939) urged us to explain compulsive behavior in terms of superego dysfunction. But what, in neurobiological terms, *are* these states—will power, moods, personality, ego, and superego? Are some of these categories like the categories of now-defunct but hitherto "obvious" Aristotelian physics, categories such as "impetus" and "natural place"?

Given scientific progress in general, along with specific evidence about the brain and how it works, our shared conventional story structures may come to be modified where they prove less successful than experimentally tested theories. The details of theory modifications are essentially impossible to predict in advance. Already, however, we can see some story modification.

In the last fifty years, we have come to realize that epilepsy is best understood in neurobiological terms, not in terms of the divine touch. Hysterical paralysis is not a dysfunction of the uterus, but of the brain. In subjects' who are compulsive handwashers, possession by spirits or superego dysfunction explains and predicts far less than neuromodulator levels. The discovery that highly addictable subjects have a gene implicated in the quirks of their dopamine reward system begins to hint that we will want to reconsider what exactly having or lacking will power comes to. None of this is surprising, for what the history of science reveals is that *some* theory revision is typical and pretty much inevitable, no matter what the domain of inquiry—astronomy, physics, biology, or the nature of our minds. That the story structure giving shape to traditional philosophical inquiry may itself evolve, perhaps quite profoundly, accordingly presents an even deeper challenge to those who wish to isolate philosophy from science.

The overarching theme of this book is that if we allow discoveries in neuroscience and cognitive science to butt up against old philosophical problems, something very remarkable happens. We will see genuine progress where progress was deemed impossible; we will see intuitions surprised and dogmas routed. We will find ourselves making sense of mental phenomena in neurobiological terms, while unmasking some classical puzzles as preneuroscientific misconceptions. Neuroscience has only just begun to have an impact on philosophical problems. In the next decades, as neurobiological techniques are invented and theories of brain function elaborated, the paradigmatic forms for understanding mind-brain phenomena will shift, and shift again. These are still early days for neuroscience. Unlike physics or molecular biology, neuroscience does not yet have a firm grasp of the basic principles explaining its target phenomena. The real conceptual revolution will be upon us once those principles come into focus. How things will look *then* is anybody's guess.

Selected Readings

Basic Introductions

Allman, J. M. 1999. *Evolving Brains*. New York: Scientific American Library.

Bechtel, W., and G. Graham, eds. 1998. *A Companion to Cognitive Science*. Oxford: Blackwells.

Osherson, D., ed. 1990. *Invitation to Cognitive Science*. Vols. 1–3. Cambridge: MIT Press.

Palmer, S. E. 1999. *Vision Science: Photons to Phenomenology*. Cambridge: MIT Press.

Sekuler, R., and R. Blake. 1994. *Perception*. 3rd ed. New York: McGraw Hill.

Wilson, R. A., and F. Keil, eds. 1999. *The MIT Encyclopedia of the Cognitive Sciences*. Cambridge: MIT Press.

Zigmond, M. J., F. E. Bloom, S. C. Landis, J. L. Roberts, L. R. Squire. 1999. *Fundamental Neuroscience*. San Diego: Academic Press.

Additional Selected Readings

Bechtel, W., P. Mandik, J. Mundale, and R. S. Stufflebeam, eds. 2001. *Philosophy and the Neurosciences: A Reader*. Oxford: Oxford University Press.

Bechtel, W., and R. C. Richardson. 1993. *Discovering Complexity*. Princeton: Princeton University Press.

Churchland, P. M. 1988. *Matter and Consciousness*. 2nd ed. Cambridge: MIT Press.

Churchland, P. S. 1986. *Neurophilosophy: Towards a Unified Understanding of the Mind-Brain*. Cambridge: MIT Press.

Crick, F. 1994. *The Astonishing Hypothesis*. New York: Scribners.

Damasio, A. R. 1994. *Descartes' Error*. New York: Grossett/Putnam.

Kandel, E. R., J. H. Schwartz, T. M. Jessell, eds. 2000. *Principles of Neural Science*. 4th ed. New York: McGraw-Hill.

Moser, P. K., and J. D. Trout, eds. 1995. *Contemporary Materialism: A Reader*. London: Routledge.

History

Brazier, M. A. B. 1984. *A History of Neurophysiology in the 17th and 18th Centuries: From Concept to Experiment*. New York: Raven Press.

Finger, S. 1994. *Origins of Neuroscience: A History of Explorations into Brain Function*. New York: Oxford University Press.

Gross, C. G. 1999. *Brain, Vision, Memory: Tales in the History of Neuroscience*. Cambridge: MIT Press.

Young, R. M. 1970. *Mind, Brain, and Adaptation in the Nineteenth Century*. New York: Oxford University Press.

Journals with Review Articles

Annals of Neurology

Cognition

Current Issues in Biology

Nature Reviews: Neuroscience

Psychological Bulletin

Trends in Cognitive Sciences

Trends in Neurosciences

Websites

BioMedNet Magazine: http://news.bmn.com/magazine

Encyclopedia of Life Sciences: http://www.els.net

The MIT Encyclopedia of the Cognitive Sciences: http://cognet.mit.edu/MITECS

Neuroanatomy: http://thalamus.wustl.edu/course

Science: http://scienceonline.org

The Whole Brain Atlas: http://www.med.harvard.edu/AANLIB/home.html

I Metaphysics

2 An Introduction to Metaphysics

1 Introduction

As a label for a subject, the term "metaphysics" has an odd origin. The story is worth telling because it helps explain the miscellany of topics herded together as metaphysical. The term was first used about 100 B.C. by an editor, probably Andronicus of Rhodes, of Aristotle's works. Aristotle's corpus covered a vast range of topics, for he had something to say on virtually everything, including logic, physics, the weather, the heavens, ethics, and reproductive processes in animals. A problem for the editor was that Aristotle had failed to give a title to the material the editor regarded as following sequentially after *Physica*, Aristotle's book on physics. To solve the problem the editor entitled this material, unpretentiously, "The Book after the Physics," that is, *Metaphysica*. Thus was born metaphysics.[1] How, then, did metaphysics acquire the status of a subdiscipline in its own right? One clue comes from the topics Aristotle had discussed in *Metaphysica*.

"Physica" means nature, and in the *Physica*, Aristotle addressed questions about the nature of things. He asked why some things fall, for instance, rocks, but other things, such as smoke, do not. He asked why a rolling ball eventually comes to a stop, why the planets move as they do, and why fire is hot. In *Metaphysica*, by contrast, he addressed questions of somewhat greater generality, such as what basic things exist, whether are there ultimately different kinds of basic things, and if so, what accounts for the differences. He discussed the view that earth, air, fire, and water are basic, Democritus's contrasting view that atoms are basic, and Pythagoras's rather strange idea that everything is ultimately made of numbers. Because Plato had argued for the otherworldly existence of mathematical objects and logical truths, Aristotle also subjected those views to close criticism. Additionally, he theorized about causality: the nature of different types of causes, whether there is a causal origin of the universe, and the fact that different sciences may give different causal explanations of related phenomena. In discussing what might be the fundamental stuff of reality, he also made some suggestions about what it *means* to say of something—anything—that it actually does exist.

The collection of subjects in Aristotle's *Metaphysica* is a bit of a hodge-podge, but he regarded them as relevant to all sciences, and hence alike in that respect. Because of their general relevance, Aristotle used the expression "first philosophy" to signify the generality of the topics discussed in *Metaphysica*. The shared generality did not, of course, entail that the topics delimit a unified natural phenomenon of any kind, and it is fairly evident that Aristotle was under no illusion about that.

Moreover, Aristotle did not suppose that the topics in *Metaphysica* were beyond the methods of science or different in *kind* from the questions of the particular sciences. Later philosophers commonly did, however. That metaphysics not only has its proprietary subject matter—the fundamental nature of reality—but also has its own distinct methods for getting true answers became philosophical orthodoxy, but not because of any endorsement from Aristotle.

For convenience, I use the expression "pure" metaphysics to refer to the school of thought that assumes that metaphysical answers are beyond the reach of scientific methods and scientific discoveries and that the job of metaphysics is to lay the absolute foundations for all the sciences. Pure reason and reflection, perhaps with the addition of introspection and meditation, are, according to this perspective, the proper methods for making progress on metaphysical questions. This view considers the very status of science itself—ultimately sound or wrong—to depend on how the metaphysical answers turn out, and hence ultimately to depend on the beyond-science methods of metaphysics. Moreover, Aristotle's rather innocent expression "first philosophy" came to acquire a more self-important significance associated with suprascientific methods and principles.

What is the status of metaphysics now? Briefly, its domain has shrunk in tandem with the maturing of the various scientific disciplines. With the development of modern physics and chemistry, theories about atoms, subatomic particles, and force fields came to dominate serious discussion of the fundamental nature of reality. Following Newton's discovery in the seventeenth century of the laws of motion and the explanation of planetary movement, the nature of space and time have been most productively pursued by physicists, theoretical as well as experimental.[2] Especially in the last century, physicists pursuing cosmology made stunning scientific progress on such issues as the nature and origin of stars, planets, and galaxies; the age of the universe; and its changes through time. Geologists have learned a great deal about the origin and history of the Earth, and biologists about the origin and history of species. In general, the various scientific disciplines have been spectacularly successful in making progress on Aristotle's metaphysical questions.

In view of this sort of scientific progress on various classical metaphysical questions, some philosophers recognized that metaphysics, as construed by the purists, is probably misguided. American pragmatists, beginning with Charles Sanders Peirce (1839–1914), cautioned against the idea that there is a rock-bottom foundation to *all* of science, where metaphysical reflection is the single tool for laying that foundation. According to Peirce, there is, for better or worse, nothing more adequate or basic than the method of science itself: observation, experiment, hypothesis formation, and critical analysis. That, as one might say, is just a fact of the human condition. We use reason and science to reexamine our earlier assumptions and make revisions where necessary, in effect bootstrapping our way to a better and better understanding of our world. As Clark Glymour put it, we have to start with whatever we *think* we know, and work backwards and sideways, as well as upwards, to improve upon it.[3]

In the later part of the twentieth century, the central figure to attack the pure, a priori conception of metaphysics was W. V. O. Quine (1908–2000). In the spirit of C. S. Peirce, he defended the idea, scandalous to philosophers even in the 1960s, that there is *no* first philosophy. There is nothing firmer and more fundamental than science itself.[4] What he meant was that we use science to bootstrap our way to a better and better understanding of the world. Beyond the scientific method, broadly conceived, there is no independent method for discovering the nature of reality. Quine was not denying a role to common sense, for he took science and common sense to be elements of the *same* enterprise: making sense of the world through experimenting, theorizing, and thinking things through. Science, in Quine's view, is actually rigorous and systematic common sense in the context of cultural evolution.

If we are persuaded by the pragmatists, we have a choice: either we abandon metaphysics as misguided, or we break with the purists and update our characterization of the subject matter. On the latter option, metaphysical questions are best *re*characterized as those questions where scientific and experimental progress is not yet sufficient to found a flourishing explanatory paradigm. This implies that "metaphysical" is a label we apply to a *stage*—an immature stage, in fact—in a theory's scientific development, rather a distinct subject matter with distinct methods. Until rather recently, theories about the self, consciousness, and free will, for example, were at a very immature stage, since neuroscience and cognitive science were not sufficiently advanced to get very far in addressing these matters experimentally. Because of this relative immaturity, these topics may still be regarded as metaphysical, but when scientific success comes, that status will eventually be cast off as uninformative and burdensome.

Redescribing metaphysical questions as questions in their prescientific phase puts them on a very different footing from that favored by a priori philosophy. It implies, for example, that whether substance dualism is probably true is fundamentally an *empirical* issue, not an issue than can be resolved by pure reason and reflection independently of scientific exploration. It implies that whether conscious decisions lack all causal antecedents in the brain is fundamentally a question of empirical fact that no amount of beyond-science hand wringing can alter.

The more we understand about brains, their evolutionary development, and how they learn about their world, the more plausible that the pragmatists are on the right track concerning the scope and limits of metaphysics. The explanation is quite simple: We reason and think with our brains, but our brains are as they are—hence our cognitive faculties are as *they* are—because our brains are the products of biological evolution. Our cognitive capacities have been shaped by evolutionary pressures and bear the stamp of our long evolutionary history. If humans, and only humans, have a special, suprascientific, "metaphysical" faculty, its origin and existence should be consistent with the facts of evolutionary biology and neural development. Yet such a faculty looks *inconsistent* with the facts of evolutionary biology and neural development. Let us take a closer look at the matter.

If, as seems evident, the main business of nervous systems is to allow the organism to move so as to facilitate feeding, avoid predators, and in general survive long enough to reproduce, then an important job of cognition is to make *predictions* that guide decisions. The better the predictive capacities, the better, *other things being equal*, the organism's chance for survival. In a population of organisms, those who are predictively adroit do better than those who are predictively clumsy, other things being equal.

When an organism survives long enough to reproduce, its offspring inherit its genes, and thus inherit the capacities whose structures are organizationally dependent on those genes. Occasionally an offspring has tiny changes in its genes, a *mutation*, that results in the organism being structurally somewhat different from its parents. Usually such mutations are disadvantageous. On rare occasions, however, a mutation will give the offspring a change in brain or body structure that, relative to the organism's environment, ends up conferring a bit of an edge in the struggle to survive. If an organism with the advantageous mutation does survive and reproduce, its offspring will inherit the modified capacity. This is descent with modification.

For the pure metaphysical approach to the mind, the implications of descent with modification are troubling. For example, it implies that a fancy visual system will not emerge just for the sheer excellence of having fancy perception. Unless improvements in visual capacity make a net contribution to the organism's overall capacity to survive, they will tend to vanish along with the organism. *When* an offspring happens to have a mutation in its genes that dictates a structural change in the nervous system that gives the organism a perceptual capacity that allows it to make better predictions than its competitors can make, *then* that organism is more likely to survive and pass its genes on to its offspring. Importantly, however, if the mutation comes at a cost to the organism—if, for example, there is a trade-off between speed of processing and sophistication of perceptual images—then a given mutation may carry a net loss, even though the higher degree of accuracy of perception is predictively useful when considered alone.

From the perspective of Darwinian evolution, therefore, any beyond-science metaphysics has to face a tough question: Would there have been evolutionary pressure for the emergence of a special faculty with a unique route to Absolute Metaphysical Truth? What could have been the nature of such pressure? Is there a plausible account consistent with natural selection that can explain how humans could come to have such a capacity? Relative to what is now known, it is doubtful that any such account is forthcoming, even if one can envisage what such a capacity would be like. Consequently, we do best to resign ourselves to the probability that there is no special faculty whose exercise yields the Absolute, Error-Free, Beyond-Science Truths of the Universe. All we can do, though it is certainly no small thing, is to learn what the best available science says, mindful that it may embody errors, both large and small, and then subject it to criticism, refinement, and extension via more of the same—experimenting, theorizing, and thinking things through (see also chap. 6, pp. 245–254).[5]

Still, it may be urged that one's feeling of having made progress in suprascientific metaphysics should count for something, and the conviction that such progress has been made does indeed exist. More exactly, feelings of certainty may be cited as the benchmark for having discovered a Beyond-Science

Metaphysical Truth. For example, feelings of unshakeable conviction or absolute certainty may accompany consideration of the hypothesis that the mind is a nonphysical substance. Descartes, as we saw in chapter 1, seems to have enjoyed such certainty and to have believed it warranted a specific conclusion.

Feelings of certainty, however, are no guarantee of truth. They can, of course, motivate *testing* a hypothesis for truth. They can motivate continuing a research project even in the face of scoffers. But feeling certain that a hypothesis is true is, sadly, all too consistent with falsity of the hypothesis. Everyone knows of occasions in his own life when certainty and falsity were happy bedfellows. Moreover, the historical record is painfully clear on this matter. At various times, people have been completely certain that the Earth did not move, that space is Euclidean, that atoms are indivisible, that insanity is caused by possession of demons, that they can see into the future, and that they can communicate with the dead. Yet all of these propositions are probably false. That falsity and conviction coexist should not surprise us. Certainty, after all, is but a cognitive-emotive state of the brain, one such state among many other cognitive-emotive states of the brain.

The pragmatic conception of metaphysics may seem a bit of a disappointment, for much the same reason that it may seem disappointing that our universe has is no such thing as Absolute Space or Lady Luck or Guardian Angels. Having to muck on as best one can, Glymour-like, seems a lot less romantic, perhaps, than being on a quest for suprascientific Metaphysical Truth. Nevertheless, in making progress, we abandon romantic notions when their wheels fall off.

What metaphysical questions still remain to be resolved? On the topic of causality, impressive mathematical and scientific progress has indeed been made. Notably, there has been relatively little progress in the pure metaphysics of causality. We shall look a bit more closely at this in the next section. One subfield in physics where fundamental issues about the nature of reality remain very much alive is quantum mechanics. On the significance and interpretation of quantum mechanics, there is fruitful interaction between physics and the philosophy of physics.[6]

Beyond these matters, the remaining metaphysical questions, traditionally classified, are about the *mind*: What is the nature of consciousness, the self, free will? Is the nonphysical mind perhaps *the* fundamental reality? The *only* fundamental reality? How can we come to understand the mind if we have to *use* it to understand it? The three topics—consciousness, the self, and freedom of the will—constitute the three chapters in the metaphysics part of this book. From the pragmatist's perspective, we shall explore questions about consciousness, free will, and the self as questions about the mind/brain, and we will see that a young science is discovering things about the nature of the mind/brain that we could never have discovered through reflection and introspection alone. Whether any uniquely metaphysical work on these topics is left for the pure metaphysician and whether they will go the way of questions about the origin of the Earth and the nature of life are issues we can reconsider toward the end of the book.

As part of the groundwork for those discussions, we need to revisit the mind-body problem raised in chapter 1. Note that there is a mind-body *problem* only if the mind is *non*physical and the body is physical. The nub of the problem is how the two substances can interact and have effects on one another if they share no properties whatever. How, for example, can mental decisions have an effect on neurons, or how can directly stimulating the cortex with an electrode result in feeling one's leg being touched? On the other hand, if the mind *is* activity in the brain, then *that* particular problem, at least, does not exist. Other problems of exist, to be sure, but not the problem of the interaction between soul stuff and brain stuff.

2   Metaphysics and the Mind

How can we come to an informed opinion on the question of the existence of soul stuff? The pragmatist suggests that we use the science we have to compare the strengths and weaknesses of competing hypotheses, design good experiments, and test the hypotheses. Were a soul-brain interaction to exist, there should be *some* evidence of the interaction. This has not been forthcoming. The laws of physics, as we currently understand them, include the law of conservation of mass-energy. An interaction whereby a nonphysical mental event causes some physical effect, such as a change in the behavior of neurons, would violate the law of conservation of mass-energy. So far, no such violations are seen in nervous systems. This is not to say we are certain none exist, but only that there is no convincing reason to believe that they do exist. Deflecting criticism by postulating a *shyness effect*, according to which it is just the nature of souls to shield themselves from experimental detection, is, needless to say, not going to fool anybody. Since there is no independent evidence for a shyness effect, postulating shyness is a blatant cheat to avoid facing the implications of the absence of positive evidence.

Powerful reasons for doubting substance dualism accumulate with the increasingly detailed observations of the dependencies between brain structure and mental phenomena. The degeneration of cognitive function in various dementias such as Alzheimer's disease is closely tied to the degeneration of neurons. The loss of specific functions such as the capacity to feel fear or see visual motion are closely tied to defects in highly specific brain structures in both animals and humans. The shift from being awake to being asleep is characterized by highly specific changes in patterns of neuronal activity in interconnected regions. The adaptation of eye movements when reversing spectacles are worn is explained by highly predictable modifications in very specific and coordinated regions of the cerebellum and brainstem. And example can be piled upon example.

One of the most metaphysically profound discoveries in this century showed that a human's mental life is disconnected if the two hemispheres of his brain are disconnected. In the 1960s, a group of patients with epilepsy so intractable that it resisted control with drugs underwent a surgical procedure that separated the two cerebral hemispheres by cutting the nerve bundle joining them. The purpose of the surgery was to prevent the seizures from propagating from one hemisphere to the other, and it was successful in achieving this aim (figure 2.1). In careful postoperative studies of the capacities of "the split-brain" subjects, Roger Sperry, Joseph Bogen, and their colleagues found that each hemisphere could have perceptual experiences or make movement decisions independently of the other.[7]

To illustrate the disconnection effect, consider the following experiment: A picture of a snowy scene is flashed to the right hemisphere, and a picture of a chicken's claw is flashed to the left (figure 2.2).[8] An array of pictures is placed before the subject, who is to select, with each hand, the picture that best matches the flashed picture. In this setup, the split-brain subject does this: his left hand (controlled by the right hemisphere) points to a shovel to go with the snowy scene, and the right hand (controlled by the left hemisphere) selects a chicken's head to go with the chicken's claw. This is described as a *disconnection* effect, since each of the disconnected hemispheres seems to be able to function in perception and choice much as a single person does. In another example, Joseph Bogen reports observing a split-brain subject seated in an easy chair. His right hand picked up a newspaper, and he began to read. The left hand took the newspaper and tossed it to the floor. The right hand picked it up again, and he resumed reading, only to have the left hand pull the paper away

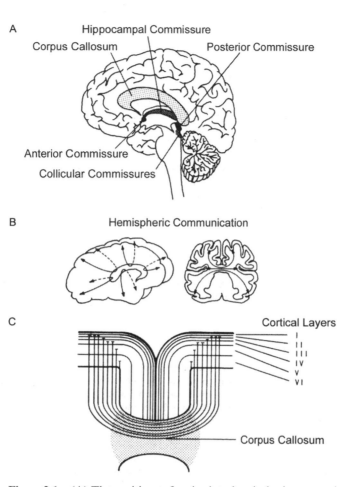

Figure 2.1   (A) The positions of major interhemispheric connections in the human brain as seen in sagittal section. (B) Interhemispheric fibers largely connect homologous areas in the two half-brains. (C) In addition, they terminate mostly in the cortical laminae from which they arose in the opposite hemisphere. (From Gazzaniga and LeDoux, *The Integrated Mind.* New York: Plenum, 1978.)

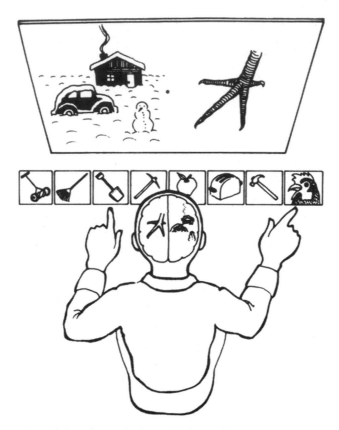

Figure 2.2 The method used in presenting two different cognitive tasks simultaneously, one to each hemisphere. The left hemisphere was required to select the match for what it saw (the chicken claw), while the right hemisphere was to select the match for what it saw (the snowy scene). After each hemisphere responded, the subject was asked to explain the behavior. (From Gazzaniga and LeDoux, *The Integrated Mind*. New York: Plenum, 1978.)

and drop it to the floor. In light of this behavior, we can conjecture that each hemisphere has its own integrated, coherent awareness.[9]

These remarkable results demonstrate that the unity of mental life is dependent on the anatomical connections in the brain itself. This seems reasonable enough on the hypothesis that mental life is activity in the brain. If the hemispheres are disconnected, the activity subserving mental function in the two hemispheres is disconnected. On the other hand, if mental life is activity in a nonphysical substance with *no* physical properties whatever, then why should splitting the brain split the mind? One could cobble together some story, perhaps, but a story that is consilient with what else is known about mental phenomena and neural phenomena—a story that has at least a modicum of plausibility—is very hard to come by. So far, none has been able to get off the ground.[10]

In general, as a hypothesis about the nature of the mind, how does substance dualism stack up against physicalism? The short answer is that substance dualism chronically suffers from the lack of any *positive* description of the nature of the mental substance and any *positive* description of the interaction between the physical and the nonphysical. The content of the hypothesis is specified mainly by saying what the soul is *not*: that is, it is *not* physical, *not* electromagnetic, *not* causal, and so forth. Negative characterizations can be useful, and they may be fine as a place to *start*. Evaluation of the hypothesis cannot proceed, however, without *some* positive elaboration: we need to hear something about *what* the proposed interaction is, *where* the interactions occur, and under *what* general conditions. Were someone to proclaim a new theory of light that says only that light is *not* electromagnetic radiation, it would be difficult to know how to test it. Because the soul-brain hypothesis lacks a substantive, positive characterization, it too is hard to take seriously, especially at this stage of science.

To compete with a brain-based explanation of, say, face recognition or obsessive-compulsive disorder or dementia, some positive claims—even the bare-bones of some positive claims—should be on the table. The slow degeneration of memory and cognition generally seen in Alzheimer's patients, for example, is currently explained within neuroscience as the progressive loss of neurons in the cortex. How, according to its adherents, might a soul-based story go? We are not told.

More generally, there appears to be no progress—not even significant experimental effort to make progress—in revealing the existence or properties of soul-brain interactions. One neuroscientist, John Eccles, did briefly entertain the conjecture that a soul-brain interaction is mediated by a special entity that he called a "psychon." Psychons, he believed, are the mediators of brain-soul interactions.[11] He predicted that they might work at certain synapses. But what are the properties of psychons? On what, in the synapse, do they exert an effect? Is the alleged effect mediated chemically? Electrically? Are psychons themselves material entities? No answers, let alone answers consilient with neuroscience, have been forthcoming. The psychon research program looks like a nonstarter.

The competing hypothesis—that mental phenomena are brain phenomena—stands in a completely different evidential condition. By contrast with dualism, it does have a rich and growing positive account, an account that draws on the entire range of neurosciences, as well as on cognitive science and molecular biology. Selected features of this positive account will emerge in the individual chapters on consciousness, self, and free will, and also in the later chapters on representation and learning.

As a preliminary to later discussion, notice that Descartes's particular version of dualism identifies *the mind* with the *conscious* mind. If there are in fact nonconscious mental states, this identification is on the skids. Notice that if some mental events, such as visual-pattern recognition, can be nonconscious, we do not have the alleged "direct access" to such mental states; i.e. we do not know about them just by having them.

There is overwhelming evidence that nonconscious *cognition* plays a critical role in memory retrieval, belief consolidation, judgment, reasoning, perception, and language use. To evaluate the evidence, we need to touch on a range of examples of nonconscious cognition in normal subjects, leaving aside for now examples of nonconscious cognition in clinical subjects.

The first example is well known to all of us. When we talk, we are aware of what we are saying, but we are not normally aware in detail of exactly what we are going to say—exactly what words, phrases, grammatical structure—until we say it. This is often true of writing as well, and many authors say that they sometimes find themselves surprised by what they write. The brain's decisions governing specific choices in words and sometimes even in content are typically nonconscious.

The second example of nonconscious cognition is also well known. In making a judgment about someone's approachability or attractiveness, based simply on a view of his or her face, one makes use of the degree of dilation of the person's pupils. If the pupil diameter is tiny, the face is judged to be less approachable and attractive than if the pupils are dilated. Surprisingly, most of us are aware neither of the role that this factor plays in our judgment nor of having detected pupil size at all. This example is one of many in which evaluative judgments are made without the subject being aware of the basis for the judgment.

In a different example, subjects are given a task of saying which of two lines, presented in the peripheral visual field, is longer. Occasionally, a word will be flashed in the very center of the visual field during the task (figure 2.3). As many as 90 percent of subjects report seeing nothing but the lines, even though the presentation of a word (for example, FLAKE) was above the subjects' sensory/perceptual threshold. Despite not being consciously seen, the word can

Task: Which line is longer—the horizontal or the vertical?

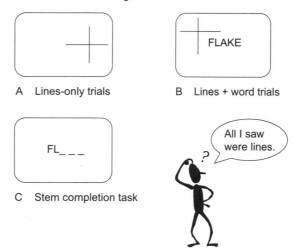

A   Lines-only trials   B   Lines + word trials

C   Stem completion task

Figure 2.3 Subliminal effects in the inattention paradigm. The task given to the subject is to report on the relative length of the intersecting lines (A). Occasionally, in addition to lines, a word will appear in the center of the screen (B). Typically subjects are attending to the task, and report no awareness of a word presented briefly under conditions of inattention. When tested on a stem completion task (C), subjects for whom the word was presented but not consciously seen are much more likely to respond with the presented word (e.g., FLAKE) than are control subjects who were not shown the word on the inattention trial. (From Palmer 1999.)

be shown to have a cognitive effect. Here is how. Subjects from the line-judging experiment as well as subjects who did not participate are given a stem completion task, in which they have to make a five-letter word given the first two letters, for example, FL_ _ _. While only about 4 percent of naive subjects make the word FLAKE, about 40 percent of test subjects make FLAKE if FLAKE was flashed. This shows that there was significant cognitive processing of the word, even though it was not consciously seen. This effect is referred to as inattentional blindsight.[13]

Consider now an example involving subthreshold stimuli. Normally, if people are asked to indicate a preference for one of two arbitrary visual patterns, such as a Chinese ideogram, they tend to choose the pattern to which they were previously exposed. The psychologist Robert Zajonc (pronounced Zy-unse) asked whether subjects would show this exposure effect if exposure were limited to a mere 1 millisecond. Not surprisingly, if a picture of an object is flashed on a computer monitor for only 1 millisecond, you will not *consciously* see anything but a blank screen. Nevertheless, the brain does detect something and does perform some basic pattern-recognition operations. This is known because when presented with two arbitrary visual patterns, people do indeed show the exposure effect and indicate a preference for the subliminally exposed image. In short, mere exposure biases choice. (*Why* this should be is another matter.) This experiment has been replicated many times, and it is an important demonstration that evaluative responses such as preferences can be generated by nonconscious exposure.[14]

Finally, one of the most intelligent ongoing behaviors is eye movements. The vast majority of one's eye movements (including tracking moving objects and saccades, occurring about three times per second) are made without anything like conscious decision or choice, and mostly in ignorance that one's eyes are moving at all (figure 2.4). Yet when tracked over time, saccadic eye movements reveal themselves to be organized around discernible goals, directed to solve visual disambiguation problems, and sensitive to attentional demands and task complexity. For example, regions with maximum relevance are fixated early in scanning and are frequently revisited. In walking, the gaze shift is typically a few steps ahead; in steering a vehicle on a variably curved path, gaze shifts forward at appropriate times to that distant point on the curve where the line of sight is tangent to the inside curve, with the result that each segment maintains constant curvature (figure 2.5).[15] These examples are but a few of many showing that if we think of the mind as intelligent, as perceiving, recognizing, and problem solving, then the mind cannot be equated with *conscious* experience, though conscious experience is part of the mind.

In addition, there are many examples from clinical research that lead to a similar conclusion. Before moving on to these topics, a further preparatory but brief comment on causation rounds out this introduction to metaphysics.

3   Causation

The traditional list of metaphysical topics typically gives a prominent place to causation. No obvious connection links causation as a metaphysical topic to causation as a topic of interest to neuroscience. There are, however, two areas of common concern: (1) How can neuroscience get beyond mere correlations of events in order to confirm causal hypotheses? That is, what conditions have

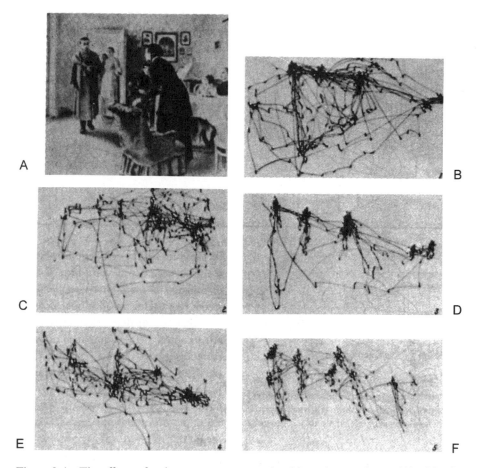

Figure 2.4   The effects of task on eye movement. A subject views a picture (A) while the experimenter monitors the subject's eye movements and direction of gaze. In each of the five cases, the instructions were different: freely view (B), estimate the economic level of the people (C), judge their ages (D), guess what they had been doing before the visitor's arrival (E), and remember the clothes worn by the people (F). A saccadic movement is represented by a line, and a momentary resting position is represented by a small dot. (From Yarbus 1967.)

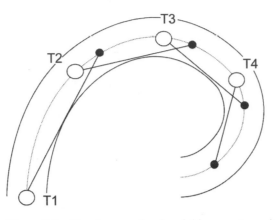

Figure 2.5   Steering a path of variable curvature. A driver (open circle) can merge trajectory segments by shifting point of gaze (black circle) at appropriate times (T1–T4) so that the line of sight is tangent to the inside curve. Each segment can meet the requirement of constant curvature, but the resultant overall trajectory can have a series of curvature variations. (From Wann and Land 2000.)

to be satisfied to establish real causal dependencies between functions such as consciousness and decision making? (2) What are the neurobiological mechanisms whereby any organism, including us humans, acquires a systematic causal map of the environs it inhabits? This is a puzzling matter, because background knowledge is essential to distinguish mere correlations from causal connections. On the assumption that nervous systems represent certain events as causally connected, and not as merely coincidentally correlated, the second question can be rephrased thus: how in fact does the nervous system deploy relevant background knowledge—together with current observations, manipulations, and interventions—to achieve a predictively powerful causal mapping of its world?

The first question is basically a *methodological* question—a question about reliable analytical or statistical tools, usable in any science, for assessing the significance of data for a hypothesis and hence in formulating adequate explanations of phenomena. These tools help us understand the importance of such matters as controls, confounds, standard deviations, measurement error, dependence and independence of variables, and sample-selection bias. They allow us to sharpen experimental design in order to extract more meaningful results. Work by philosophers, statisticians, and others has yielded an exuberant body of important results available for any science, including neuroscience.[16]

The second question is very different. It concerns the *cognitive neuroscience* of causal understanding; that is, it pertains to the nature of the actual processes and operations that underlie a brain's causal mapping of its world. Because this is fundamentally a question about learning and knowledge, the topic best fits into chapter 8, where it can be more productively discussed within the wider context of learning *in general.*

As formulated, these two sets of problems seem straightforward enough. Nevertheless, there is a version of these problems that is metaphysical—in the beyond-science sense of "metaphysical"—and this version addresses the ostensibly deeper matter of the fundamental reality of causes. Although these two sets of problems can be readily distinguished from their metaphysical companions, discussions of causation have a tendency to drift into the metaphysical realm. To forearm against unnecessary confusion, therefore, I shall outline the basic problem in the *metaphysics* of causation and suggest how its dangers can be avoided when neuroscientists address questions concerning either methodological tools or the neural mechanisms of causal inference.

Causal explanations have to do with how something came to happen or came to be as it is. We want to understand why some people get gastric ulcers, whether acidity in lakes reduces fish populations, or why the car has a flat tire. We want to understand what causes a goose to begin its southern migration, or to molt, or to imprint on the first large moving thing it sees after hatching. Metaphysics, now and for the past two thousand years, includes causation as a topic largely because it is not obvious what makes something a cause as opposed to a coincidental ride-along, or what exactly in a connection makes for a *causal* connection.

Causes are part of the universe, but not in the same way that rabbits and waves and electrons are part of the universe. A rabbit can be the cause of something, such as the footprints in the mud, and rabbits can be caused by things, such as other rabbits. Yet if all the entities in the universe were listed, "causes" would not be an item in the list. The reason is not that causes are spooky. On the contrary, causality is about as real as anything gets. If the dentist needs to do a root-canal procedure, we want him first to cause something, namely that the nerves innervating the tooth cease to respond to stimuli.

Being a cause means acting in a certain role, and we usually distinguish three types of causal roles: (1) a *precipitating* cause (lightning caused the forest fire), (2) a *predisposing* cause (having high blood pressure predisposes one for a stroke) and (3) *sustaining* cause (proximity to the ocean and a southerly location cause the moderate climate of San Diego). Any of these three types of casual roles may be *productive* (lightning caused the forest fire) or *preventative* (the rain prevented the forest fire). Depending on interest, on what we already do and do not know, as well as on the available possibilities for manipulation or intervention, one or another of these roles can assume prominence in a discussion, and thus one event or one variable may be selected as "the cause."

Are causes just self-evidently distinguishable from correlated occurrences of independent factors? Not at all. It can be very difficult to nail down which conditions are causal and which are independent. The history of science has many stories that illustrate the point, but one will suffice. For many decades it was firmly believed that stomach ulcers were primarily caused by stress, along with ingestion of irritating foods such as coffee and beer. This was not unreasonable, since most patients who had pyloric ulcers were under stress and their symptoms were made worse by coffee and beer. In the 1980s a pair of Australian physicians, Robin Warren and Barry Marshall, discovered a new strain of bacteria, later named *Helicobacter plyori*, in the stomach tissue of patients with pyloric ulcers (the pylorus connects the stomach to the duodenum, the first segment of the small intestine). Because the stomach is highly acidic, physicians naturally assumed it to be a hostile environment for bacteria, so this discovery was astonishing. Even after the discovery, most physicians assumed that the presence of *H. pylori* in patients with gastritis was entirely coincidental; that is, it was noncausally correlated with ulcers and hence independent of the disease.

In proving the causal role of *H. pylori* in the formation of pyloric ulcers, Marshall showed that if patients with pyloric ulcers were given antibiotics, their ulcers soon cleared up.[17] He then used himself as a guinea pig. Having first established that his own body tested negative for *H. pylori*, he then infected himself with it. Shortly thereafter ulcers appeared in his pylorus. He then cured himself with antibiotics. This intervention showed that *H. pylori* is probably the cause of pyloric ulcers. Anxiety and stress probably do not play a causal role, though the discomfort of ulcers may cause anxiety, which then occurs concurrently. People with frequent ear infections rarely have ulcers, since they frequently take antibiotics for their ear infections, which kill any *H. pylori* that happen to be present. Notice, however, that although frequent ear infections do not *cause* ulcer protection, they are correlated with ulcer protection via the common cause—antibiotics. This sort of example, simplified though it is, reminds us that distinguishing causes from coincidental correlations is not always obvious.

Given these and related examples, one may wonder what is it about the relations between events or conditions that makes for a *causal* relation? What in general distinguishes an event or process that is a cause from an event that is only coincidentally connected to it? As a first pass, one might assume that causes and their effects are *necessarily* connected, whereas coincidental events are only *contingently* (accidentally) connected. That is, we think of the cause as *making* the effect happen, or as *producing* the effect, or as being a special kind of force—a causal force.

This general answer seemed more or less adequate until David Hume in the eighteenth century pointed out that the *necessity* or *productive force* that supposedly explains causality is itself as mysterious as the causal connection it is meant to explain. What sort of property is this necessity? If necessity is just the property of causally determining, the answer fails to move us forward but rather merely moves us round in a circle. Moreover, Hume pressed on, necessity does not appear to be an observable property of events in the world, in the way that "being heavier than" or "being next to" are relations in the world. So far as the observable evidence is concerned, all we can determine is that first one thing happens then the other—first *H. pylori* gets into the system, then ulcers begin to form in the pylorus. Unless we can explain what it is for necessity or causal force to be in the world, opined Hume, we may have to conclude that appeals to necessity and causal force *as features of the world* are just metaphysical tomfoolery.

Since Hume's first unflinching formulation of the problem, legions of philosophers have struggled to answer him. Hume's challenge could not be dismissed as a joke or an idle problem, since causal explanations are at the heart of science. Not understanding what it is *in the world* that underwrites the differences between causal connections and coincidental connections is troublesome. If causality is not an objective feature of the world, how can a causal explanation be a real explanation? How can it be exploited to predict and manipulate other events?

Roughly speaking, two Hume-answering strategies have been deployed, with many clever, but ultimately unsatisfactory, twists on each. The first aims to find some plausible way to show how necessity really *is* in the world. And one way to do that is to consider event *A* as causing event *B* as an instance of a natural law. If the *H. pylori* in John's pylorus is in fact the *cause* of the ulcer, then there must be a natural regularity connecting *H. pylori* and ulcers such that, in general, if *H. pylori* is in someone's stomach, ulcers will form. Moreover, this lawlike regularity implies a counterfactual statement: had John been free of *H. pylori* in his stomach, he would not have gotten ulcers. If we take stress as an independent variable, notice that this counterfactual does *not* follow: had he been stress-free, he would have been ulcer-free. The *necessity* we conventionally attribute to causal connections therefore reduces to the fact that there are objective *regularities* in nature. Genuinely causal connections are capturable by natural laws, such as "Bacteria cause ulcers," "Nails puncture tires," "Iron readily combines with oxygen to produce iron oxide," and "Copper expands when heated." The idea is that whereas causes are governed by natural laws, coincidental connections are not.

To critics of this view, it seems that the regularities exist *because of* the causal powers of objects, such as the puncturing potential of nails. The natural-law strategy seems to imply that things go in the opposite direction; the causality derives from the lawlike regularity. Moreover, trying to give a *noncircular* and scientifically coherent account of a natural law ended up having most of the same problems as explaining what makes an event a cause. What is it that makes "Copper expands when heated" a natural law but "All cubes of gold in the universe are less than 1,000 miles on each side" *not* a natural law? Both are true (presumably), both are generalizations, both are testable, both support counterfactuals.

Another effort to identify the difference could take this form: "because heating really *causes* the expansion of copper, whereas nothing about gold makes it necessary to have the sides of any gold cube be less than 1000 miles." Alas, that is the one answer you cannot give, since going around in circles is not progress. And what of the *necessity* alluded to? Can we compose a sentence expressing a truth that is not a natural law but is a necessary truth? Easily. The sentence "All cubes of pure uranium 238 in the universe are less than 10 feet on a side" *is* necessarily true, because that much U238, we know, is a critical mass, and would explode before we could ever get our $10' \times 10' \times 10'$ cube made. So does that sentence express a natural law? Surely not.

Few seriously doubt that there are natural laws, but hammering out a satisfactory—and *noncircular*—account has so far been exceedingly difficult. Citing examples of agreed-upon natural laws is typically sufficient to teach students the difference between causes and coincidences, since they can then generalize on the basis of learned prototypes. But what metaphysicians want to know is what the prototypes have in common that enable students to generalize. Put another way, they would like to understand what lawful connections in nature amount to.

More or less out of desperation, some philosophers decided it might be worthwhile to explore the second option, namely, that *necessity is not really in the world, but in the mind.* Needless to say, getting an even remotely acceptable story on this option is difficult, since causal explanations for why the dinosaurs disappeared or why a star exploded or why the average temperature of the planet is increasing are surely about the world, not the mind. Moreover, they seem to be about a world before there were humans to think about causality. Most simply, the objection to this approach is that causal statements are statements not about *us*, but about the way the *world is*.

Kant (1724–1804) is the watershed for a hybrid in-the-mind and in-the-world approach. He well recognized that he needed to avoid the obvious objection to making causality an entirely subjective matter, yet he also saw the force of Hume's arguments. To a first approximation, Kant aimed to figure out how necessity could be a real feature of events, yet be *in* the subject—as part of the "lens" through which we see the world. Not surprisingly, he had a tricky problem of explaining how causal necessity was not *merely* subjective. If this sounds like an impossible goal, that is because at bottom it likely is. Although Kant wrestled long and brilliantly with the problem, his project his was probably doomed from the start.

A semi-Kantian strategy rooted in evolutionary biology might hypothesize that brains have evolved the capacity to infer causality from certain patterns of regularity observed in experience. Because of the need to make good predictions about food sources, predators, and so on, this is a reasonable hypothesis, and it can be empirically explored. Partly *because* it can be empirically explored, this hypothesis is regarded by some philosophers as fundamentally irrelevant to the genuinely metaphysical problem as outlined above. They still want to know what the property is *in the world* that brains can detect.

In sum, neither strategy for answering Hume has produced universally accepted results. Although some progress has been made, causation as a *metaphysical* issue remains an unsolved problem. As indicated earlier, certain *non*metaphysical issues regarding causation have, in contrast, permitted considerably more progress. This work clarified causal reasoning by demonstrating that a given effect can have multiple causes, that events may be independent but have a common cause, that statistical analyses are essential in cases where we are trying to identify causally relevant factors, that certain sampling techniques help eliminate confounds, and so on.

In view of the value of this kind of progress, a pragmatic approach counsels putting Hume's problem aside, at least for now. The pragmatist will suggest that we adopt the working hypothesis that there are genuinely causal laws and that we predict the course of nature better when we have discovered what they are. Having that hypothesis in place, we can redirect our energy into improving techniques for identifying causal factors, judging the objective probability of the occurrence of a given event relative to specific conditions, and figuring out how brains actually make reasonable causal inferences. With luck, some of these results may end up bringing the metaphysical issues to heel. At the very least, they may help us understand why the metaphysical questions seem compelling and how they might be reinterpreted.

Selected Readings

Bechtel, W., and G. Graham, eds. 1998. "Methodologies of cognitive science." Part III of *A Companion to Cognitive Science*, pp. 339–462. Malden, Mass.: Blackwells.

Churchland, P. M. 1988. *Matter and Consciousness*. 2nd ed. Cambridge: MIT Press.

Churchland, P. S. 1986. *Neurophilosophy: Towards a Unified Understanding of the Mind-Brain*. Cambridge: MIT Press.

Hacking, I. 2001. *An Introduction to Probability and Inductive Logic*. Cambridge: Cambridge University Press.

Rennie, J. 1999. *Revolutions in Science*. New York: Scientific American.

Skyrms, B. 1966. *Choice and Chance: An introduction to Inductive Logic*. Belmont, Calif.: Dickenson.

Williams, G. C. 1996. *Plan and Purpose in Nature*. London: Weidenfeld and Nicolson.

Wilson, E. O. 1998. *Consilience*. New York: Knopf.

Websites
BioMedNet Magazine: http://news.bmn.com/magazine

Encyclopedia of Life Sciences: http://www.els.net

The MIT Encyclopedia of the Cognitive Sciences: http://cognet.mit.edu/MITECS

3   Self and Self-Knowledge

1   The Problem and the Internal-Model Solution

1.1   What Is the Problem?

Sliding out of the MRI tube, I noticed Dr. Hanna Damasio studying the lab's display screen as my brain's images appeared. I stood by her and watched the image on the screen. "Is that *me*?" (figure 3.1). Well, yes, in a certain sense, up to a point. What I was looking at was an image of the thing that makes me *me*. Somehow, starting in infancy, my brain built stories about its body, its history, its present, and its world. From the inside, I know those stories—or perhaps I should say, "I *am* one of those stories." Surely, though, I am not *just* a bit of fiction. I am about as real as things get in my world. So how do I make sense of all this? What exactly is it that the brain constructs that enables me to think of myself?

Descartes proposed that the self is not identical with one's body, or indeed, with *any* physical thing. Instead, he concluded that the essential self—the self one means when one thinks "I exist"—is obviously a *nonphysical, conscious thing*. To the eighteenth-century Scottish philosopher David Hume, however, Descortes's answer was anything but obvious. Hume proceeded to examine whether there is evidence for something that is the self apart from the body. He came to realize that if you monitor experience, there does not seem to be any self *thing* there to perceive. What one can introspect is a continuously changing *flux* of visual perceptions, sounds, smells, emotions, memories, thoughts, and so forth.

Among all those experiences, however, there does not exist a single, continuous felt experience that one can attend to and say, *"That's* the self," as one

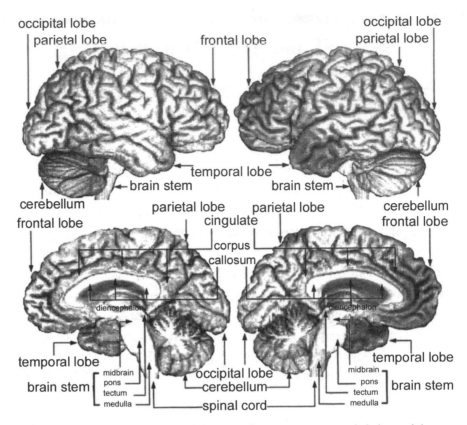

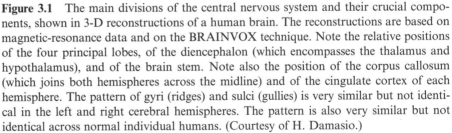

Figure 3.1 The main divisions of the central nervous system and their crucial components, shown in 3-D reconstructions of a human brain. The reconstructions are based on magnetic-resonance data and on the BRAINVOX technique. Note the relative positions of the four principal lobes, of the diencephalon (which encompasses the thalamus and hypothalamus), and of the brain stem. Note also the position of the corpus callosum (which joins both hemispheres across the midline) and of the cingulate cortex of each hemisphere. The pattern of gyri (ridges) and sulci (gullies) is very similar but not identical in the left and right cerebral hemispheres. The pattern is also very similar but not identical across normal individual humans. (Courtesy of H. Damasio.)

can attend to a felt experience and say, "That's a headache." One can remember events in one's past, but active recollections are yet more current experiences, albeit experiences where the pronoun "I" figures prominently. Nor is there a single continuous spatial object that one can attend to and say, "*That* is the self," as one can attend to one's body and say, "That is my neck." Because there seems to be more to *me* than my body, observations of my *body* are not simply equivalent to observations of my *self*. Thus, Hume concluded, there does not seem to be a *thing* that is the self, at least not in the way we unreflectively suppose there is.

Of course, Hume realized very well that nothing *seems* more evident than the statement "I exist." In reflection, we take for granted that a single thread of "me-ness" runs through the entire fabric of one's experience. If a brick falls on my foot, I know the pain is *mine*. If I scold myself about jaywalking, I know that it is *me* scolding *myself*. We generally awake from a deep sleep knowing who we are, even if we are confused about when and where we are. We know, without pausing to figure it out, "*This* body is my own," and "This hand and this foot are both parts of my body." We know very well that if we fail to plan for future contingencies, our future selves may suffer, and we care *now* about that *future* self. Hume too knew all that. But he also thought that these reasonable beliefs did not amount to an *answer* to his question "What is the self?"

So here is Hume's conundrum: I think I am some*thing*, yet my self is not anything that I can actually observe—at least not in the way that I can observe pains or fatigue or my hands or my heart. So if my self is not an identifiable experience, if it is not something I can observe, what is it? If the "self" is a mental construction—a mode of thinking about my experiences—what are the properties of this construction, and where does this construction come from?

In this century, we have the advantage of addressing Hume's questions within the framework of neuroscience. *Thinking*, we are reasonably sure, is something the brain does. Therefore, *thinking of oneself as a thing* enduring through time is also something the *brain* does.

At least in *very* general terms, therefore, we have an answer to Hume's question concerning where the constructed "self" comes from: *the brain*. Such unity and coherence as there is in my conception of myself *as a self* depends on, among other things, these neurobiological facts: (1) my body is equipped with one brain, (2) body and brain are in close communication, and (3) activity in diverse parts of the brain is coordinated at a range of time scales, from milliseconds to hours.

Evolutionary biology, moreover, suggests a *very* general answer to the question of *why* brains might construct a self-concept: it plays a role in the neuronal organization used to coordinate movement with needs, perceptions, and memories. Such coordination is essential to an animal's survival and well-being. Coordination of functions ensures that inconsistent behaviors—fleeing and feeding, for example—are not attempted at the same time. It ensures that a hungry animal does not eat itself. For organisms with high-level cognition, self-representational capacities constructed on the more fundamental platform help us to think about the future, make useful plans, and organize knowledge (see also section 1.3).

Still, these terms are *very* general, and much more detail is required to explain how brains work so that I can reflect on my motives, imagine myself swimming, remember myself riding a bicycle, fall into deep sleep during which my conscious sense of self vanishes, dream about flying, and wake up knowing who I am. Much of the detail remains to be discovered, though what is known so far permits us to sketch a basic framework for entertaining some reasonable answers. It is also enough to allow us to design experiments that may unearth more detailed answers concerning how the brain generates the *I* that I am.

In specifying the range of self phenomena to be addressed by neurobiology, it may be useful first to consider how we routinely conceptualize the self. In the ground-clearing stages of our inquiry, determining what we *believe* about the self by examining what we *say* about the self is a probe into the role of self concepts in "coherencing" our inner life. How much of what we believe is *true* is, of course, a distinct, *empirical* matter.

Frequently we use "self" to mean *body*, as in "I cut myself" and "I weighed myself"; on other occasions, we mean to distinguish self from body, as when you are exhorted, for example, to "talk to yourself." This ambiguity in the word "self" rarely causes misunderstandings, since we share rich background knowledge concerning when the word "self" does and does not refer to the body.

In conversation about the self, metaphors are the standby. Sometimes we use *object* metaphors, as when we say we pushed ourselves to finish, pulled ourselves together, fell apart, or tied ourselves in a knot. On the other hand, when we say "I annoyed myself" or "I deceived myself" or "I talk to myself," the *person* metaphor is invoked.[1]

Using the self-as-person metaphor, people commonly describe themselves in terms of a cluster of selves, such as one's good self and bad self, one's shy self and extrovert self, or one's social and private selves, all of which are selves belonging to "me." My good self and my bad self are sometimes conceived of as *parts* of the one thing, myself; sometimes as two persons in a group of many. One may bemoan losing control of oneself or of being controlled by one's superego.

In describing character traits, one may refer to one's *real* self, which one can consider as hidden or revealed or transformed or inaccessible. What one considers one's *real* self is partly a cultural and a conventional matter, though only partly. We do not usually talk about our "unreal self," though we do admit to masking or covering our true selves. Sometimes the self is conceived of as a *project*, for example, when we undertake self-improvement or self-discipline. Sometimes one's self is analogized as a *process*, such as becoming mature or wise.

Thus juxtaposed, these commonplace metaphors are strikingly diverse. A space alien would be unable to extract from them an underlying coherent and consistent prototheory about the self. What the *nonsystematic* character of metaphorical language suggests is that *the self* is not a thoroughly coherent, single, unified representational scheme about which we have thoroughly coherent, unified beliefs. Rather, the self is something like a squadron of capacities flying in loose formation.[2] Depending on context, it is one or another of these capacities, or their exercise, to which we refer when we speak of the *self*. Some of these capacities involve explicit memory, some involve detection of changes in glucose or CO_2 levels, others involve imagery in diverse modalities or emotions of diverse valence. The *fundamental* capacity, however, probably consists in coordinating needs, goals, perception, and memory with motor control.

1.2   Self-Representational Capacities

These considerations motivate recasting Hume's problem in terms of *self-representational capacities*. This removes the temptation to lapse into supposing that the self is a *thing*, or if it is a representation, that it is a *single* representation. Self-representations may be widely distributed across brain tissue, coordinated only on a "as needed" basis, and arranged in a loose hierarchy. We do not understand yet exactly how all this works. But despite the large gaps in our knowledge, adopting the terminology of representational capacities facilitates the formulation of specific questions about the neural components that play a role in some particular self-representational capacity or other.

What are representations?

On the hypothesis that "the self" is actually a loosely connected set of representational capacities, the chief workhorse in the account is *representation*. Hence, we need to know what, in terms of neuroanatomy and neurophysiology, representations are. How, in general, do brains represent? How can neural states be representations *of* anything, in the sense that they point beyond themselves to the thing they represent? These issues are addressed more fully in chapter 7. In the meanwhile, we shall make do with a simple sketch to tide us over.

To a first approximation, representations are states of the brain, such as *patterns of activity* across groups of neurons, which carry *information*. For example, a pattern of neuronal activity can embody information that something hot touched the left hand, or that the head is moving to the right, or that food is needed. We may consider a representational *model* to be a coordinated organization of representations embodying information about a connected set of objects and what happens to them across time. Thus a brain might have a representational model of the body or of one's hunting territory or of one's clan and the pattern of social relationships within it. A brain can also have models of its own processes. If some neuronal activity represents a motor command to reach for an apple, other neuronal activity represents the fact that a specific command has been issued. If some neuronal activity represents a light touch on the left ear, higher-order neuronal activity may represent the *integration* of many lower-order representations (light touch on the left ear *and* buzzing sound to left, which means that there is a mosquito, etc.).

The brain not only represents the sensations of one's limbs; it specifically represents the sight and feel of the limb *as belonging to* oneself (there is a mosquito on *my* left ear). Yet further neuronal activity may represent *that* representation as a mental state (I *know* I feel a mosquito on my left ear). One's brain also has a model of one's preferences (I know I prefer beets to cabbage), one's skills (I know how to tie a trucker's knot but not how to play squash), one's memory (I do not know the names of my second cousins), even when one is not now exercising those preferences and skills.

Self-representation, evidently, is not an all-or-nothing affair; it is not the sort of thing that you either possess in its full glory or in no amount. Rather, self-representation comes in grades, degrees, shades, and layers. The various self-representational capacities are undoubtedly dependent on the task and the context. For example, people normally express themselves very differently when they are with family than when they are negotiating with business associates. Certain self-representational capacities may wax or wane, depending on neurochemical and endocrine conditions (e.g., depressed during abnormally low serotonin conditions), behavioral state (being awake, being in a deep sleep, or dreaming), task demands (during battle versus during rest), and immediate history.

The multidimensional character of self-representation glimpsed in the array of commonplace metaphors is well supported by neuropsychological and cognitive data. Before tackling the neuroexplanatory task, therefore, it will be useful to have a closer look at some of this data to understand a bit more about how the multiple capacities can dissociate, malfunction, or deteriorate.

Autobiography and self

Memories of what I saw, felt, and did are part of the story of my life, part of my autobiography. For each of us, one's life story is an important part of who one is now. As we shall see below, having an autobiographical memory is not necessary for having a body representation. But is autobiographical memory necessary for the conscious representation of oneself as an agent, as having desires and goals, as being a person? The situation is complicated, as always in biology, but the first-pass answer is "No." This conclusion is based on studies of patients who have lost essentially all autobiographical memory.

R.B., a patient studied in the Damasio lab in Iowa City, has profound amnesia.[3] Owing to an attack of herpes simplex encephalitis, R.B. suffered massive destruction of both temporal lobes, including the overlying cortical areas, as well as the deep structures including the amygdala and the hippocampus. He has no recollection of his past, save for one or two facts such as that he has lived in Iowa. This aspect of his condition is known as "retrograde amnesia." Everything else—whether he was married and had children (he did), whether he was in the army or went to college or owned a house—is beyond his ken.

He has also lost the capacity to learn new things (and thus also has anterograde amnesia). He has a short-term memory of only about 40 seconds, less if distracted. Undoubtedly, his sense of himself is different before and after the onset of the disease, at least in the respect that he cannot recall anything about himself or his life. Nevertheless, it is striking that R.B. does have important features of self-representation as a self among selves. That some self-representational capacity endures is made evident by his being able, with no apparent effort, to refer to himself with the pronoun "I." For example, he might say, "I would like some coffee now," or in response to a question about the weather, "I think it is still snowing." That some capacities are lost while others remain reinforces the point that self-representation is a *many-dimensioned* phenomenon, not an *all-or-nothing* phenomenon.

R.B. can attribute intentions and feelings to others, though his attributions tend to be somewhat routinized. They are also slanted toward the positive emotions, perhaps because he has lost tissue in a region of prefrontal cortex known to have a role in negative feelings such as depression. Shown a picture of a happy family at a birthday party, he will correctly describe it. Shown a picture of a man striking a woman, who is shrinking from the blows, he described the man as loving the woman very much and trying to help her stand up. Although mistaken about their specific feelings, he does ascribe feelings to them. Nor does R.B. ascribe negative feelings to himself. He always says he feels just fine—not sad, lonely, disappointed or angry. Just *fine*! This Pollyanna bias may indicate some decrement in his self-representation insofar as these and related data suggest that his ability to have those feelings is impaired. Insofar as he is thus impaired, it is reasonable to say that his sense of himself as a person is also impaired.

R.B. is a remarkable patient, and he does demonstrate, however impossible it might have seemed antecedently, that one can have a basic sense of self despite an essentially complete loss of autobiographical memory. Obviously, however, his loss *is* truly devastating. He can neither reflect on his past nor wonder whether some of his choices were regrettable, whether he has been self-deceived about some things, or whether he squandered opportunities for self-realization. He cannot reminisce about his children or even his own childhood; he cannot strive to make up for lost time or make good past wrongs. He is, moreover, unaware of his deficits. These capacities—to reminisce, self-reflect, know that you have undergone a change—are very important aspects of self, and R.B. has lost them all. He does *not* have a normal human sense of himself, but what is remarkable is that the fundamentals of self-representation do persist, despite the loss of life memories.

Depersonalization phenomena

A contrasting profile can be seen in certain schizophrenic patients. During florid episodes, a patient may have good autobiographical memory, but may suffer what are called *depersonalization* effects, where he is confused about self/

nonself boundaries. In recalling a florid episode during which she kept notes, one computer scientist described her confusion as "not knowing where I stopped and the world began; not knowing what, physically or mentally, was *me*." Afflicted with depersonalization, a schizophrenic may respond to a tactile stimulus by insisting that the sensation belongs to someone else or that it exists somewhere outside of *him*.

Auditory hallucinations, often considered diagnostic of schizophrenia, may be a particularly striking example of an integrative failure in a self-representational capacity. The hypothesis is that the "voices" heard by some schizophrenics are in fact the subjects' own inner speech or even their own whispered speech not recognized as such.[4] A subclass of schizophrenics may be quite deluded about their personal identity—about who in fact they are. For example, a patient might be utterly convinced that he is Jesus, and he habitually conforms to his conception of Jesus' demeanor, dress, and behavior. Aristotle, in pondering this phenomenon, accurately described such as person as not knowing who he is.

Certain drugs can also trigger depersonalization phenomena.[5] Surgical patients given the anesthetic ketamine, for example, are susceptible to depersonalization effects. A patient awaking from ketamine anesthesia may be convinced she is dead or possessed or separated from her body or separated from her own feelings. Similar depersonalization effects may also occur in subjects who have taken phencyclidine (PCP) or LSD. These effects have prompted some researchers to wonder whether some of the so-called "out of body" and "near death" experiences of patients who are otherwise asymptomatic might have fundamentally the same neurophysiological origin as disturbances caused by ketamine or LSD (see chapter 9).

Parietal cortex lesions

A very different kind of abnormality in self-representational capacities may be observed in some patients who suffer loss of sensation and movement in the left-side of the body following a stroke in the region of the parietal cortex of the right hemisphere. Such a patient may be adamant in denying that her left hand or left leg is in fact hers, insisting that the limb really belongs to someone else. This is termed "limb denial." As one otherwise normal stroke patient remarked about her left arm, "I do not know whose it is. Perhaps it belongs to my brother, since it is hairy." On occasion, a patient with limb denial has been known to try to throw the arm or leg out of the bed, believing it to be alien.

In a somewhat different profile, the patient with right parietal cortical damage may recognize her left arm as her own, but deny that it is paralyzed. This condition is called "anosognosia" (unawareness of illness). Ramachandran studied one patient who, though very normal in other respects, believed that her motor functions were entirely normal, and specifically that she could move her paralyzed left arm and leg.[6] She nonchalantly explained her presence in the hospital as owing to some minor problem. When asked to move her left hand, she would cheerfully agree to comply, and a moment later when queried about not complying, she would reply that indeed she just *did* move it. If asked to point at Ramachandran's nose, she would agree to do so, and later reply that yes, she could *see* her hand pointing directly at his nose.

This was not a psychiatric effect in the traditional sense, but a compromise of right parietal function. Remarkably, in some patients the denial can be made temporarily to disappear using a minor intervention that increases the activity in the right vestibular system. Using a technique developed by Eduardo Bisiach, Ramachandran put cold water into the left inner ear of the patient, thereby stimulating the right vestibular nucleus. For reasons we do not understand, in these conditions, the patient's anosognosia disappeared. During this brief time, she acknowledged that she was in the hospital for a stroke, that her left side was paralyzed, and that she could not move her left arm. As the effect of the cold-water irrigation wore off, the anosognosia returned. Nor did she remember her lucid description during the intervention.

Significantly, limb denial and anosognosia are rarely seen following a lesion in the *left* parietal region, even though such a stroke results in comparable loss of movement and feeling of the right side of the body. Nor is it seen with spinal cord injuries, despite whole-body loss of sensation and movement. Christopher Reeve, for example, is a quadriplegic and knows full well that his arms are his, and knows he can neither move nor feel them.

Why is integrity of the parietal cortex of the right hemisphere necessary for these aspects of self-representation? Although neuroscience cannot yet answer this precisely, convergent evidence favors the hypothesis that an *integrated* body representation may be fundamentally connected with integrated spatial representations more generally. Because of a loss of movement and feeling, and because of a breakdown of spatial integration, a patient's brain may have no basis for identifying the arm in her bed as hers. Evidence supporting this connection to spatial representation derives from an array of sources, including independent studies on split-brain subjects. These tests have shown that the right parietal cortex in particular has a crucial role in spatial capacities, including spatial memory, recognition of spatial configurations, and spatial problem solving. The nature of this connection between normal body/self representation and spatial representation is not yet understood, though as we shall see in section 1.3, it would not be surprising if it were rooted in the brain's solution to the problem of generating appropriate movements to intercept objects in space. (For further discussion of parietal-lobe symptoms, see chapter 7.)

The dementias

Dementia (Latin *de + mens*, meaning *mind*) is an acquired loss of intellect. The dementias are diffuse in their effects, meaning that widespread brain areas are involved. There are many forms of dementia, and they differ in their causes (e.g., infective agents, blows to the head, intoxicants), initial region of damage, temporal course, and treatability.

It is the progressive forms of dementia that are particularly relevant to this discussion. These diseases include Alzheimer's, Pick's, Creuztfeldt-Jakob, kuru, HIV dementia, and Korsakoff's (alcoholic dementia). In these dementias, all capacities, including self-representational capacities, degenerate. Memory losses are typical, and more recent autobiographical memories are lost before very old memories. Patients tend to lose physical vigor, show gait disorders, and have diminished language abilities. As the disease progresses, patients' autobiographical memory fades, along with knowledge of their own lifelong preferences. Personality changes are common, and are unpredictable in their direction. There is relentless decline of specialized skills (e.g., carpentry, cooking), social skills, and ultimately ordinary, everyday skills (e.g., buttoning a shirt, tying shoelaces). Toward the end, patients become deeply confused about who they are, as well as when and where they are. From observing an Alzheimer's patient over many years, it is reasonable to conclude that the "self" progressively vanishes as the various self-representational capacities disintegrate.

Anorexia nervosa

One very puzzling body misrepresentation is typical in subjects with severe anorexia. An emaciated female may insist that she looks chubby and that she needs to lose a few more pounds to look acceptable. No amount of reasoning and explaining convinces her otherwise. What happens if you ask her to look at her body in a mirror and make a judgment about whether she is fat? Even then patients will honestly and forthrightly size themselves up as plump, chubby, tubby, and so forth. This seems impossible, given the unambiguous observational cues. Collectively, the data suggest that the disease involves a significant impact on body representation. The etiology of anorexia, bulimia, and other body dysmorphias (pathological distortions of body image) has not been established but is under active investigation.[7] There does appear to be a genetic predisposition, but other factors are involved in precipitating the onset of anorexia. One possibility under discussion is that in anorexic subjects, the nervous system has an impaired ability to monitor internal milieu (see below, pp. 71–76), resulting in a heightened anxiety that leads to loss of self-integration when the brain's standard strategies for reducing anxiety are ineffective. Whether this is a cause, an effect, or even a consistent feature of anorexia nervosa is still unsettled.

This discussion has touched on a fragment of the data relevant to the proposition that self-representation is multidimensional. There are many other kinds of cases I have not discussed, including brain-lesion subjects who have lost the capacity to recognize faces and cannot recognize their own face in a mirror or photograph, patients with focal brain damage who can no longer tell you which digit is their index finger and which is the pinkie (finger agnosia), patients with akinetic mutism, who have lost all inclination to say or do anything. My aim, however, has been to illustrate the multidimensionality of self-representation through a sample of cases of fragmentation and dissociation of self-representational capacities. The next matter to address is the neurobiological mechanisms supporting self-representational capacities.

1.3 Self as Agent

The key to figuring out how a brain builds representations of "me" lies in the fact that first and foremost, animals are in the *moving* business; they feed, flee, fight, and reproduce by moving their body parts in accord with bodily needs. This *modus vivendi* is strikingly different from that of plants, which take life as it comes. If an animal's behavior is haphazard or incoherent, the animal tends not to live long enough to reproduce. Consequently, an overarching demand on any nervous system is that it appropriately *coordinate* the body: its movable parts, its needs, its stored information, and its incoming signals.[8] This demand is a powerful constraint on the evolution of neural organization.

Swimming or running, swallowing food or building a nest, stalking prey or hiding from predators—smooth performance of any of these activities requires tightly timed coordination of spatially dispersed muscle cells. Sometimes the coordination must extend over long time periods, as in stalking and hiding. Sometimes it can be handled by a reflex, such as ducking when a projectile approaches your head. Because individual muscles move at the behest of motor neurons, motor-neuron activity must be appropriately orchestrated. But to serve survival, behavior must also be coherent relative to the animal's needs (don't feed if you should flee), suitable to current given sensory signals (the berries are too green to eat), and appropriate in view of relevant past experience (porcupines should be avoided; cover bee stings with mud) (figure 3.2).

Coordination can only be performed by *neurons*, since there is no intelligent, extraneuronal "mini-me" inside who puts it all together. The intelligence of the system has to emerge out of the *patterns* of neuronal connectivity, the *response properties* of particular types of neurons, the activity-dependent *modifiability* of neurons (learning), and a neuronal *reward system* for strengthening neuronal connectivity when things go well and weakening connectivity when they go awry. Given this very broad construal of coordination, this problem, one might say, just *is* the problem of how the brain works. Perhaps that is true. Nevertheless, in addressing the nature of self-representational capacities, we shall aim more modestly to characterize only gross aspects of the coordination problem, leaving the vast wealth of related detail to be mined from the suggested readings.

To depict the problem in its most fundamental aspects, we shall consider first how the brain sets the animal's basic goals and then how the brain solves the basic problems of sensorimotor coordination so that it can achieve those goals.

Internal milieu, needs, and goals

In the nineteenth century the French physiologist Claude Bernard was intrigued by the seemingly trivial distinction between an animals' external environment and its internal environment. He was struck by the entirely *non*trivial fact that while the external environment can fluctuate a great deal, its *internal* condition is kept relatively constant. For example, human body temperature stays about 37° C, and a mere five degrees either way brings us death. Homeostasis—the maintenance of a largely constant internal milieu—is a buffer against environmental fluctuations. The brain keeps track of levels of blood sugar, oxygen, and carbon dioxide, as well as blood pressure, heart rate, and body temperature, in order to detect perturbations to the internal milieu that are detrimental to the animal's health. Deviation from the normal set

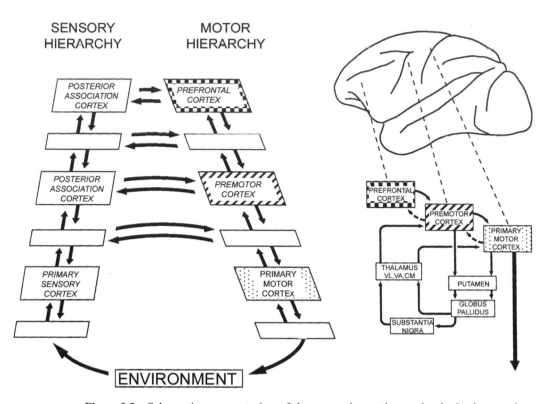

Figure 3.2   Schematic representation of the perception-action cycle: the basic organization of pathways at the cortical level. Notice that there are both forward projections *and* back projections in *both* the sensory and motor cortical areas, and that beyond the primary sensory regions, there are connections *between* the sensory and motor regions. Right: The basic organization of cortical motor connectivity and its subcortical connective loops. The complex, looping connectivity, including both cortico-cortical pathways and cortico-subcortical pathways, undermines simple ideas about modularity and rigidly staged feedforward processing, and suggests instead that the functional architecture of nervous system "hierarchies" is actually very heterarchical. (From Fuster 1995.)

points cause an orchestrated set of neuronal responses that ultimately cause the animal to seek either food, water, warmth, a hiding place, or the like, thereby restoring deviant values to their normal values.

Homeostatic functions—and, in particular, the ability to switch between the different internal configurations for *fight and flight* from that needed for *rest and digest*—require coordinated control of heart, lungs, viscera, liver, and adrenal medulla in a set of interconnected structures. In all vertebrates, the brainstem is the site of convergence of afferents (input neurons) from the viscera and the somatic sensory system, and it contains also nuclei for the regulation of vital functions. In addition, the brainstem houses neuronal structures that regulate sleep, wakefulness, and dreaming, as well as structures mediating attentional and arousal functions (figure 3.3). Antonio Damasio (1999) has emphasized that this anatomical proximity of structures is an important clue to the coordinating role of the brainstem and its pivotal role in self-representational capacities (table 3.1).

Maintaining a constant internal milieu means that the nervous system has to "know," in some sense, what the internal set points *should* be. This scare-quoted sense of "know" can be cashed out in terms of patterns of neuronal activity to which the system is rigged to return when perturbed. (More about such patterns of activity will be discussed in chapter 7.) Additionally, the system has to "know" what motor behavior would be effective in returning the body to normal after changes in critical values. That is, the system has to be rigged so that if low blood sugar is detected, for example, the animal's nervous system should prompt it to begin looking for food, not fleeing, unless fleeing is currently necessary for survival. Pain signals should be coordinated with withdrawal, not with approach. Cold-temperature signals should be coordinated with shelter seeking, not with sleeping. Body-state signals have to be integrated, options evaluated, and choices made, since the organism needs to act as a *coherent whole*, not as a group of independent systems with competing interests.

By making some effects pleasant and some not, the nervous system directs the animal's choices. Emotions are the brain's way of making us do and pay attention to certain things. That is, they are assignments of value that direct us one way rather than another, and they seem to have a role in every aspect of self-representation, and certainly in body representation. Brief periods of oxygen deprivation give rise to overwhelming feelings of needing air; extreme hunger and thirst can make us feel so desperate as to banish all thought of anything but water and food. Satisfaction is felt after feeding, sex, and

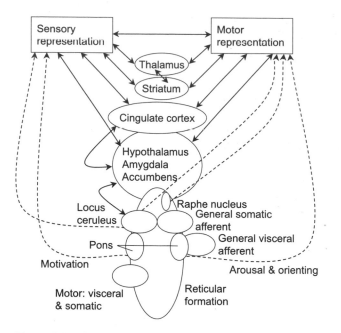

Figure 3.3   A schematic representation of the main structures involved in coordinating motivation, arousal, orientation, innerbody signals, musculoskeletal signals, and evaluations of perceptual signals. The axis along the brainstem, hypothalamus, and cingulate cortex constitutes the basic coordinating platform. The *hypothalamus* figures in basic drives, such as sex, hunger, and thirst; the *amygdala* figures in processing fear evalutions and responses; the nucleus *accumbens* is critical in feeling pleasure. The broken arrows from brainstem structures to the sensory and motor corteces represent *diffuse but very broad* modulating projections; the solid arrows represent more specific "information-bearing" projections. For simplicity, only some of the pathways are indicated.

successful predator avoidance. More generally, self-preservation is underpinned by powerful feelings.[9]

As neuroscientists have emphasized, this part of the system probably plays a role not only in emergency situations, but also in providing assignments of hedonic value in more humdrum categorizations, as when objects and events are classed as desirable, nasty, familiar, novel, safe, dangerous, and what have you.[10] If you come into a shed and encounter a nasty smell, it will be recognized first and fundamentally as dangerous, as the basic fear circuits respond well before the cognitive niceties get deployed and long before "cool" reason kicks in for impulse control.

Table 3.1 Main cell masses of the mesencephalon

Cell masses	Connections		Possible functional associations
	Afferent	Efferent	
Tectum			
Tectum opticum (called "superior colliculus" in mammals)	II, cord, bulb, sensory nucleus of V, isthmus, torus semicircularis or inferior colliculus, pretectum, thalamus, telencephalon	Cord, bulb, periaqueductal gray, reticular formation, nucleus isthmi, thalamus (especially birds and mammals), retina (teleosts, amphibians)	Correlation of visual, auditory and somesthetic; feature extraction; localizing stimuli formulation of higher reflex commands; eye and head movements, especially in orientation
Tegmentum			
Torus semicircularis (called "inferior colliculus" in mammals)	Lateral line nuclei (fish), cochlear nuclei (tetrapods), vestibular nuclei (fewer in higher groups), cord, V sensory nucleus	Tectum, thalamus, reticular formation	Correlation of information on equilibrium and near-field aquatic displacements (and electric fields); sound sources; localization
Nuclei III, IV (including general somatic and general visceral efferent)	Vestibular nuclei, cerebellum, tectum (indirectly), reticular formation	Extraocular muscles, iris, and ciliary muscle (parasympathetic)	Movements of eyes; accommodation; pupillary constriction
Periaqueductal gray matter, tegmental nuclei, interpeduncular nuclei	Complex, including tectum, hypothalamus, habenula, cord, telencephalon	Complex, including nuclei of III, IV, VI, pons, thalamus, hypothalamus	Limbic system; affect, visceral control
Isthmo-optic nucleus	Tectum	Retina (in birds only)	Horizontal cell response
Nucleus isthmi (in nonmammalian forms)	Tectum, probably torus semicircularis	Tectum, torus semicircularis tegmentum, thalamus	Correlation of optic, equilibrium, acoustic influences
Reticular formation, including tegmental reticular nuclei	Cortex, pallidum, reticular formation of other levels, cerebellum, vestibular nuclei, cochlear nuclei, tectum, cord	Reticular formation of other levels, thalamus, cord	Motor control; pupil; many other functions; reticular activating system

Table 3.1 (continued)

| Cell masses | Connections | | Possible functional associations |
	Afferent	Efferent	
Red nucleus	Dentate, interposed nuclei, precentral cortex (somatotopically organized)	Cord, bulbar reticular formation, inferior olive, cerebellum, thalamus (especially from small-celled newer part of red nucleus)	Motor coordination, especially righting; flexor activity; well developed in carnivores, poor in primates
Intermediate zone			
Substantia nigra (large in man, small in other mammals; only a forerunner in reptiles)	Caudate, putamen, subthalamus, pretectum	Striate, pallidum, thalamus	Extrapyramidal motor; inhibition of forced movements; pathologic in Parkinsonism

Source: Bullock 1977, table 10.5.

Moving, causing, and surviving

A brain that efficiently and accurately detects needs, but cannot orchestrate the body to move in order to satisfy those needs, is a brain destined to be some creature's next meal. So how can a brain make successful limb and body movements? How can sensorimotor coordination, both in short-term and in long-term actions, be achieved by neurons? Bits of the story are known, many of the details are not, and in this context, simplification of what is known is unavoidable.

If you are a simple tube, such as a worm, with only circular and longitudinal muscles and a few sensory neurons, the solution to the problem of how to move is rather straightforward: you move down the gradient of good odors to get food and away from noxious stimuli to avoid injury. Your behavioral repertoire and equipment is limited. For animals such as mammals and birds, however, the story must be gloriously complicated, given the range of components that are coordinated by the nervous system and the complexity of the coordination needed to make a many-limbed body move in just the right way, at just the right time, and over just the right time.

For engineering reasons, it behooves a nervous system to have an internal representation of the body that is a *kind of simulation* of the relevant aspects of a body's movable parts, the relations between them, the relations to its sensory input, and its goals. In this context, we shall talk in terms of an inner *model* rather than an inner *representation*, since model talk allows us to interface with research in control theory. This engineering subfield concerns how to organize a complex system, such as automated take-off and landing controls in the Airbus, so that given the variable parameters of the system, the goals of the system are reliably achieved.

Very roughly, the idea introduced by Daniel Wolpert is that one strategy brains use to solve the coordination and control problem involves neuronal simulations—inner models of the body.[11] Rick Grush calls these models *emulators*.[12] The engineering value of neural emulators springs from three main sources. The first and most basic source of value derives from the fact that input neurons, such as visual-system neurons, map the world in terms of sensory structures, such as the retina, whereas the motor system maps the world in terms of the body's movable equipment—joint angles, muscle configuration, and so on. Emulators can help make the sensory-to-motor transition. Emulators also help you intercept a target you can no longer see and allow you to imagine possible solutions to a problem. Finally, feedback from an emulator can be many milliseconds faster than feedback through sensory systems, and when time is of the essence, that can be a boon. We shall consider these more closely.

Consider a sensorimotor problem. You see a plum on a tree, you are hungry, and you want to grasp the plum with your hand. Simplified, the problem for a nervous system is this: the visual system has a *retina-based story* about where the plum is, but the motor system has to have a *joint-angle story* about where the plum is, since it is the arm that must reach and the fingers that must grasp the plum. So the motor system needs to know what joint-angle combination will serve to achieve the goal. Consciously, one never worries about this, since the brain has the wherewithal for solving the problem without our conscious attention to it.

The easiest way to think of this problem is that the visual system represents the spatial position of the plum in retinal coordinates, while the motor system represents the plum's position in joint-angle coordinates (figures 3.4 and 3.5). On this construal of the problem, the brain's task is to transform the position of the plum in retinal coordinates into the position of the plum in joint-angle coordinates so that the motor system can issue a command that will result in the hand grasping what the eye sees.[13]

More succinctly and more generally, the brain needs to be able to make coordinate transformations so that the body is in the right configuration to get the desire satisfied. The coordinate-transformation problem is referred to as the

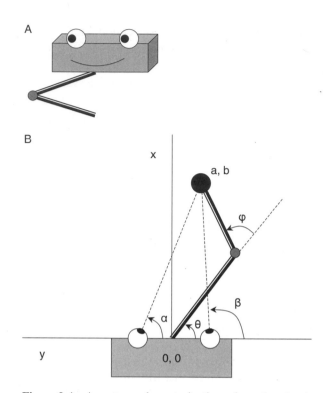

Figure 3.4   A cartoon characterization of an ultrasimple problem of sensory-motor co-ordination. Consider a device with two rotatable "eyes" and an extendable "arm" with one joint (A). In panel (B), as the eyes triangulate a target (dotted lines) by assuming angles (α, β), the arm joints must assume angles (θ, φ) so that the tip of the forearm makes contact with the target.

kinematic problem, as it concerns only the path the arm and hand should take and does not take into account such matters as the changes in momentum of the arm, friction on the joints, or whether there are additional loads on the arm, such as a bag hanging from the wrist. The part of the problem that does take forces into account is called the *dynamics*, and will be set aside here as we focus solely on the kinematic question.

The general form of the kinematic problem is well known to engineers. The solution is to construct an *inverse model*, that is, a model internal to the system that says (for goal *g*), "If I managed to get *g*, what command *y* would I have used to get it?" A good inverse model will specify *y*, which then becomes the motor command of the moment, and if all goes as planned, the plum is successfully grasped. So now the question is this: how can a brain construct a

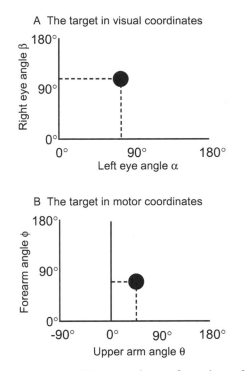

Figure 3.5   The respective configurations of the sensory and motor systems can be represented by an appropriate point in a corresponding coordinate space, as shown in (A) for the eyes and (B) for the hand. The position of the target in *visual space* is not the same as its position in *motor space*. Consequently, to make the arm go to the right place, a coordinate transformation from visual space to motor space is needed.

successful inverse model to generate motor commands for a range of different actions, including grasping the plum?

A computationally direct solution would be to completely specify all transformations by a neuronal look-up table. For animals like us, alas, this solution would involve excessive amounts of wiring and hence an excessively large head. This is because the arm can have many different starting points, it can take any one of many different adequate paths to the desired object from any given starting point, and reaching the target may require moving the body as a whole, and thus require appropriate leg movements and postural adjustments.

In addition to all that, life involves more than grasping plums. We sometimes want to kick a ball, catch a fish, or climb the plum tree so we are within grasping distance of the plum. And not only do we sometimes want to grasp the object we see, but we may need to do it while running, perhaps over rough terrain. While running, we may need to throw a heavy object, such as a spear, at another moving object, such as a deer. Moreover, the body changes its size and shape during development or after accidents or with use of tools such as knives and skis. So the look-up table would have to be bigger than gigantic. Efficiency of wiring and flexibility of performance, therefore, demand a compact, modifiable, accurate inverse model. How can a brain come by such a desirable device?

One elegant engineering solution is to hook up a somewhat sloppy inverse model with an error-predicting *forward* model and let the two converge on a good answer.[14] If, for example, the goal is to reach a plum, the inverse model gives a first pass answer to the question, What motor command should be issued to get my arm to contact the plum? Taking the command proposal, the forward model calculates the error by running the command on a neuronal emulator, and the inverse model responds to the error signal with an upgraded command. The command from the inverse model need only be good enough to get the hand very close, since on-line feedback can take over to make minor corrections for the final few inches. If the forward model is also capable of learning, this organization can be very efficient in acquiring a wide range of sensorimotor skills (figure 3.6).

Brain circuits with forward models organized to work with inverse models are emulators in Grush's sense. With sufficient access to background knowledge, goal priorities, and current sensory information, emulators can make a wide range of relevant predictions. They can not only predict that on command y your hand will miss the plum, but also that you will fall over, or that your hand will contact nettles, or that if you grasp the plum you will pitch forward, and so on. Probably, predictions as fancy as this will not be featured in a leech's nervous system, for example, but the bet is that they are found in the brains of mammals and birds, among other animals.

The second value of the emulator is that it allows the brain to make an appropriate movement even after the target has become invisible. This could happen because, for example, the lights have suddenly gone out, or because the early stages of executing a plan require a whole-body movement, during which the target becomes occluded. It might routinely occur when an animal looks into a cavity for birds' eggs or into a hole for gophers and then uses its forelimbs to go after what it can no longer see. More generally, it can occur whenever you have a plan for the future where the target is not currently visible.

The third important point about emulators is that they can be engaged "off-line" in evaluating very abstract behavioral options, such as shooting the rapids

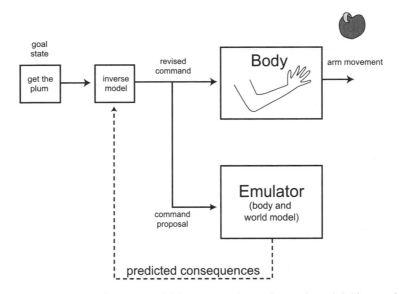

Figure 3.6   An inverse model is connected to a forward model (the emulator). The inverse model gives a first pass answer to the question, What motor command will get my arm to the plum? The inverse model proposes an answer and sends out a command proposal to the forward model, which then calculates the error by running the command on the neural emulator. The inverse model then responds to the error signal with an upgraded command.

or portaging around them. Off-line imagining yields an advanced peek at the likely consequences of pondered actions, which permits undesirable consequences of contemplated actions to be foreseen and avoided.[15] So, for example, one may envision the risk of capsizing the canoe in rough water, as against the many hours portaging up a steep grade and through dense bush. Eventually, one's brain settles on a decision, whereupon more detailed actions can be planned, such as pulling out the canoe, hoisting it up on one's shoulders, and so forth. In the planning phase, the motor signals generated by the inverse model are merely "what if" motor commands, not full-blown commands to move.[16] Off-line planning also permits an animal to prepare to intersect targets that do not currently exist but are expected at some point in the future. Thus a bird can build a nest, or a wolf pack can plan to intercept the annual migration of caribou across a certain point of the Alsek River.

It is evident that humans regularly use sensory and motor imagery to work out in their brains solutions to problems, both highly abstract and somewhat concrete, before implementing the solutions in the world. Contemplating a steep, icy ski slope, one's emulator will make motor predictions about the likelihood of losing control. In building a shelter, one envisions before construction what would be a suitable location, what materials are available, how it should be structured to withstand wind and rain, and so on. As Grush has stressed, this form of problem solving is essentially the brain manipulation of a body image.[17] Envisioning how to answer questions in an interview may be little different, but probably draws on many of the same operations.

The final point concerns speed and the fact that in a competitive world, speed matters. It is not the only thing, but it is an important factor. Feedback concerning the consequences of the execution of a plan will come faster from the emulator than from the body itself. It takes time for a motor-command signal to reach the various muscles, for the muscles to change, and for feedback signals from the muscles, tendons, and joints to return to the brain. If visual feedback is used, it takes time for signals to be processed in the visual system, which is relatively slow, since the retina takes about 25 milliseconds of processing time. Especially when the animal is large and the distance between limb and brain is on the order of meters, (as in humans, whales, and elephants), feedback that comes faster than what is available via the perceptual route is desirable. This shortcut may give the brain an additional 200–300 milliseconds, and when getting the timing exactly right is important, those milliseconds can make the difference between success and failure.

So far emulators have been discussed in terms of their engineering virtues.[18] What is the evidence that brains do in fact uses emulators? Neurobiological studies at the level of the single neuron and the network strongly suggest that posterior parietal cortex and area VIP do execute transformations from visual to motor coordinates.[19] More correctly, it seems likely that this region takes information from a range of sensory systems—visual, auditory, vestibular, somatic sensory—and converts it into eye-centered coordinates, head-centered coordinates, body-centered coordinates, and world-centered coordinates, depending on the body's starting configuration and the brain's goals (see figures 3.7 and 3.8). Pouget and Sejnowski have constructed a convincing artificial neural network showing exactly how this could be done.[20] In view of the supporting physiological evidence, they propose that real neural nets in this region are disposed to represent "where perceived objects are in my-body [egocentric] space," as well as where objects are in allocentric space.[21] (See pp. 309–312.)

Additionally, in this region and also in the dorsolateral region of the frontal cortex, to which the posterior parietal region projects and from which it gets signals, there are neurons that hold a target location on-line even when the

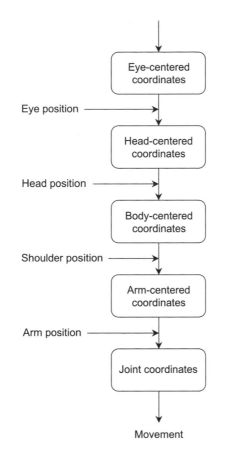

Figure 3.7   Coordinate transformations required to specify an arm movement toward a visual target. The position of the target on the retina is specified in retinotopic coordinates. This position needs to be remapped in joint coordinates to move the arm to the corresponding spatial location. This transformation can be decomposed in a series of subtransformations in which the target position is recoded in various intermediate frames of reference. (From Pouget and Sejnowski 1997.)

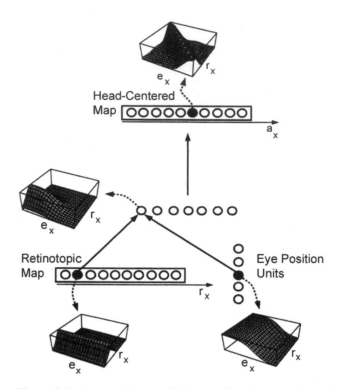

Figure 3.8 A neural network for transforming a retinotopic map to a head-centered map. The input contains a retinotopic map of the visual input, and the output consists of a head-centered map. The eye-position units have a sigmoidal tuning to eye position and a range of thresholds. The function represented by the network is nonlinear, as illustrated by the fact that the response to r_x and e_x of the units in the output layer is clearly not a plane. This mapping could be implemented by middle-level units that compute the product of a Gaussian of r_x with a sigmoid of e_x. Such units would provide basis functions of the input variables and would respond like gain-modulated neurons found in the parietal cortex. (From Pouget and Sejnowski 1997.)

target itself has disappeared, as the emulator hypothesis predicts.[22] Moreover, lesions to parietal cortex cause misreaching and other disturbances of visually guided grasping, such as misshaping the hand to a target shape. Other structures directly involved in emulator function include the cerebellum and the basal ganglia.

Additional evidence for the existence of brain emulators derives from psychological experiments concerning eye movements. Here is how the story goes. Without conscious commands, our eyes constantly scan the environment, moving about three times per second along paths that maximize task-relevant visual information. These eye movements are known as saccades. Other eye movements involve tracking an object, when the object is moving or the subject is moving, or both. Such tracking is known as smooth pursuit. Even though the retina registers huge shifts in light patterns owing to all this eye movement, stable objects in the visual scene appear to remain stable. That is, the brain interprets retinally detected motion as motion of *our eyes*, not motion in the world. Moreover, if things in the world *are* moving, the brain can distinguish between motion due to object movement and motion due to eyeball movement. So as I move my eyes around a scene, I can tell the difference between movement of the dog and movement of my eyes. Although the computations responsible for this result must be exceedingly complex, at a conscious level the achievement is effortless. How does the brain make these very important distinctions?

The brain undoubtedly uses emulators. It knows from a copy of the eye-movement command (*efference copy*), sent to the forward model among other places, whether or not the eyeballs were commanded to move, and in what direction. Here is one small piece of evidence for this hypothesis. Suppose that the brain used only *feedback* from the eyeball *muscles* to know whether the eyeball moved. On this supposition, as Helmholtz (1867–1925) rightly reasoned, if you close one eye and *passively* move the open eye by gently pressing on it, you should still see stationary objects as stationary and see the movement as due to eye movement. This is not what happens. As you can test for yourself, stationary objects actually appear to move when you gently press the eyeball. This simple experiment provides evidence in favor of efference copy: in the passive-movement condition, no eye-movement command from the brain exists to "explain" the stimulus movement with respect to the retina, so world movement is perceived.

In a more decisive, but also more invasive, experiment, John Stevens and colleagues reported in 1976 that they had used a pharmacological agent to paralyze the eye muscles. This experiment is a control condition for the Helmholtz passive-movement condition, for here the intention to move the eyes exists, but the eye muscles cannot move. Three subjects (Stevens and two colleagues) sit and look at an object, say a coffee cup. At some random time, the subject looks to the right, or rather, he *intends* to look to the right. Because of the paralysis, the eye muscles cannot respond to the command, and hence the eyeballs do not move. Thus he continues to see the coffee cup. As each subject reports, however, something interesting does happen: the subject *visually experiences the whole scene jumping to the right*. Why?

This stunning perceptual effect is at least partially explained on the efference-copy hypothesis, and hence on the emulator hypothesis. Crudely speaking, the brain thinks this: "I issued a command to move the eyes to the right, yet the coffee cup is still in full view. That can only be because the whole scene—coffee cup included—moved when the eyeballs moved." In short, the brain makes a prediction about a change of scene based on the eye-movement *command*, which hitherto has always been followed by real eye movement. When the prediction fails, the brain grabs the "best explanation." Stevens's experiment is thus not only evidence for the role of efference copy; it is also an important illustration of how the brain's eye-motion emulator can have a powerful effect on sensory experience itself. Incidentally, if one supposes that sensory systems essentially mirror reality, with no top-down coloration, Stevens's result is a brilliant falsification of that supposition.

Is there evidence of emulators used for off-line problem solving? A rather striking example of problem solving that probably involves off-line manipulation of the body image is seen in ravens. The ethologist Bernd Heinrich tightly tied a piece of meat to one end of a length of twine (about three feet) and tied the other end to a trapeze.[23] One at a time, hungry ravens were released into the room. A bird's only successful strategy for getting the meat is to sit on the perch, draw up a length of twine with its beak, step on the twine, and repeat the procedure about seven times until the meat is level with the perch. In other words, this problem cannot be solved in a single step, and no reward is obtained until all seven steps are complete. So a simple *response-reward learning device* will not find the solution. This is not a problem the birds encounter in the wild, and hence the problem is novel.

When Heinrich did this experiment with a crow, invariably the crow would fly at the meat and try to snatch it. This strategy is hopeless, and the crow suffers the discomfort of a jerked neck. Heinrich observed a dozen crows, one by one, stuck on this hopeless strategy, never managing to figure out how to get the meat. So the solution is not obvious (whatever *that* means), even to a bird as bright as a crow.

Ravens are legendary for their cleverness, and they did indeed respond in a very different fashion. Of six ravens, one was string-shy and would not approach string in any condition. (Like many intelligent animals, ravens apparently have irrational fears and phobias.) Five ravens solved the problem within five minutes of being allowed into the area, and their strategies for solving the problem followed much the same order. First, they spent a little time just looking at the setup. Second, they pecked at the string where it was attached to the trapeze as if trying to sever the string. No raven performed this act on string to which no food was attached. Third, they grabbed the top of the string and twisted it violently from side to side as if trying to break it off. Fourth, they reached down to pull up a length of string, stepped on it, and repeated the procedure until the meat was at their feet. This fourth procedure took 10–20 seconds. If Heinrich shooed them off the trapeze after they had performed the pull-up, they dropped the meat and flew nearby. As soon as it was safe, they returned and straightaway repeated the pull-up procedure. If, out of sight, Heinrich rearranged the string with a pulley so that the raven had to pull *down* on the string to get the meat to come *up*, they easily switched modes. If the string and meat were merely laid on the trapeze but not attached, the birds directly snatched the meat and flew off.

That none of the ravens got its neck jerked by going for the attached meat while flying suggests that their brains expected what would happen were they to do that and decided against it. That the ravens turned to the pull-up strategy within minutes and were successful in pulling up the meat *in one trial* strongly suggests that the ravens used body-image manipulation in causal problem solving. As Heinrich argues, "The simplest ... hypothesis is that the birds anticipated at least some consequences of the behaviors before overtly executing them."[24] The emulator hypothesis gives a very plausible explanation of this remarkable problem-solving behavior, especially in the context of independent evidence for neural emulators of the body.

Off-line emulation also appears to have a significant effect in skill acquisition. For example, covertly practicing a golf swing—going through the movements in imagination—does improve the swing at a rate greater than doing nothing, and almost as well as actually practicing.

Yet another bit of psychological evidence for the existence of emulators comes from the difficulty of tickling yourself. Being tickled by someone else feels very different from tickling oneself. As in the paralyzed-eye-muscle experiment, here too something about the brain's internal representation of the motor-intention signal affects the *feeling itself* that results from the touch. Moreover, this is true even when the touching device is not your own hand, which would provide sensory feedback and thus clue the brain in, but a lever with a feather that you can move. When the subject moves the lever, the touch still feels different from when someone else moves the lever, even though you get the very same stimulus.

There is, however, a way to fool the brain. Sarah Blakemore and her collaborators rigged a self-touching device so that the experimenter can put a *delay* in between when the subject pushes the lever and when the subject is touched.[25] The experimenter can also perturb the trajectory of the lever. The protocol is to interleave *self-touching* trials with *other-touching* trials. When the experimenter inserts a delay and/or the trajectory of the lever is perturbed, it feels to the subject as though someone else were touching him, even when it is his movement that causes the tickle.

Why should we be able to feel the touch as an other-touching stimulus under these conditions? The most likely hypothesis is that in normal conditions the brain's action emulator says, to put it crudely, "Got a copy of the intention-to-tickle-left-foot, so the left-foot-touch is my own." When there is a delay or a perturbation, the brain thinks, "Well, that can't be me, because my command would have been executed earlier." This representation of the intention, along with representation of the *normal time* for execution of the intention, affects the actual feel of the stimulus. This is extremely important, since it shows that the brain's body model includes temporal parameters. Notice that this effect also demonstrates again that experience itself can be altered by the cognitive representation of an intention.[26]

Other experiments tapping into the brain more directly indicate that *in general*, intentions to move are integrated into the brain's ongoing self/body model. Suppose you raise your left hand. A number of brain areas contribute to achieving the effect. These include the supplementary motor area (SMA), the premotor cortex (PMC), the primary motor area, parts of the cerebellum, and the somatosensory cortex (see figure 3.9). Studies using activity-sensitive magnetic resonance imaging technology (functional MRI) show that when you merely *imagine* that same action, the same motor areas (the SMA and PMC) are active.

Not surprisingly, activity in the *somatosensory* cortex is then much diminished, since there are no afferent signals from the extremities to indicate changes of muscles, joints, and tendons. Incidentally, other areas that show

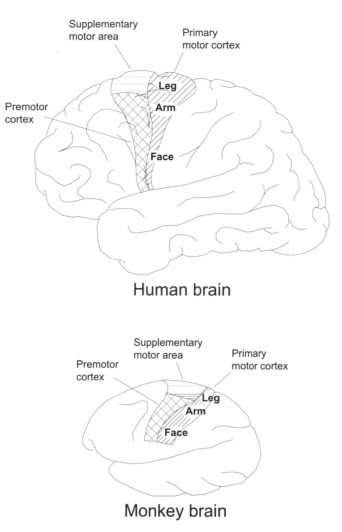

Figure 3.9   The location in the monkey and human brains of primary and supplementary motor areas of the cortex and posterior parietal cortex.

heightened activity during *visual* imagery, such as parts of the visual cortex, were not above baseline in the *motor* imagery task. To control for nonmotor effects, subjects were trained to avoid all visual images when imagining their movements, attending only to kinesthetic images (arm-moving feelings). To control for actual motor signals activating muscles, subjects were also trained to keep their muscles relaxed when imagining a hand movement.[27]

This range of data fits well with the hypothesis that the brain has a model integrating body configuration, movement decisions, and expected results of intended movements, all of which are time-sensitive. In other words, the data support the hypothesis that neural emulators in the sense discussed exist in the brain and are a watershed for self-representational capacities in general. This is not to suggest that the emulators are *the self*, that they are the little person in the head we jokingly envisage. Rather, emulators are one component in the story of our self-representational capacities.

In animals with large brains, such as humans, there will be coordination on a grander scale than in rats. Highly sophisticated coordinative functions ultimately yield fancy results, such as impulse control, long-term planning, richly detailed autobiographies, and imaginative explorations that stir emotions. At this level, where there are representations of representations of representations, and so on, we come upon those human self-representational capacities about which we typically converse. These high-level networks embody one's long-terms plans, as well as one's preferences, skills, attitudes, and temperament. At bottom, however, what anchors self-representational capacities is the neuronal organization serving coordination and coherence in "making a living," so to speak.

In this section I have stressed the role of intentions-to-move, while helping myself to the assumption that the emulator has available to it a rich supply of signals regarding the soma (Latin: body)—its postural configuration, its location relative to other objects, its sensations and perceptions. Obviously, these signals are extremely important. If I need to flee, my motor system needs to know what my current body configuration is, since the motor commands will be different depending on whether I am starting from a sitting, standing, or crouching position. If I am to learn skills such as being able to climb a tree or throw a rock, my brain needs feedback from the joints, tendons, and muscles. If I am to avoid bodily injury, I need to know when and where it hurts, whether and where it is hot or cold. All this requires a sensory system that informs the brain about what is going on bodywise. Now we need to look in more detail at the nature of the sensory information the brain gets about the body.

2 Inner Models of Body, Self, and Others

2.1 Sensory Systems Representing the Body

The nervous system is generally considered to have two main systems whose function is to represent the body: the *somatic sensory system*, which has receptors in the muscles, joints, tendons, and skin, and the *autonomic system*, which innervates the cardiovascular structures; the bronchi and lungs; the esophagus, stomach, and intestines; the kidney, adrenal medulla, liver, and pancreas; the urinary structures; and the sweat glands in the skin. The genitalia are innervated by both, but the labor is divided. For example, the autonomic system stimulates erection and ejaculation, the somatic system carries signals of touch, pressure, and so on.

The two systems follow different pathways from the extremities to the brain, and they appear also to be different in their effects on conscious awareness. For example, while both the tongue and the stomach have movement receptors, one can be aware of the movement of one's tongue, but one is not aware of the stomach's peristaltic movements. The visceral system has a motor subsystem that functions, for example, in sweating, secreting tears, and changing the heart rate. By contrast, motor control for the skeletal muscles is a system distinct from the somatic sensory system, though of course the two are integrated at various levels from the spinal cord to the cortex.

In the next two sections, we shall consider the somatic sensory and visceral systems to see in a bit more detail what is known about how they contribute to one's sense of oneself.

The somatic sensory system

Patients with damage to their right parietal cortex teach us that although normally nothing could be more obvious than that this arm is mine, nevertheless this is a judgment that the brain has to construct. How does my brain know my body's position? How does my brain know whether something touched my body or whether it touched itself? The rough answer is that nervous systems have highly specialized structures for detecting and transmitting signals; they have highly organized wiring for connecting body to brain and brain to body. The body-to-brain wiring keeps the brain informed about what is happening to the body, while the brain-to-body wiring allows the brain to control the body.

The patterns of connectivity yield representational models of the body that keep track of the schedule of motor commands along with changes in body configuration, body contact, and body needs.

The somatic sensory system is the nervous system's primary device for telling the brain how the body is configured, whether it has been harmed, whether it is in contact with other objects, and what the features are of any contacted objects. It is actually a rather diverse system comprising four submodalities, each specialized for detecting a distinct signal type. The basic subdivisions are light touch and pressure, temperature, proprioception (from joints, muscles, and tendons), and pain (nociception), which has various subsystems of its own.

Each submodality can signal the intensity of the stimulus, its duration, and its location on the body surface. Complex stimulus properties, such as textures (e.g., rough or smooth), spatial configurations (e.g., curved or straight), and tactile recognition (e.g., feels like a paper clip) depend on combinations of neuronal responses. One particular combination of signals will represent that there is something fuzzy crawling up my left ankle; a different combination will represent that something cold and hard is pushing on my left ankle.

Each submodality has its proprietary pathway leading from the location of the receptor in the body to the spinal cord. Maintaining their submodality specificity en route, spinal neurons project to regions in the brainstem, the thalamus, and the cortex (figure 3.10). Within the thalamus, each submodality has a proprietary region where it makes synaptic contact. The next set of projections goes from the thalamus to the cortex, with axons from each submodality clustering together in a typical path.

Distinct pathways of fibers carrying signals about body parameters are mapped in an orderly way in the spinal cord, brain stem, hypothalamus, thalamus, and several cortical regions (the insula, S2, S1, and the cingulate). Adjacent neighborhoods at the periphery are mapped to adjacent neuronal neighborhoods; e.g., the arm representation is next to the hand representation, the middle-finger representation is between the index-finger and ring-finger representations, and so on. In this sense there are maps—literal maps—of the body in the brain stem, with successive remappings at a series of higher-level structures (figure 3.11).

Specialized receptors in the skin perform different jobs and give rise to distinct sensations. Hairy skin, such as that on the back of the hand, contains receptors that wrap around the hair follicle and respond to movement of the hair. This is the principal device for signaling very light touch on hairy skin. In some animals, muzzle whiskers are highly sensitive and provide

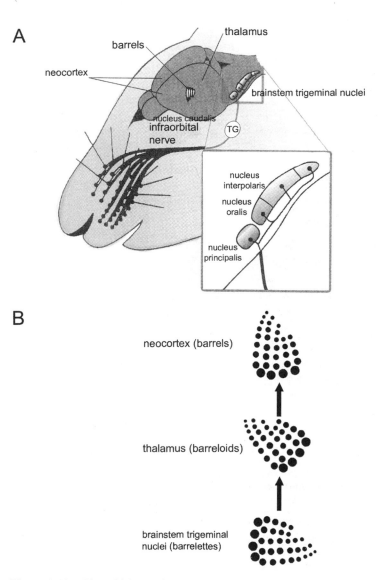

Figure 3.10   The whiskers of the rats are represented at many stages in the nervous system. (A) The afferent pathways from whiskers to the brainstem, to the thalamus, and then to the neocortex. (The cerebellum is removed to allow the other structures to be visible.) (B) At each stage the order and arrangement of the whiskers on the face is preserved in the order and arrangement of the neurons. In the brainstem, the neuronal groups representing individual whiskers are called *barrelettes*, in the thalamus they are called *barreloids*, and in the cortex they are called *barrels*. Abbreviation: TG, trigeminal nerve. (From Gerhardt and Kirschner 1997.)

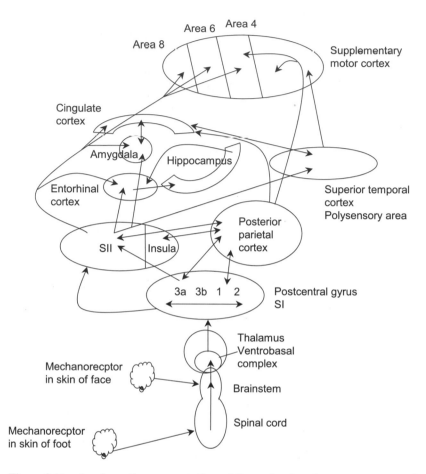

Figure 3.11 A schematic representation of the path taken by somatosensory signals to the motor system. Input signals make synaptic connections in the ventrobasal complex of the thalamus, which projects to the topographically mapped areas of somatosensory area SI. From there, signals are mapped in somatosensory area SII and the posterior parietal areas. The next stages are (1) the limbic structures (the entorhinal cortex and hippocampus), where signals engage memory functions; (2) the limbic structures (the amygdala, cingulate cortex, hypothalamus), which play an evaluative/cognitive role; (3) the polysensory cortex in the superior temporal gyrus; and (4) the motor system (the primary and supplementary motor cortex), where continuous sensory feedback to the motor system occurs.

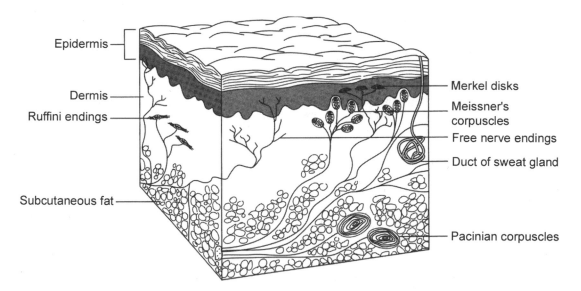

Figure 3.12 The location and morphology of mechanoreceptors in hairless (glabrous) skin of the human hand. Receptors are located in the superficial skin, at the junction of the dermis and epidermis, and more deeply in the dermis and subcutaneous tissue. The receptors are Meissner's corpuscles, Merkel disk receptors, and bare nerve endings. Subcutaneous receptors include Pacinian corpuscles and Ruffini endings. Nerve fibers that terminate in the superficial layers of the skin are branched at their distal terminals, innervating several nearby receptor organs; nerve fibers in the subcutaneous layer innervate only a single receptor organ. The structure of the receptor organ determines its physiological function. (Based on Goldstein 1999.)

important data on such things as burrow diameter. Some animals, such as rodents can also *move* their whiskers to actively reach out for additional information.

Glabrous (nonhairy) skin, such as that found on the palms of the hands, contains two types of receptors specialized for responding to touch in the absence of hairs: Meissner's corpuscles and Merkel disks (figure 3.12). These differ in their response style: A Meissner's corpuscle is fast adapting, which means that it responds abruptly to stimulus onset and then stops responding, even if the stimulus continues. By contrast, a Merkel disk is slow adapting, which means that, to a prolonged stimulus, it responds at stimulus onset and continues to respond to continued stimulation, though with a diminished frequency of firing.

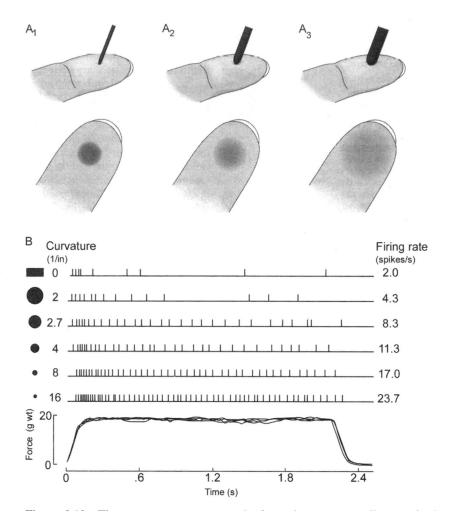

Figure 3.13 The sensory systems encode four elementary attributes of stimuli—modality, location, intensity, and timing—manifested in sensation. The four attributes of sensation are illustrated in this figure for the somatosensory modality of touch. (A) In the human hand the submodalities of touch are sensed by four types of mechano-receptors. Specific tactile sensations occur when distinct types of receptors are activated. The firing of all four receptor types produces the sensation of contact with an object. Selective activation of Merkel disks and Ruffini endings produces sensations of steady pressure on the skin above the receptor. When the same patterns of firing occur only in Meissner's and Pacinian corpuscles, the tingling sensation of vibration is perceived. (B) Location and other spatial properties of a stimulus are encoded by the spatial distribution of the population of activated receptors. Each receptor fires an action potential only

Beneath the skin are found two additional types of receptors that respond to mechanical deformation and contribute to the sensation of touch as well as to the sensation of pressure. These are the Pascinian corpuscles (fast adapting) and Ruffini endings (slow adapting). The packing density of these various receptors varies over different regions. The greater sensitivity of the finger tips relative to forearm, for example, is due to the higher density of Meissner's and Merkel receptors in the finger tips. All of the receptors also vary their response as a function of stimulus intensity (figure 3.13).

Feeling *temperature* depends on two distinct classes of receptors: those for warm stimuli and those for cold stimuli. A priori, one might have imagined that one receptor type would suffice, with the whole range of hot to cold signaled by variations in code. That is not, however, the solution evolution lit upon.

Cold receptors in the skin are very sensitive to small decreases in temperature, and they discharge in proportion to any drop in temperature from the normal baseline (34° C). Their standard detection range is between 1° and 20° below the normal baseline. Below that, their response to cold temperature falls off. Warm (higher than baseline) receptors discharge when the stimulus is between about 32° C and 45° C, falling off thereafter. How is it that we can feel very hot things (above 45° C) as hot? Mostly because there are pain receptors that activate at higher temperatures, but also because warm receptors located at some remove from the hot stimulus source will respond to the diffuse warmth. Though one cannot tell by introspection, high temperature and extreme heat are mediated by different submodalities. A chemical found in chili peppers, capsaicin, will selectively depolarize the warm receptors, and hence we feel a hot sensation, even though nothing is actually hot. Conversely, menthol selectively acts on the cold receptors, generating a feeling of coolness.

when the skin close to its sensory terminals is touched, i.e., when a stimulus impinges on the receptor's *receptive field*. The receptive fields of the different mechanoreceptors— shown as shaded areas on the fingertip—differ in size and response to touch. Merkel disks and Meissner's corpuscles provide the most precise localization of touch, as they have the smallest receptive fields and are also more sensitive to pressure applied by a small probe. (C) The intensity of stimulation is signaled by the firing rates of individual receptors, and the duration of stimulation is signaled by the time course of firing. The spike trains below each finger indicate the action potentials evoked by pressure from a small probe at the center of the receptive field. Two of these receptors (Meissner's and Pacinian corpuscles) adapt rapidly to constant stimulation, while the other two adapt slowly. (From Kandel, Schwartz, and Jessell, *Principles of Neural Science* [2000].)

There is also a phenomenon called paradoxical cold, which can be experimentally induced thus: apply a very hot stimulus (above 45° C) to a punctate region of skin containing only receptors for cold. Though the stimulus is in fact hot, it will be felt as cold. This is because cold receptors will respond to a very hot stimulus. Since they are "wired to report coldness," to put it crudely, the very hot stimulus is felt as cold.

When you put the flat of your hand against a granite cliff-face, the sensation itself may *seem* to be "holistic" or seamless, not a vector with many components. In fact, however, the responses of a variety of skin receptors are involved. Cool receptors will indicate one property, Pascinian corpuscles will discharge briefly in response to the pressure of the rock against your hand, Ruffini receptors will also respond, but only for the duration of the pressure. If you press hard, pain receptors will also respond. If you lay your hand on gently, Merkel's receptors will respond to touch, as will the fast adapting Meissner's receptors. This chorus of responses at the periphery will be conveyed to the brain and will allow you to have the feeling of roughness, coolness, and solidity that you can identify as a rock surface.

Receptors in the muscles and joints serve to update the brain on the position and movement of limbs (proprioception). These fiber pathways can be destroyed by diseases (peripheral neuropathies), and a patient whose proprioceptive system is damaged is seriously debilitated. They often have great difficulty with even simple motor tasks, such as walking, because they do not know where their legs and feet are. To walk, these patients have to use their *eyes* to determine their body configuration. If a subject with peripheral neuropathy is standing in a room when the lights go off, he will be unable to maintain posture and, unless aided, will tend to fall in a heap. In their daily business, normal subjects take all the incoming proprioceptive signals for granted. We scarcely know we have this precious modality, and some philosophers have denied that they are aware of proprioceptive signals, suggesting that they know without awareness the position of their limbs. Be that as it may, disruption to proprioception reminds us of how crucial these signals are to our body sense as well as to our ability to move our limbs and whole body as we intend.

Representations of head movements are rather special, because they include signals from a very specialized structure in the inner ear, the semicircular canals. The three semicircular canals, roughly at right angles to each other, detect head movement and are crucial to maintaining balance and posture. The canals are filled with fluid, and fine hairs project into the fluid. When the head

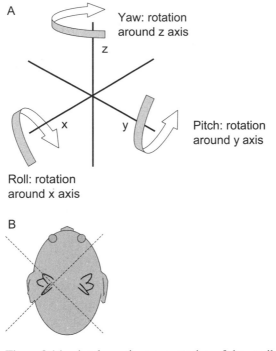

Figure 3.14   A schematic representation of the vestibular organs of the inner ears. Each organ consists of three semicircular canals oriented approximately 90° with respect to each other. The canals are rigid tubes filled with fluid, and movement of the fluid is detected by hair cells in a membrane stretched across the tube.

moves, the canal moves relative to the fluid, which tends to stay put due to inertia. Hence, the hairs move in the fluid, and their resulting deflection depolarizes the receptor in which each hair is embedded (figure 3.14). The integrated signals from the three canals tell us whether the head is moving, and in what direction, relative to absolute space. Receptors in the neck muscles also contribute to head-position representation, this time, relative to the trunk.

Adaptive effects are commonplace. As is well known, if you put one hand in ice water and one hand in hot water for a few minutes and then plunge them both into a pail of tepid water, to each hand the very same water feels a different temperature. It feels quite warm to the hand originally immersed in ice water and quite cool to the hot-water hand. Adaptation effects also take place over a long time period. Normally, one always depresses the clutch on a car with the left foot, and the feel of the resistance of the clutch becomes deeply familiar. If you now try to depress the clutch with your *right* (naive) foot, the feeling is completely different. In a middle-range time period, skates initially feel heavy when laced on, whereas removing them after a few hours skating makes one's feet feel unusually light. Similarly, one gets used to a heavy backpack and feels a little like a moonwalker when it comes off at the end of the day. The various adaptive effects reinforce the point that what we experience is always mediated by nervous-system structures, with their own peculiar response patterns and organization. These species-specific features are shaped by evolutionary pressures.

How much body representation do newborn humans have? Observations of newborns have shown a consistent order of the emergence of hand-to-face movements in the first hours after birth. The median values are as follows: movements to the mouth, 167 minutes after birth; then the face, 192 minutes; the head, 380 minutes; the ears, 469 minutes; the nose, 598 minutes; and the eyes, 1,491 minutes.[28] In the first weeks of life, infants use proprioceptive signals to control posture, and they explore their bodies, especially their mouths, toes, and fingers. Infants show some hand-eye coordination in reaching, which steadily improves. The mouth anticipates the arrival of the hand, and the hand can take any one of many paths to the mouth, from many different starting points, and does not need visual guidance.

Remember, however, that the fetus does not just sit idly in the womb, but is busily moving about, from about the tenth week of gestation. As well as kicking and waving movements, it puts its hands to its mouth and makes whole body movements, such as turning. These movements, along with the sensory feedback, are part of what is needed to get the motor system and the somatic-sensing system properly wired up. Many of the movements the fetus has been practicing in utero provide the basics for bootstrapping to more sophisticated skills in the postnatal world. (Development will be considered in chapter 8.)

One revealing dimension of infant body representation was discovered by developmental psychologist Andrew Meltzoff. Even very young infants will stick out their tongues in response to seeing another human stick out his tongue.[29] Meltzoff found that as early as he could test—forty-two *minutes* after birth—newborns will gaze fixedly at his face as he sticks out his tongue, and then, slowly, haltingly, out would come the infant's tongue. Infants will also mimic a gaping mouth and a scrunched up face (figure 3.15). Interestingly, the infants do not respond well, if at all, unless they see the whole movement. A static protruding tongue does not evoke the neonate's imitation.

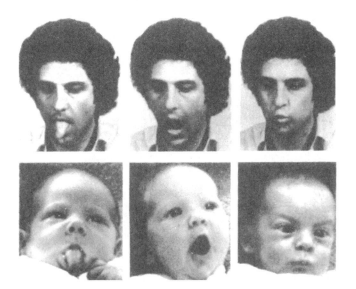

Figure 3.15 Photographs of two- to three-week-old infants imitating facial acts demonstrated by an adult. (From Meltzoff and Moore 1977. Reprinted in *The MIT Encyclopedia of the Cognitive Sciences*, s.v. "Imitation.")

This behavior implies that the brain, even at this very early stage, is able to map what it sees of another's facial movements onto its own sensorimotor representations. In a loose sense, the infant brain "knows" that what it sees ("your tongue moving out") corresponds to what is in its mouth ("my tongue"), and that by moving a set of mouth and tongue muscles, "I can look like you." Here again, the terms "know" and "I" are emphatically in scare quotes, since the infant does not know these things in the way a three-year-old child does. The infant's self-representation is more fragmentary and less connected than that of the three-year-old, but even so, the capacity to mimic simple facial expressions betokens a rudimentary coherence and the wiring that supports it.

This capacity may be mediated by a special class of neurons in the prefrontal cortex referred to as "mirror neurons." First discovered in the 1990s by Rizzolatti and his colleagues in the monkey, they are neurons that respond either when the monkey himself makes a particular hand movement, such as picking up a raisin, or when he sees another make exactly that hand movement.[30] Although the function of these mirror neurons in self-representation has not yet been established, their unique response pattern does suggest that they might

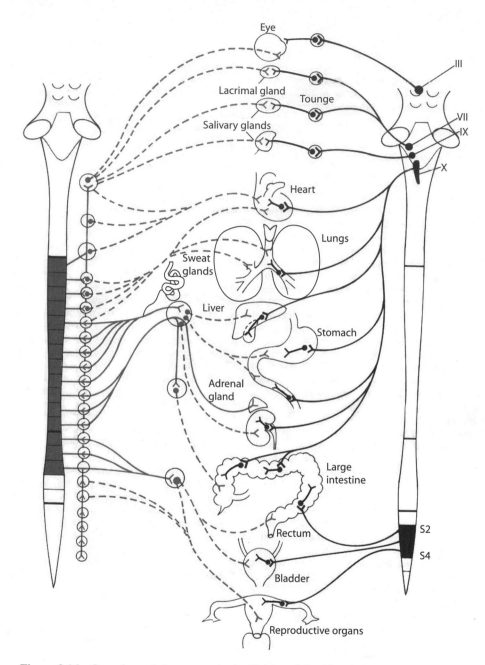

Figure 3.16 Overview of the sympathetic division (left side of the figure) and parasympathetic division (right side of the figure) of the visceral motor system. The parasympathetic system can constrict the pupil, stimulate salivation and tears, constrict

well play a role in imitation, me/not-me distinctions, and social cognition more generally. (These neurons and their possible role in imitation is discussed below, pp. 108–110).

The visceral system

The other part of the story of body representation concerns the autonomic nervous system, which regulates what we loosely call our "innards." The dimension of self-representation anchored by neurons regulating visceral functions is probably shared by all animals of varying complexity. Without our conscious control, the autonomic nervous system tends to our vital functions. We breathe, our hearts beat, our stomachs digest, our bladder muscles contract. Among other things, we secrete saliva, insulin, and digestive enzymes; we vasodilate our skeletal muscles when fleeing and vasoconstrict them when digesting. These are all motor functions, as surely as walking or whistling are motor functions, but they operate mainly on structures hidden from view. The autonomic system acts on smooth muscles (e.g., in the blood vessels and intestines), cardiac muscles, and glands (e.g., the adrenal gland, salivary glands, lacrimal gland).

The autonomic system also has afferent pathways, carrying signals from our innards to the brain and spinal cord. Among other things, these feedback signals appear to provide the input for a range of generalized feelings, such as feeling well or ill, feeling energetic or fatigued, feeling relaxed or on the alert.

The autonomic nervous system has two major divisions, the *sympathetic* system, which mobilizes the body to act in challenging conditions, and the *parasympathetic* system, which allows the body to recover from strenuous activity. The two systems tend to counterbalance each other (figure 3.16). For example, if a predator is attacking, its pupils dilate, and its heart rate increases; there is vasodilation of the bronchi and coronary artery, sweat secretion,

airways, slow the heart beat, stimulate digestion, dilate blood vessels in the gut, stimulate the bladder to contract, and stimulate sexual arousal. The neurotransmitter for this division is acetylcholine (Ach). The sympathetic system has the opposite profile. It can dilate the pupil, inhibit salivation and tearing, relax airways, stimulate glucose production in the liver, stimulate secretion of epinephrine and norepinephrine from the adrenal medulla, relax the bladder, and stimulate orgasm. It uses norepinephrine (NE) for some of its functions (indicated by broken lines), and Ach for others (indicated by solid lines). Abbreviations: III, oculomotor nerve; VII, facial nerve; IX, glossopharyngeal nerve; X, vagus nerve. (Based on Heimer 1983.)

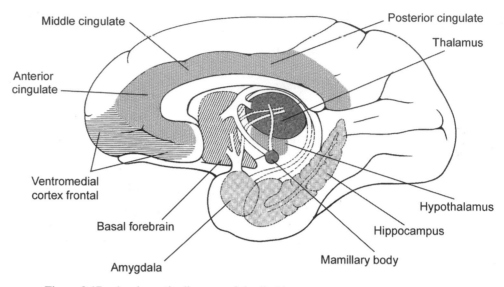

Figure 3.17   A schematic diagram of the limbic structures.

secretion of catecholamines from the adrenal gland, and inhibition of smooth-muscle activity in the digestive tract. If the predator's attack is complete and the prey caught, it settles down to its meal: its pupils constrict, secretion of saliva returns, motor activity in the digestive tract resumes, digestive enzymes are secreted, and the heart rate is reduced.

Neural networks in the brainstem, medulla, and hypothalamus play the central role in such coordination. Signals from the brainstem also travel to the amygdala via the thalamus into such cortical regions as the somatosensory cortex, parts of the cingulate cortex, and the orbital frontal cortex. Integration of inner body signals with signals from the somatic sensory system occurs at many levels, from the (phylogenetically more ancient) brainstem to the (phylogenetically more recent) frontal regions of the cortex (figure 3.17).

Cortical representation, coordinated with cohort thalamic signals, may be a necessary condition for awareness of these visceral feelings.[31] Some afferent signals, such as those representing duodenal distension and blood pressure, seem to be inaccessible to conscious awareness. How much of the activity in the autonomic pathways informs behavior without reaching the level of awareness is not known, nor is it really understood what makes some signals, such as bowel and bladder load, seem introspectively vivid and salient, while others, such as feeling tired or full, seem more subtle and backgroundish. What explains these differences in the conscious status of autonomic signals is an unanswered, but researchable, question.

The autonomic nervous system is pretty much left to itself in the everyday business of life, so long as it runs smoothly. Indeed, at a first pass, this part of the nervous system might seem to have little to do with how one *self-represents*. Why, one might ask, should regulation of such functions as peristalsis, heart rate, glucose levels, and so forth, have anything to do with *self*-representation? It seems obvious that autobiographical memory has a role in what makes me *me*, but visceral perception seems to be a less likely player.

Nevertheless, the autonomic system—because of the centrality of its role in coordinating vital functions, biasing behavior choice, and giving emotional color to ongoing experience—constitutes the core of what makes an animal a coherent biological entity. It is by no means the whole story of self-representation, but it is a crucial component, both in the individual and across species. The autonomic system and the somatic sensory system—along with their connections to the brainstem, cingulate cortex, hypothalamus, and amygdala—embody a model of an animal: its drives, its current parameter settings, and its state of arousal. Although the self-representational capacities we frequently talk about, such as consciously recollecting one's earlier life events or consciously wondering about one's motives or preferences, seem to be the obvious center of the *self*, they are likely evolution's extensions and elaborations of the rudimentary self model rooted in the autonomic and somatic sensory systems.

The main points of sections 1.3 and 2.1 are these: our basic self-representation capacities are tied to the centrality of agency and inner regulation in an animal's survival. Fancier self-representational capacities likewise have their roots, long and winding though they may be, in agency and inner regulation. Cognition and regulation of the inner milieu can thus be thought of as regions on *one and the same* capacity continuum. Roughly speaking, inner regulation is essentially low-level cognition with a narrow plasticity range; high-level cognition is essentially fancy regulation, with a much broader plasticity range. Although it may not be immediately obvious how being able to add and subtract, for example, has anything, ultimately or immediately, to do with survival-promoting behavior, a moment's reflection reverses that intuition. By and large, fancy cognitive capacities pay their way in the nervous system of a species by permitting the animals with those capacities to be smarter or faster or otherwise able to outcompete rivals in the survival game.

Some self-representational capacities involve awareness; some do not. Some incorporate high level cognition; some do not. The body seems to be represented many times over in the brain, at different time scales, in different degrees of generality, with different levels of computational goals, and with different blends of motor sequences. A long list of questions remain unanswered, including how integration of information is handled, how evaluation of goals and motor options is achieved, how past experience influences forward models, how learned skills play a role, and so on. What we have on the table is merely an outline. It is, moreover, an outline highly simplified for purposes of exposition.

2.2 Myself among Other Things

Representation of body parameters, sensory and motor, is just the beginning of the representational adventures of the complex brain. Guided by its rich postnatal experience, the brain constructs a systematic representation of the *external* world: for humans, the world of pillows and toys and grandmothers and cookies; for robins, the world of grubs and hawks and leafy bushes in which to hide. Think of this as elaboration from the protoself level, where the brain's categorizations are more or less of the form "Ouch, hurting here" and "Ooh, smelling good," to the level of computational sophistication where the brain begins to identify objects in terms of their causal properties: "That wasp can sting me" or "Those cookies taste good" or "I can catch that bird."[32] Much of learning consists of constructing a causal map of one's world.

What sort of *causal* knowledge do baby humans have?[33] Developmental psychologists have learned quite a lot about this. For example, if you tie a ribbon around a neonate's foot and tie the other end to a mobile hanging over the crib, the infant soon learns to make the mobile move by kicking. It has some understanding, therefore, that its own leg movement can make something happen. But its understanding of the causal situation is limited. For example, if the ribbon is detached from its foot, the infant will continue to kick expectantly, apparently not realizing that the ribbon must be connected to the mobile to get the effect.[34]

With experience and maturation, babies come to have an increasingly competent causal understanding of the world. Suppose that you put a toy on a cloth so that baby can get the toy only by grabbing the cloth and pulling on it. One-year-olds will successfully do this when the toy really is on the cloth, and they will not bother pulling the cloth if the toy merely sits alongside the cloth. Younger babies will pull on the cloth even if the toy merely sits alongside the cloth, and may get frustrated when the toy fails to come along with the cloth. At eighteen months, babies can use a toy rake to pull an object towards them, but one-year-olds do not.

The world of bottles and toys is important, but there is still more to represent. Especially in gregarious creatures like ravens, wolves, monkeys, and humans, the brain also comes to understand and represent the complex social world in which it finds itself. This is a world not just of other objects but also of other *selves*, that is, other articulated bodies with complex perceptual skills, motor skills, and their own representational capacities and practical agendas.

In the social world, it is vital to comprehend what others intend and feel and want. Such cognitive comprehension seems to depend on modeling, in some manner and to some degree, the internal cognitive states of others, such as what objects they can see from their position, what they are planning during the hunt, or what they are feeling about a threat. The advantage of such cognitive representation is that it permits the animal to anticipate and manipulate the behavior of these other cognitive creatures, and to navigate the social world that, collectively, they constitute.

This level of representational capacity is more complicated than the protoself representation of the body's internal parameters in an "aah-feels-nice-here" sort of framework. To a first approximation, the brain is now representing the representational activities of *brains in general*; it is now capable of representing, at least to some degree, its *own* activities as a *representational system*. Such representation need not be very sophisticated or penetrating, from a scientific point of view, in order to be useful. Thinking "She likes me," "He is afraid of me," and "She intends to hit me" is the stuff of successful social navigation for raven flocks and grade-school playgrounds alike.

Notice that if my brain represents you as wanting to be groomed, fearing a snake, seeing me, or the like, this involves my seeing your facial expressions and bodily behavior as *resulting from something that I do not directly observe*, namely your *feeling* fear, *desiring* to be groomed, or the like. I can see your face blanch and your eyes widen, but your fear is *your* brain state. But I think of you as having internal states that cause these effects, and I think of your state as like mine when I am afraid. In *this* respect, representational models of other selves and the external world are more akin to using a scientific hypothesis, such as Newton's law of gravity, to explain why things fall, than they are to generalizations embodied in the wiring supporting classical conditioning.

The analogy between scientific theories and a scheme to represent conspecifics *as other minds* was largely invented by the American philosopher

Wilfrid Sellars.[35] Sellars realized, of course, that there are important dissimilarities; for example, scientific theories are initially *explicitly* proposed as hypotheses; "folk theories" are not. "Theories" of other minds would not have emerged as a Cro-Magnon clan sat around the evening fire while Krong explained his new idea that we folks have mental states. Sellars certainly was not imagining anything as dopey as that. His real point was this: in our representational framework for understanding minds, several features—such as the interdependence of categories, the *model's use* in observation, prediction, intervention, and explanations—are importantly analogous to the *role* theories play in science. Incidentally, Sellars's insight applies not only to folk psychology; it applies also to other domains of commonsense understanding: folk physics, folk biology, and folk medicine. Nevertheless, it was application of his insight to our inner states, our mental states, that loosened the death grip of a priori philosophy of mind on our theories of the mind.

A related way of making the same point ties the notion of understanding the intentions of others to emulator function. As we saw, the inverse model component of emulators generates a motor command (intentions), a copy of which goes to the forward model, where consequences are predicted and evaluated. If I see another person begin an action, e.g., reach towards a plum, I understand his intention by simulating that action in my own brain. To a first approximation, the forward model would predict the consequences of the observed motion, and the inverse model would produce a "what if" command that, while not itself executed, gives the brain the basis for interpreting the *observed* movement.[36] This is essentially representing others' intentions via simulation (what would I be up to if I were doing that?), and simulation, like off-line planning, is surely a function that can be performed by making minor modifications to the vanilla emulator. First proposed by Alvin Goldman, the simulation hypothesis improved upon on Sellars's hypothesis especially because it was overtly free of any notion that the simulation must be mediated either by language functions or by explicit reasoning.

The hypothesis also connects to the discovery by the Rizzolatti lab of *mirror neurons* in the premotor cortex (see above, p. 101). Rizzolatti and colleagues have identified grasping-with-the-hand neurons (which are selective for particular kinds of grips), grasping-with-the-mouth neurons, holding neurons, tearing neurons (figure 3.18). As noted earlier, mirror neurons respond either when the animal *sees* a particular movement made by another animal or when the animal *makes* that specific movement. The behavior of these neurons suggests that in seeing the other animal make the movement, the premotor cortex generates

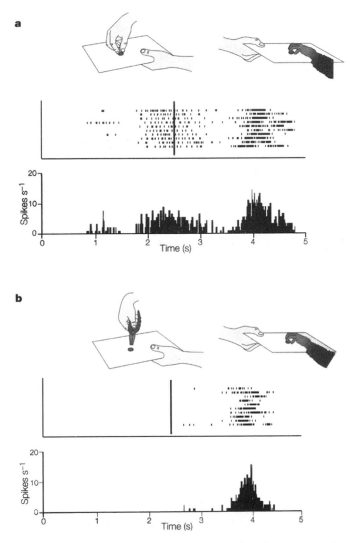

Figure 3.18 Visual and motor responses of a mirror neuron in area F5. (a) A piece of food is placed on a tray and presented to a monkey. The experimenter grasps the food, then moves the tray with the food towards the monkey. Strong activation is present in F5 during observation of the experimenter's grasping movements and while the same action is performed by the monkey. Note that the neural discharge (lower panel) is absent when the food is presented and again when it is moved towards the monkey. (b) A similar experimental condition, except that the experimenter grasps the food with pliers. Note the absence of a neural response when the observed action is performed with a tool. Rasters and histograms show activity before and after the point at which the experimenter touched the food (vertical bar). (From Rizzolatti, Fogassi, and Gallese 2001.)

incipient motor commands to match the movement. These signals can be detected as intentions, albeit inhibited or "off-line" intentions, which are then used to interpret what is seen.[37]

In infants the inhibition of the motor decision is less developed than in adults, and hence once sees infants' imitating such behavior as sticking out the tongue, waving, smiling, clapping, and so on. Moreover, even fourteen-month-old infants show sensitivity to *being* imitated and recognize whether movements do or do not match their own. As Meltzoff and Gopnik showed, playing the imitation game and experimenting within it is how infants learn about others' intentions, desires, and perspective; that is, how they acquire their folk-psychological theory.[38]

Cortical areas other than superior frontal (F1, F2, F7) and inferior frontal areas, such as the superior temporal sulcus (STS) in humans, also have a demonstrated role in social cognition. Certain neurons in this large area are involved in recognizing another's gaze as making eye contact or as averting eye contact or as looking at another object. Other neurons in STS are responsive when the subject sees mouth movements of another. Some are preferentially responsive to specific hand movements (figure 3.19).[39]

The explanatory and predictive role of our psychological understanding is so commonplace as to pass almost unnoticed. Consider a homely but useful example. I can offer a likely causal explanation of why Bill is walking towards the coffee cart at 8:30 in the morning. The explanation would advert to his *desire* for coffee in the morning and his *belief* that the coffee cart is a good place to get coffee. If I have seen Bill go to the cart for coffee on several mornings, I can predict that he will do it today as well, even if I have not yet seen him approach the cart. I can predict with reasonable assurance that if I pay Bill $100 not to drink coffee today, he will not drink coffee today. We can make generalizations such as this: if I insult my students, they will be angry and discouraged. If you have eaten nothing for 24 hours, you will feel great hunger. People who are overtired are often grouchy and have poor judgment. And so on, and so on.

Like scientific theories, a folk-psychological theory can be contemplated, tested, revised, and augmented. Carl Jung (1875–1961), for example, hoped to augment folk psychology with the notion of the "collective unconscious" to explain common themes in dreams and stories. In the end, it turned out to be a weak and unconvincing proposal.[40] Freud thought excessive hand washing could be explained in terms of sexual repression. This seemed at first to be more successful than Jung's proposal, but it too has proved to be explanatorily less effective than neurobiological explanations. Excessive hand washing is one

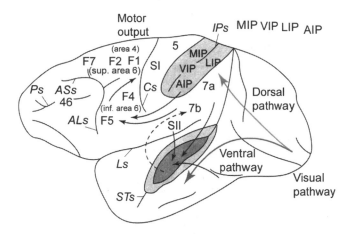

Figure 3.19 A sketch of a monkey brain and some areas hypothesized to be involved in imitation. Abbreviations: Ps, principal sulcus; ALs, inferior arcuate sulcus; ASs, superior arcuate sulcus; STs, superior temporal sulcus; Cs, central sulcus; Ls, lateral sulcus; IPs, intraparietal sulcus; MIP, medial intraparietal area; VIP, ventral intraparietal area; LIP, lateral intraparietal area; AIP, anterior intraparietal area; SI, primary somatosensory cortex; SII, secondary somatosensory cortex. F areas are related to motor function. Gray areas indicate an opened sulcus. Arrows indicate known neuronal projections between different areas of the brain; dashed arrows indicate hypothesized connections. (Based on Schaal 1999.)

typical manifestation of obsessive-compulsive disorder, which appears to have a neurobiological basis for which there is a genetic predisposition.

Developments in the neurobiology of addiction have put pressure on the folk-psychological idea that smokers suffer from "weakness of will." We now appreciate more clearly how nicotine causes changes in the brain's reward pathways that cause people to crave nicotine. Moreover, scientific theories, as W. V. O. Quine correctly noted, are *continuous* with common sense; they are common sense subjected to critical analysis, to demands for consistency and coherence, and to the increasingly well-honed standards of experimental test that are themselves solidly rooted in common sense.

However it happens that the brain *comes by* its earliest version of mind modeling, Sellars's analogy between mind models and scientific models gives us a new slant on the representational interconnectedness in our understanding of other minds. The analogy helps us understand the logic and structure of the framework of concepts that gets us around the social world. It helps us appreciate that even these familiar models of folk psychology are revisable, just as "folk physics" or "folk biology" were revisable. More strongly, it underscores the fact that representational models that wear the badge of obviousness may nevertheless be improved, sometimes in quite radical and surprising ways.

Sellars's idea is now captured in the "*theory* theory" and has been widely adopted in experimental psychology. It is used in describing what infants represent about minds, and what mature humans understand about their own and others' minds. This approach gives us a tool to raise questions about infant and adult capacities,[41] about animal capacities,[42] and about our prospects for *improving* our everyday theory-of-mind beliefs as psychology and neuroscience coevolve. It opens the door to a neurobiological understanding of the neural basis for familiar phenomena such as addiction, mood swings, eating disorders, and dreams. Perhaps the most important consequence of Sellars's idea is that it liberated philosophers from the entrenched assumption that how we think about our own and others' minds is a strictly philosophical, a priori, Platonic, and *nonempirical* matter. His proposal made it not only acceptable but *necessary* for philosophers to look outward to psychology, neuroscience, and biology in general to try to understand how the brain represents its own activities and capacities.[43]

Earlier we noted that at 14 months babies can tell whether their own movements are imitated by another person. What else do human infants understand about the minds of others? Between about 9 and 12 months, babies begin to display a cluster of behaviors that imply an early and developing concept of self and others-like-myself. If the mother gazes at some object in the corner of the room, the child will look at the mother's face, and its gaze will follow that of the mother. At this stage, the child points not only to what it wants, but also to something it wants the other person *to notice*. By 16 months, still before they acquire their first spoken words, children comprehend what someone is trying to do and can screen out what is accidental in an action. For example, suppose that the mother demonstrates how to take a new toy apart and during the demonstration she accidentally drops the toy and then resumes taking it apart. When the child imitates her actions, he omits the accidental dropping. In test after test, the child appears to distinguish between what the adult was trying to do and what was unintended or accidental. Other tests show that the child has an understanding of what the mother knows or sees or expects.

One may thus conclude that by 16 months, the child already has some understanding of what is in another person's mind, so to speak. This emergence of cognitive capacities is called the development of *perspective-based* representations. They permit the child a degree of understanding of how things look or feel from another's point of view. To a first approximation, these representations cohere as a framework for predicting and manipulating the behavior of other cognitively complex creatures. The mind-model still has much development to undergo, however. A two-year-old infant can be surprised that he can still be seen when he covers his eyes, but by three, he has a clearer sense of how to hide, given another's point of view.

Elizabeth Bates has shown that a rudimentary contrast between self and others is marked explicitly in language between 18 and 20 months.[44] As Bates notes, however, this does not mean the child has worked through all the consequences of this contrast. Children may make linguistic errors, saying, for example, "Carry you," when they mean "You carry me," though it is clear behaviorally what is intended. Because of the number of distinct personal pronouns and the complexity of the conventions governing them, it does take the child some time to sort it all out. This stage is preceded by using objects to communicate (e.g., showing Daddy the truck) at about 9 months. This merges into the period where objects are given (10 to 12 months). At around twelve months, this is followed by communicative pointing, where the child extends arm and index finger to objects he wants the adult to notice. Such behavior is clearly communicative, since the child repeats or emphasizes the pointing until the adult acknowledges the object referred to.

Three-year-olds explain and predict what other humans do mainly by referring to desires and perceptions, but they are not yet in command of the notion of beliefs. They can use counterfactuals about desires and easily answer such questions as "If Billy wanted a cookie and I gave him a crayon, would he be happy?" Not until they are about four do children begin to use the notions of beliefs and thoughts to explain and predict what others do or would do if they saw something. In a classic experiment, pencils are put in a candy box, and this is shown to the child. When asked, "What will Billy think is in the box?" three-year-olds say "pencils," and four-year-olds say "candy." The idea that someone else will have a false belief based on misleading evidence is *very* sophisticated and represents a new stage in the developments of the child's psychological theory. Notice that it requires the child to use generalizations to arrive at a likely belief, given what one would *normally* see and expect, and even when this belief is different from what she herself believes to be true. In the relevant respects, this is like using a scientific hypothesis to predict what would happen if various conditions were satisfied.

To the extent that the organism uses the perspectival model to plan and predict the organism's *own* behavior and to think about its own feelings, the model permits the organism to represent its self. Does the child first apply the frame-work to itself and then say, in effect, "Wow, mummy and Joey are just like me, so I guess they can see and feel and want things too!" Probably not. The aforementioned data, along with other data on self-referencing, imitation, and so forth, suggest that the child's development of perspectival representations proceeds in tandem with, and positively adds to, his growing understanding of his self.[45]

Whatever the precise nature of this capacity for perspectival representations, notice that having already learned a language is *not* essential. Of course, the acquisition of language can enhance and significantly *change* and *augment* the capacity, but the essential rudiments of the capacity seem to be language-independent. As the infant-development research convincingly shows, a rather rich perspectival representation system probably has to be in place for language to be acquired at all.

Do animals have a theory of mind? Does a chimpanzee, for example, know what can be seen or not seen from another chimpanzee's point of view? The answer seems to be "yes". For example, in carefully controlled experiments, Josep Call found that chimpanzees followed head direction of humans and conspecifics to find a target above and behind them. In conditions of social competition between subordinate and dominant chimps, he found that when food was placed so that from the perspective of the dominant chimp, one morsel was occluded and the other visible, the subordinate more frequently retrieved the morsel unseeable by the dominant (see figure 3.20). In a second set of experiments, the subordinate chimpanzee more often retrieved the morsel from the workspace if the workspace was baited when the dominant chimp could not see (figure 3.21).

Ethologist Frans de Waal discusses data showing that chimps may use pointing gestures when they want something, though they do not use the human style of pointing: outstretched arm and index finger. Here is one of his own observations of a chimpanzee using a gesture similar to what a human might use to indicate that a sinister character has just joined the party:

A chimpanzee named Nikkie once communicated with me through the same subtle technique. Nikkie had gotten used to my throwing wild berries to him across the moat at the zoo where I worked. One day, while I was recording data about the apes, I totally forgot about the berries, which hung on a row of tall bushes behind me. Nikkie hadn't forgotten. He sat down right in front of me, locked his red-brown eyes into mine, and—once he had my attention—abruptly jerked his head and eyes away from mine to fixate with equal intensity on a point over my left shoulder. He then looked back at me and repeated the move. I may be dense compared with a chimpanzee, but the second time I turned around to see

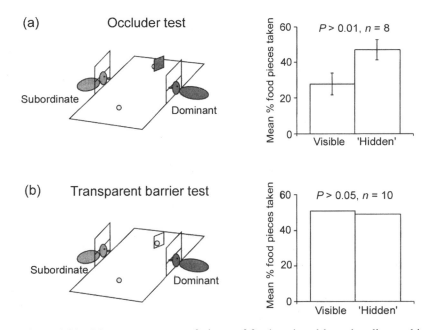

Figure 3.20 Mean percentages of pieces of food retrieved by subordinate chimpanzees as a function of whether food pieces could be seen by the dominant chimpanzee. In the occluder test (a), one of the pieces of food was hidden from the dominant chimpanzee, and this increased the likelihood of its being retrieved in preference to the visible piece. When both pieces of food could be seen by the dominant animal (b), there was no difference in retrieval percentage. (From Call 2001.)

what he was looking at, and spotted the berries. Nikkie had indicated what he wanted without a single sound or hand gesture.[46]

Others report observations in well-controlled conditions of chimpanzees and monkeys using body language to convey the location of prized or dangerous objects. These and a huge range of other experiments imply that the animals are not merely responding to specific cues but are also making use of representations of what others can see, want, intend, and feel. A chimpanzee's theory of mind undoubtedly does not map smoothly onto that used by humans or that used by baboons or dogs, especially because different animals will be different in how they make their living and what they care about. But it is entirely plausible that they have *some* measure of a theory of mind that enables them to manipulate the behavior of others by using representations of others' inner states.[47]

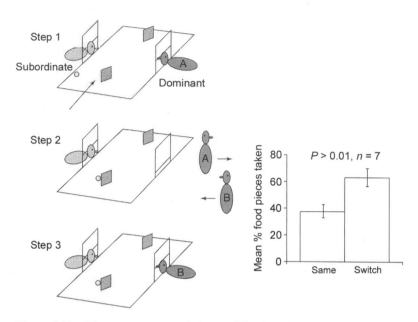

Figure 3.21 Mean percentage of pieces of food retrieved by subordinate chimpanzees as a function of whether the dominant chimpanzee who witnessed the baiting process was the same one who competed over the food with the subordinate. When the dominant animal was switched (steps 2 and 3), the subordinate was more likely to retrieve the food. This suggests that the subordinate is able to represent what its competitors can or cannot see. (From Call 2001.)

What would a human brain be like if it lacked a theory of mind? Autism, according to one prominent hypothesis, is the result. Autism is a developmental disorder whose core characteristics include impairments in socialization, communication, and imagination. Primary symptoms include failure to make eye contact, follow pointing gestures, follow gaze, and play the imagination game where you tell what someone would be feeling if x happened to him. Uta Frith notes, "Most individuals with autism fail to appreciate the role of mental states in the explanation and prediction of everyday behavior, including deception, joint attention, and the emotional states which depend on monitoring other people's attitudes, for example pride."[48] On this hypothesis, autism is a kind of "mind blindness."

Finding consistent brain abnormalities in the brains of autistics has been a challenge, and so far the data have been perplexing. What has emerged in the last few years is that there are neuronal abnormalities in limbic structures (amygdala, hypothalamus, hippocampus) and in the cerebellum.[49] The chief finding is reductions in the numbers and sizes of specific types of neurons: pyramidal cells in the limbic structures and Purkinje cells in the cerebellum. It has been intriguing to many that cerebellar abnormalities are found. This is because the cerebellum has traditionally been thought to serve mainly in sensorimotor coordination and not to play a role in cognitive functions, traditionally conceived. The cerebellar evidence makes sense, however, if simulation of the minds of others is a spin-off function of Grush emulators and Grush emulators are cerebellum-intensive.[50]

Mind models, applied to oneself and others, can get increasingly complex, at least in humans. One can engage in *self-reflection*, for example, to examine one's motives, excuses, and desires. This involves a *representation* of a *self-representation*, and hence is a recursive capacity. Memories of specific events in one's past experience are also instances of such self-reflection. For example, you can *remember* the *perception* of seeing pelicans diving for fish, or you can remember being afraid when you heard the thunder. You can also remember today that yesterday you remembered that you were hungry on the canoe trip last summer (a representation of a representation of a representation). Humans, at least, can create iterated representational structures of this kind, though the extent to which nonhuman animals can enjoy recursive representation is not determined. The recursion may be rate-limited, however, for it may not be useful to stack up representations of representations beyond four or five iterations. "I believe that I remembered that I thought that I experienced a pain in my foot" may be useful only rarely.

Although the capacity for self-reflection is important, it is not, on the Grush-emulator hypothesis, the fundamental platform of the sense of self. That platform, I have suggested, is first and foremost a matter of body regulation and body representations. Nevertheless, the capacity for self-analysis, self-reflection, and self-awareness—the capacity to know that I know—has seemed to betoken something suprabiological and even supraphysical about the mind. In the next and closing section, we return to the question of dualism and knowing what is in our minds.

2.3 Knowing Oneself: A Philosophical Problem

Descartes believed that the (conscious) mind, and only the mind, is *directly* known. The conscious mind, he was convinced, is known more certainly than anything else is—or *could be*—known. He used the alleged *epistemic* specialness of the mind (directness) to defend the *metaphysical* specialness of the mind (the thing known). His argument, in short, says that if the mind can know itself directly and with certainty, it must be a *different sort of thing* from things in the physical world. Physical objects, he argued, we know only *indirectly* and with degrees of uncertainty.

What is meant by the *directness* of self-knowledge? Boiled down, it means that one typically makes judgments about what one is feeling or hearing or seeing *without* first going through *any* explicit reasoning from evidence to conclusions. For example, you usually know without explicit inference that you feel cold or see a light or smell smoke. If you feel a pain, you just know that; you do not have to reason it out from more obvious information. These are features of the world about which you are unable to say *how* it is that you discriminate one such feature from another: *you simply can.*

Noninferential knowledge of one's own mental states, the argument goes, is evidence for the special nature of the mind, *metaphysically* speaking.[51] This argument has remained an intuitively powerful resource for many who wish to resist the explanatory advances of neuroscience into the domain of the conscious mind. This special directness in discriminating simple features, such as colors and pains, it may be insisted, will never go away. Hence there can never be a science that can be as firmly known and as deeply believed as one's knowledge of one's own conscious mind.

The logic of the situation, however, is this: *nothing* follows about the metaphysical uniqueness of the mind from the existence of discriminable *simples*, i.e., judgments made without consciousness of the computational antecedents. First, absolutely *all* knowledge involves *some* neural processing prior to conscious recognition that something is an α or a β. This is so whether the cognition pertains to the mind or to the body, whether one is aware of a stimulus as hot or as lasting for seconds or as looming towards you. *There is no such thing as unprocessed perception.*

Second, when one becomes aware of the *result* of nonconscious processing, one has no introspective (conscious) access to the processing steps that went into producing the result. It is therefore entirely inevitable that there will be some discriminations—the results of nonconscious processing—that are spontaneously, noninferentially, and, one might say, *directly* experienced.[52] That one cannot articulate how the discrimination was made is simply explained by the fact that there is a vast amount of nonconscious neural activity to which one does not—and perhaps cannot—have conscious access. For example, even feedback techniques will probably not allow me to be aware of what the amacrine cells of my retinae are now doing, anymore than I can become aware of when hormones are released from the pituitary or what my blood pressure is. I do not have introspective access to the processing that yields a stereoptic, three-dimensional representation of the visual scene. I just simply see things in stereoptic depth. I cannot tell you how I identify a melody as "Three Blind Mice"; I just do. But so what, *metaphysically* speaking?

Once the "nonconscious processing" point is on the table, the case for a metaphysically special stuff to handle direct knowledge is enfeebled. Additional arguments weaken it further. In particular, noninferential judgment is *not* confined to knowledge of one's *mind*. Normally, one also knows many things about one's *body* without relying on any explicit inferences.[53] For example, I directly know that I am sitting or standing or that my arms are folded on my chest. I directly know (*using no explicit inference*) whether my head is rotating or tilted forward or back. I directly know whether my tongue is moving and whether my feet are cold. Normally, you do not have to make any explicit, overt inferences to know that you are sneezing, vomiting, choking, suffocating, or passing water.

The hedge word "normally" fronts all of these claims, because under unusual or pathological conditions, a person may have to fall back on reasoning to figure out what is going on with his body. Someone whose arm was amputated may continue to feel an arm, which, he must remind himself, is not really there. Suffering a migraine attack, someone may feel her body to be the size of a tiny doll, but she turns on the light to check and be reassured. Affected by the anesthesia ketamine, a patient may feel he is floating above his body. In zero gravity, one feels as though one is constantly falling. These are all very unusual conditions. They are, however, instances of errors about body states that one *usually* knows about noninferentially; they are instances where a subject can "reason himself" to the more correct judgment.

Unconvinced, the dualist may try another tack. Even if I do have non-inferential (and hence direct) knowledge of my body, the dualist may argue, I can be wrong about the state of my body, whereas I cannot be wrong about the state of my conscious mind. I have noninferential *and* infallible knowledge of "discriminable simples." Such *infallibility*, the argument continues, entails something metaphysically special about the mind.

Note that for the argument make any headway, the infallibility claim has to be exceedingly strong. "Infallible" here has to mean not just that one is *usually* right, or even that *in fact* one is *always* right. It has to mean that one cannot—in principle—ever be wrong. As we shall see, this messes up the dualist.

First, let's look closely at the infallibility claim. First, *if* indeed I correctly describe my mental states, it has to be proved that this is not just a contingent fact but an a priori metaphysical truth. The favored cases for the infallibility argument are discriminable simples, for example, feeling a hot sensation. They are, after all, discriminable *simples*, so they have fewer degrees of fallibility than, for example, recognizing something as a B-17 Bomber or a chanterelle mushroom. Reliable identification of these simples is what normal nervous systems are wired to achieve, not for metaphysical reasons but for survival.

Second, if I never *consider* myself to be wrong, this is partly owed to our convention of normally giving the speaker the benefit of the doubt when he describes his inner states, as he is usually in a privileged position. This is not a *metaphysical* privilege, but the privilege of being the one whose brain has produced the sensation. It is an *epistemological* privilege: because *my* sensations happen in *my* brain, I am likely to know about them before, and better than, you.

The third and perhaps most important point is that just as there are conditions, usually somewhat abnormal conditions of course, where I err in my noninferential judgment about the body, so there are abnormal conditions where I err in my noninferential judgments about my conscious states. Let us canvas a few of these cases. As novelists such as George Eliot have rightly observed, especially in censorious societies, a female may misread her feelings of sexual attraction in one way or another: as repulsion, shyness, anger, fear, or nervousness. A particularly inhibited person may need to learn to recognize her own sexual feelings via inference from her flustered behavior in the presence of a particular man. More generally, all those feelings we allegedly inhibit when in denial are instances of fallibility.

The infallibilist, however, may want to dismiss these sorts of cases on grounds that they are not the sorts of cases, like feeling something hot, that he has in mind. In particular, they are not discriminable simples. Why not? Suppose that he replies, "Because those are mental states you can be wrong about, just as you say. I am talking about the ones you *cannot* be wrong about." This response makes his argument circular, since he is rejecting any counterexample on the grounds that his infallibilist conclusion *must* be true. So this response logically imperils the position. We can be generous, however. For the sake of argument, we can allow that the Freudian counterexamples do not falsify the infallibilist claim. Let us grant that the cases involving misidentification of moods and emotions are off limits. There are other examples where squirming off the hook is even more difficult.

Sensations can, on odd occasions, fail to be correctly apprehended. Expecting a very hot stimulus, one may at first believe that one feels a burning sensation, only to quickly realize that one is actually experiencing an icy cold sensation. Expecting a pain, I have been surprised to realize that the sensation is actually not pain at all but only pressure. The infallibilist will, of course, insist that in these instances heat really was felt, pain really was felt. But we can be sure of this only if we assume, with circularity, that the infallibilist is right, that we can never be wrong about what are feelings are. Even if it is only an *open question* whether we are right or wrong, the claim for infallibility as a metaphysical truth has lost ground.

Sometimes when the signal is faint or the subject is anxious, he can be unsure whether he feels something or not. Can I be wrong about whether I hear a sound at all? Yes, for example, as I wake up, or when I have been paying close attention to a book, or when I am in a state of great anxiety. There are other obvious cases where we can be wrong or unsure about certain of our mental states. Young children are sometimes unsure, even when queried, about whether they feel the need to empty the bladder. When very tired, children, and adults too, may not recognize the feeling of being tired.

One could, of course, adopt a convention whereby if a subject says he feels heat, as opposed to cold, then he really does. Adopting such a convention is fine, but it fails to yield what the infallibilist wants, namely a metaphysical truth about the special nature of the mind. Another line of defense is to say that the cases supporting the infallibilist claim are those where conditions are normal, the stimulus is well above threshold, the sensations are simple, the subject is fully awake and attentive, and he is not under the influence of drugs. Fine, but this defense also looks circular, for it looks like identifying the cases as a function of whether or not the subject is in fact wrong. That the subject is not wrong in these cases is a function of how we have picked them out, not of some metaphysical truth about the ethereal etiology of these cases. Moreover, if the infallibilist can use this strategy, so can we. I can identify cases of *physical* knowledge (e.g., knowing whether I am standing up) where I am not wrong: conditions are normal, the stimulus is well above threshold, the subject is fully attentive and awake, and he is not under the influence of drugs. If such cases can show that physical knowledge can be infallible, then mental knowledge is not special in this regard.

To move on to other counterexamples to infallibilism, it is interesting that one is routinely and regularly wrong about what one thinks one *tastes*. As neuroscience and psychology have demonstrated, most of what we regard as a sensation of taste is actually owed to our sense of *smell*, however convincingly it otherwise appears. The "taste" of barbecued pork ribs is actually mostly the smell of the ribs. Taste space is limited to five dimensions: sweet, salty, bitter, sour, and umami (stimulated by monosodium glutamate). Smell space, by contrast, runs into may hundreds of dimensions. The "taste" of a Chardonnay wine is largely the complicated *smell* of that wine. It probably does not matter for survival that smell and taste are not kept strictly separate in awareness, the way that sight and smell, for example, normally are. Hence, the brain is not equipped with mechanisms for the effortless and noninferential detection of the separate components of taste and smell.

Pathological conditions give quite another dimension of error in the self-reporting of mental states. A patient with a sudden lesion to his primary visual cortex may fail to realize that he is blind, even when this is pointed out to him, and even when he repeatedly stumbles into the furniture. Described as blindness *unawareness*, Anton's syndrome is a rare, but well-documented deficit. In patients with Anton's syndrome, the blindness may be transient, though after recovery of some vision, patients are likely to say that nothing has changed in the visual capacity. There are reports of unawareness of blindness that persist indefinitely.

Are the patients with Anton's syndrome really just mistaking visual *imagery* for actual vision? Drawing on anatomical data and behavioral tests, most clinical neurologists believe not. For one thing, the cortical regions needed for vision are also the regions believed to be needed for visual imagery, and these are the very ones destroyed by stroke. Not implausibly, Paul Churchland has argued that these patients have lost the very mechanisms for knowing whether one is seeing or not. Since the brain has no information to indicate otherwise, it goes with the *standard* state of affairs.[54] Thus these patients say, "Of course I can see" and they will smoothly confabulate a reasonable story when asked what they see. If asked whether the doctor is wearing glasses, the Anton's patient will answer with confidence, but the answer is mere guesswork. It is also significant that confabulatory responses in Anton's patients are restricted to the topic of visual experience. They will be entirely frank and forthright in response to questions on nonvisual topics. By contrast, patients with Korsakoff's syndrome (alcoholic dementia) freely confabulate about any subject.

The mystery of Anton's syndrome is worth dwelling on because visual experience seems *so* self-evident. If anything seems dead obvious, it is that one *can* or *cannot* see, and it is hard to imagine being wrong about which is which. Nevertheless, the patients with Anton's syndrome present us with a compelling case where the brain is simply in error about whether or not it has visual experiences. To insist that such subjects must be having visual experiences if they think they are, because one cannot be wrong about such things, is of course, to argue in a circle. The question precisely at issue is *whether* one can ever be wrong about such matters. Prima facie, at least, Anton's patients present evidence that one can be wrong and that there is a neurobiological reason why they are wrong. More than a mere a priori conviction of infallibility is needed to reverse the hypothesis or reinterpret the data.

From the point of view of cognitive neuroscience, whether or not someone's recognitional skills deploy *explicit* reasoning appears less important than certain other properties, such as the neural pathways involved, the contribution of affective components, the nature of cross-modal and top-down effects, how much learning has gone on, and how the brain automates cognitive skills. The predilection, most evident in British Empiricism and German Idealism, for taking the differences between inferential and noninferential judgments to be a momentous *metaphysical* division looks about as misguided as believing, as pre-Galilean physicists did, that the difference between the sublunary realm and the supralunary realm marks a momentous metaphysical division concerning the structure of the cosmos.

Of course, there *is* a difference between superlunary space and sublunary space, and the difference means something to humans, because of the proximity of the Moon to Earth. But it does not mark a metaphysical difference, or even a difference in what principles of physics apply. Similarly, there *is* a difference between inferential and noninferential judgments, but we should hesitate to attach profound *metaphysical* significance to these two types of neural processing. (See also pp. 130–133.)

Dualism is implausible at this stage of our scientific understanding. In the business of developing an ongoing research program, dualism has fallen hopelessly behind cognitive neuroscience. Unlike cognitive neuroscience, dualist theories have not even begun to forge explanations of many features of our experiences, such as why we mistake the smell of something for its taste, why amputees may feel a phantom limb, why split-brain subjects show disconnection effects, why focal brain damage is associated with highly specific cognitive and affective deficits. In truth, dualism does not really even try.

To be a player, dualism has to be able to explain *something*. It needs to develop an explanatory framework that experimentally addresses the range of phenomena that cognitive neuroscience can experimentally address. While it is conceivable that this can be done, the bookies will give long odds against its success. Until at least *some* distinctly dualist hypotheses are on the table, dualism looks like a flimsy hunch still in search of an active research program.

3   Conclusions

The brain makes us think that we have a self. Does that mean that the self I think I am is not real? No, it is as real as any activity of the brain. It does mean, however, that one's self is not an ethereal bit of "soul stuff." But it is as real, for example, as the coherent neuronal activity that yields your capacity to walk or think about global warming or find your way back from a hike in the bush. Brain activity is an entirely real thing.

But, one might say, that is not how I am used to thinking of myself. Why would my brain lie to me? Think of it this way. Fundamentally, your brain's task is to allow you to make your way in the world, and that means it needs to be able to make reasonably good predictions, and to make them in a timely manner. One's scheme of representational devices need not be the *best possible* in order to have practical and predictive value. It just has to be *good enough* so that you can make a living, in the broadest sense of the term. In particular, for most of the business of surviving on the planet, the details of *how the brain actually works* need not be explicitly known by the brain. Brains manage reasonably well by using such categories as "wants," "fears," "sees," "is angry," etc., as the representational apparatus for understanding its own activities. For much of the business of everyday life, human brains can manage without such categories as "neuron," "DNA," "electrical current," and so on.

Nevertheless, humans, for neurobiological reasons we do not yet understand, have the stunning capacity to play the "ratchet game."[55] That is, children can learn the best their culture has to offer and can improve upon it. And *their* children can start where they left off. Unlike chimpanzees, where each chimp starts at essentially the same place where all of his ancestors started, human children can start well ahead of where their parents started, and vastly far ahead of where our stone-age ancestors started. They can build on what their culture already knows. Hence in the general business of trying to understand the reality behind appearances, humans can develop science and technology, and can pass it on to their offspring. This gives us the unique opportunity to use technology and science to develop increasingly abstract, scientifically penetrating categories, such as "atom," "valence," "DNA," and "neurotransmitter."

We have discovered that brains permit us to see, plan, walk, and wonder. And now the ratchet game opens up the possibility of going beyond the familiar categories, though they work reasonably well in the everyday business of explaining and predicting human behavior. It allows us to ask, for example, how a brain is organized so that by means of two-dimensional light arrays from two retinae, we see a single image in three-dimensional depth. We can ask how a brain organizes its information so that it has self-representational capacities. Here, as elsewhere, scientific discoveries give us surprising new ways of looking at familiar phenomena. For brains, as well as for the stars, fire, and the heart, there *is* a reality behind the appearances, and the exciting thing is to figure out how to think about that reality in a way that improves upon the old ways.

In this century, modern neuroscience and psychology allow us to go beyond myth and introspection to approach the "self" as a natural phenomenon whose causes and effects can be addressed by science. Helped by new experimental techniques and new explanatory tools, we can pry loose a real understanding of how the brain comes to know its own body, how it builds coherent models of its world, and how changes in brain tissue can entail changes in self-representational capacities. Neurobiology is beginning to reveal why some brains are more susceptible than others to alcohol or heroin addiction, and why some brains slide into incoherent world models. We can see progress on our understanding of the staged emergence of self in childhood, as well as of the cruel inch-by-inch loss of self in dementia.

Though well short of full answers, neuroscience has discovered much about the effects of localized brain lesions on higher functions, such as complex decision-making, speech, and voluntary behavior. Perhaps some questions will forever exceed the neurobiological reach, though it is impossible at this stage to tell whether such problems are just as *yet* unsolved or whether they are truly unsolv*able*. In any case, incomplete but powerful answers anchored in data can often provide a foot-hold for the next step. And that, in turn, for the next step thereafter. But this is just how science proceeds—one step at a time.

Suggested Readings

Damasio, A. R. 1999. *The Feeling of What Happens*. New York: Grossett/Putnam.

Dennett, D. C. 1992. The self as a center of narrative gravity. In F. Kessel, P. Cole, and D. Johnson, eds., *Self and Consciousness: Multiple Perspectives*, pp. 103–115. Hillsdale, N.J.: Lawrence Erlbaum & Associates.

Flanagan, O. 1996. *Self Expressions: Mind, Morals, and the Meaning of Life*. New York: Oxford University Press.

Gopnik, A., A. N. Meltzoff, and P. K. Kuhl. 1999. *The Scientist in the Crib*. New York: Morrow.

Hobson, J. A. 2001. *The Dream Drugstore: Chemically Altered States of Consciousness*. Cambridge: MIT Press.

Jeannerod, M. 1997. *The Cognitive Neuroscience of Action*. Oxford: Blackwells.

Kosslyn, S. M., G. Ganis, and W. L. Thompson. 2001. Neural foundations of imagery. *Nature Reviews: Neuroscience* 2: 635–642.

Le Doux, J. 1996. *The Emotional Brain*. New York: Simon and Schuster.

Panksepp, J. 1998. *Affective Neuroscience*. New York: Oxford University Press.

Rizzolatti, G., L. Fogassi, and V. Gallese. 2001. Neurophysiological mechanisms underlying the understanding and imitation of action. *Nature Reviews: Neuroscience* 2: 661–670.

Schacter, D. L. 1996. *Searching for Memory: The Brain, the Mind, and the Past*. New York: Basic Books.

Schore, A. N. 1994. *Affect Regulation and the Origin of the Self*. Hillsdale, N.J.: Lawrence Erlbaum & Associates.

Tomasello, M. 2000. *The Cultures and Origins of Human Cognition*. Cambridge: Harvard University Press.

Websites

BioMedNet Magazine: http://news.bmn.com/magazine

Comparative Mammalian Brain Collections: http://brainmuseum.org

Encyclopedia of Life Sciences: http://www.els.net

Living Links: http://www.emory.edu/living_links

The MIT Encyclopedia of the Cognitive Sciences: http://cognet.mit.edu/MITECS

Neurosciences on the Internet: http://neuroguide.com

4 Consciousness

1 The Problem and Empirical Directions

1.1 Introduction

When you wake up, you become aware of sights and sounds, of feelings in your body, perhaps of limb movements. You may become aware of thoughts about the movie you saw the previous night, of emotional residue from an earlier dream, of the smell of breakfast cooking. From a hubbub of many voices, you may follow only that of your child. You will be unaware other many other events, such as changes in blood pressure and the decisions guiding eye movement as you watch the birds flying outside. Dreams occurring just before waking may be remembered, if only in fragments, while dreams occurring early in the sleep cycle will escape conscious recall. If you are attending to what the birds are doing, other events may go unattended or unnoticed, such as the music playing softly in the next room, the movement of your tongue in your mouth, the pain in your knee. Even unattended or subliminal events, however, can have an effect on your behavior, present and future.[1]

From the inside, so to speak, it is the *conscious* plans, decisions, memories, and so forth, that seem to make me *me*. This presumption is almost unavoidable, since that is the only me I am aware of. In fact, however, the conscious events are only a miniscule part of the story of my inner life. So what is going on here? What happens when I shift attention and become aware of an irritating mosquito on my leg, and what happens when I am so preoccupied with putting up the tent that I fail to notice the mosquitoes biting my arms and legs?

Why is it that no amount of trying to attend to peristaltic movements in the small intestine results in awareness of those movements, though attention to my heartbeat yields awareness? How is it that I can be aware of understanding what you are saying, but I have no awareness of the processes underlying that understanding? What happens when I learn a task such as riding a bicycle well enough that I no longer need to pay much attention to my balance? What happens when I am in deep sleep, unaware of the somatic, auditory, and other signals that continue to percolate through the nervous system? In sum, what constitutes the difference between conscious states and unconscious states?

There are basically two attitudes that one can have toward these questions. One attitude is, roughly speaking, pragmatic. It emphasizes the search for revealing experiments, perhaps by understanding what happens to the brain in a coma or during anesthesia, or how awareness changes after specific kinds of brain damage. In other words, the pragmatist adopts the position that we try to make scientific progress on all the aforementioned questions, while subjecting all hypotheses to criticism and comparing the merits of competing theories.

The opposing attitude, which Flanagan refers to as "mysterian," takes the view that these questions cannot be answered *scientifically* and, indeed, cannot be answered *at all*.[2] The mysterians emphasize lack of progress rather than actual progress, the mysteriousness of the various phenomena at issue rather than tools for reducing the mystery, and the hopelessness of opening up experimental avenues rather than the opportunities presented by new advances. Whereas pragmatists tend to emphasize that consciousness is a *natural* phenomenon of the brain, mysterians favor the idea that it is a *supernatural* phenomenon, or at least is *beyond the physical*, in some sense or other.

Pragmatism seems the better counsel to me. At least, I favor an attitude that says, "Let's *try* for a neuroscientific explanation," over one that is not prepared to try. This is not dogma or an article of faith. It simply draws on past scientific successes to predict that progress can often be made even when a problem looks unsolvable. Nevertheless, it is essential to analyze those arguments that profess to demonstrate the impossibility of a scientific explanation of consciousness, the better to assess whether those arguments have greater force than the arguments favoring the try-and-see approach. One cannot tell a priori where the probabilities lie, and thus a balanced examination is necessary. The main aim of the next section is to lay the groundwork for approaching the problem and then to delineate several promising empirical approaches. At the end of this chapter, in section 2.2, I shall set out and analyze the main objections to empirical approaches to the assorted problems of consciousness.

1.2 Definitions and Science[3]

In its everyday use, the term "consciousness" can describe a range of somewhat different things: not being in a coma, not being in a deep sleep, not being under anesthesia, being aware of feelings and thoughts, and so forth. If we are to explore a phenomenon, surely we had better know what the phenomenon is, or we shall end up in confusion and pointless debate. To address the vagueness of the term "consciousness" it will be tempting to propose that we defer investigation until we have first determined precisely the proper definition of the term. So perhaps we should stop here and precisely define our terms before we plunge ahead, building and testing theories.

Although well intentioned, this recommendation is decidedly ill conceived, especially in the early stages of inquiry. Let me explain.

Prescientifically, we classify things on the basis of their gross physical and behavioral similarity, or on the basis of their relevance to our particular needs and interests. Plants may be classified as edible or poisonous, and some may be weeded by farmers in one locale but cultivated as cash crops in another. Likewise, animals that are docile or dangerous are more likely to be grouped with others that are docile or dangerous, respectively. Highly unusual or distinctive features may also call for distinct classification. So all birds with interesting vocalizations are referred to as songbirds, even though they may come from species as diverse as mockingbirds and nightingales. Rare, polishable substances get called gems, even though diamonds, rubies, amber, and opals differ radically from each other in their chemical composition and nature.

Developed sciences tend to bootstrap themselves up from such early classification schemes. As we come to understand the reality behind the appearance, classifications are drawn according to different sorts of principles. Properties such as "edible" or "makes a nasty smell" are not necessarily abandoned, but they no longer serve as the basis for the taxonomies that we use in articulating the deeper explanatory principles. The taxonomies current at a given stage of scientific development do not, of course, seem at all superficial to us. They seem to us to be a true and faithful reflection of how things really are.

Terms may change their range of application as new discoveries are made. These changes in turn have an effect on perceptual recognition. The history of the term "fire" provides a striking example of how the boundaries of a familiar category get redrawn. Not so very long ago, the category "fire" included anything that emitted light or heat, and the presence or absence of this property could be determined just by looking or feeling. "Fire" was used to classify not only burning carbon stuffs, such as wood, but also activity on the sun and various stars (which we now know is not fire at all, but nuclear fusion), lightning (actually, incandescence following an electrical discharge), the northern lights (actually, spectral emission), and the flash of so-called fireflies (actually, biophosphorescence). Moreover, these phenomena were thought to share something deep in common—their *essence* or *essential nature*—which allegedly made them all instances of fire.

As modern science slowly came to realize, burning wood involves oxidation, and this process has nothing in common with the processes underlying the other assorted phenomena. That fact, however, is not something you can know *just by looking*. The development of our understanding of fire as oxidation also led us to see a deeper connection between fire on the one hand and iron rusting and biological metabolism on the other. These processes were not originally considered to share anything with burning. Because detectable heat was taken to be an essential feature of the class that included burning wood, the sun, and lightning, it would never even occur to someone to suppose that rusting might be an instance of fire. Since you cannot feel any heat from rusting iron, it took an understanding of the hidden reality of oxidation to reveal that rusting and burning of wood are in fact the same process. As for metabolism, our bodily heat was thought to be just *how we are*. The suggestion that heat in animal bodies involves the same process as burning of wood struck some as obviously ridiculous (figure 4.1).

Why does science tend to reject our everyday folk criteria in favor of others that are arcane and of little apparent relevance to everyday life? One answer is that the scientific categories more accurately reflect the structure of reality itself. We consider the categories more accurate because they enable more powerful explanations, predictions, and manipulations of the world. For example, our production and manipulation of fire was aided by understanding the chemical process of oxidation. But oxidation is of little use in understanding what makes the sun hot, since nuclear fusion involves events at the *subatomic* level. Additionally, the development of modern scientific categories permits scientists to connect and unify their understanding in ways that the primitive categories do not. Moreover, science and technology develop together, which means that our everyday life changes as well, sometimes quite radically.

Now consider a classification fundamental in science for thousands of years and easily observable by anyone: the distinction between the *sub*lunary realm (the universe below the level of the moon) and the *super*lunary realm (every-

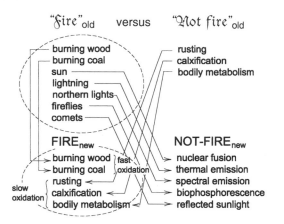

Figure 4.1   In the early stages of a scientific investigation, a thing's category membership is determined largely by similarities in easily observable properties. Thus the category "fire" initially embraced a range of phenomena involving the emission of heat or light or both. As physics and chemistry progressed, the category fragmented, and similarities based on theoretically informed properties became a more useful basis for new groupings. The upper panel shows items in the old classification of "fire," and the lower panel shows the modern classifications. Calxification is oxidation of nonferrous metals.

thing beyond that) (figure 4.2). Completely different principles were assumed to govern each domain. The superlunary realm was thought to be immutable, perfect, and governed by divine principles, such as the constant circular motions of the planets. Here on sublunary Earth, in contrast, things change unpredictably, they can become rotten and worn, perfectly circular motion is rare, and *Earthly* principles such as "Nothing moves unless it has a force acting on it" and "Everything moves to its natural place" prevail. Thus spake medieval physics.

Rending all this asunder, Newton proposed that *one* set of laws could explain motion *wherever* in space it occurred. The planetary motions, the trajectory of an arrow, the movement of the moon, the falling of an apple—all are embraced by a single set of laws. In developing this new framework, Newton dumped the sublunary/superlunary distinction entirely.

The apparently indispensable and completely intuitive notion of Natural Place also dropped out of the picture. On the old theory, rain falls *down* because it had "gravity," and things with gravity have their *Natural Place* in the center of the universe, namely Earth. Smoke, on the other hand, rises, because it has *levity* and things with levity have their Natural Place away from the

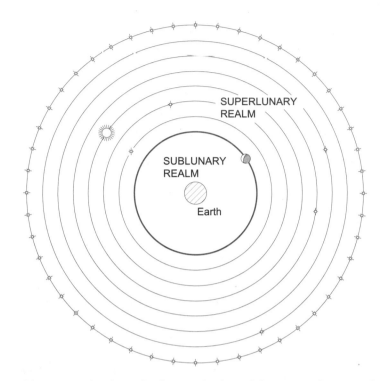

Figure 4.2 A schematic characterization of the geocentric conception of the universe, viewed looking down on Earth, the Moon, and the embedded series of crystal (transparent) spheres. The realm inside the first of the crystal spheres (the *sublunary* realm) was presumed to be governed by very different physical laws than those governing bodies and events in the *superlunary* realm. The "fixed" stars are attached to the outermost crystal sphere, which does not move, whereas the planets, Moon, and Sun are attached to the intermediary spheres, whose rotations were believed to explain the movement of these bodies. A major problem for medieval physics was to explain what caused the huge glass spheres to move. This problem was abandoned with the advent of Newton's radically different explanation of the movements of the planets, Moon, and Sun. (Courtesy of P. M. Churchland.)

center of the universe. Newton replaced the old conception of gravity with a completely new conception: *a reciprocal force between any two masses*. The seemingly obvious idea of Natural Place, comfortably entrenched for roughly two thousand years, thus found *its* natural place in the scrap heap.

The more general lesson is this: *theories* about certain things and *definitions* as to *what in the world count* as those things evolve together, hand in hand. Firm, explicit definitions become available only fairly late in the game, as the science that embeds them firms up and matures.[4]

What, then, about defining "consciousness"? If we cannot begin with a solid definition, how do we get agreement on what phenomenon we are trying to study? Roughly, we use the same strategy here as we use in the early stages of any science: delineate the paradigm cases, and then try to bootstrap our way up from there. Using common sense, we begin by getting *provisional* agreement on what things count as *unproblematic* examples of consciousness.

First in the set of prototypically conscious states are a range of *sensory perceptions*, such as seeing a bird fly, feeling the pain of a burn, hearing a police siren. The *somatic* sensory experiences pertaining to touch, vibration, pressure, limb position, body orientation, and body acceleration are also included in the prototype. Smells and tastes round out the list of sensory perceptions.

Second, we can include in our list states that, as are not usually considered sensory experiences per se because they are not so closely tied to a specific sensory organ. This list includes such states as *remembering* what you had for breakfast, *knowing* that you can ride a bicycle, *imagining* a six-legged dog, *attending* to the feeling in your big toe, *wondering* whether to eat a mango, *surprise* that an expected event did not happen, and so forth. Likewise, *emotional states*, such as feeling fear, anger, sadness, and elation, as well as *drive states*, such as hunger, thirst, sexual desire, and parental love belong on the list. In this context, we also need to distinguish between *capacities*, which are *dispositions*, and the current exercise of those capacities. The contrast is between the capacity to remember what you had for breakfast (though you are not thinking about that now) and your remembering *now* that you had sausages for breakfast.

Occupying a still less central location in the *conscious awareness* prototype space are a host of other cases. Probably we are at least somewhat aware during dreaming states, even when they are not recallable. We are not sure whether we are aware at all during *deep sleep*, or whether a kind of low-level awareness persists throughout. For example, Navy SEALS are trained to react to a threat even before they are awake. We are not sure when the fetus's nervous system is sufficiently developed that it becomes aware of sensory stimuli such as sounds. Further, it is uncertain how we should think of conscious states such as recognizing that something is unfamiliar or odd, or that something is intellectually satisfying, morally unsettling, musically harmonious, or esthetically jarring.

Fortunately, we need not worry too much at this stage about these cases. By identifying prototypical examples of conscious states, we gain lots of scope for designing revealing, interpretable experiments. With some progress in hand, less central examples may come to assume greater importance, perhaps even gain recognition as *the* prototypical cases.

Cognizant of the possibility that these ostensibly obvious categories may be reconfigured later under the pressure of new discoveries, perhaps we can agree that this rough-and-ready delineation of prototypes provides us with a reasonable way to get the project off the ground. Because the neuroscientific approach to consciousness is young, the reasonable hope is for discoveries that will open more doors and suggest fruitful experimental research. In the long haul, of course, we want to understand consciousness at least as well as we understand reproduction or metabolism, but in the short haul, it is wise to have realistic goals. It is probably not realistic to expect, for example, that a single experimental paradigm will solve the mystery.

1.3   Experimental Strategies

Although there are many proposals for making progress experimentally, for convenience the strategies targeting the brain can roughly be grouped as one of two kinds: a *direct approach* or an *indirect approach*. These strategies differ mainly in emphasis. In any case, as will be seen, they are *complementary*, not mutually incompatible. To see the strengths and weaknesses of each, I shall outline the somewhat differing motivations, scientific styles, and experimental approaches.

The direct approach

It is possible, for all we can tell now, that consciousness, or at least the sensory component of consciousness, may be subserved by a physical substrate with a distinctive signature. In the hope that there is some distinct and discernible physical marker of the substrate, the direct strategy aims first to identify the substrate as a *correlate* of phenomenological awareness, then eventually to get a reductive explanation of conscious states in neurobiological terms. The physical substrate need not be confined to one location. It could, for example, consist in a pattern of activity in one or two structurally unique cell *types* found in a particular layer of cortex across a range of brain areas. Or it could consist in the synchronized firing of a special cell population in the thalamus and certain cortical areas. On these alternatives, the mechanism would be *distributed*, and hence would be more like the endocrine system, for example, than the kidney. For convenience, I shall refer to a postulated physical substrate as a *mechanism* for consciousness.

Notice also that the distinctive mechanism could reside at any of a variety of physical levels: molecular, single cell, circuit, pathway, or some higher organizational level not yet explicitly catalogued. Or perhaps consciousness is the product of interactions between these myriad physical levels. The possibility of a distributed mechanism, together with the opened-ended possibility concerning the *level* of organization at which the mechanism inheres, means that hypotheses are so far quite unconstrained. The lack of constraints is not a symptom of anything otherworldly about this problem. It is merely a symptom that science has a lot of work to do.

Discovering some one or more of the neural correlates of consciousness would not *on its own* yield an explanation of consciousness. Nevertheless, in biology the discovery of which mechanism supports a specific function often means that the next step—determining precisely *how* the function is performed —suddenly becomes a whole lot easier. Not *easy*, but easier. Were we lucky enough to identify the hypothetical mechanism, the result would be comparable in its scientific ramifications to identifying the structure of DNA. That discovery was essentially a discovery about structural embodiment of information. Once the structure of the double helix was revealed, it became possible to see that the order of the base pairs was a code for making proteins, and hence to understand the structural basis for heritability of traits. In the event that there is a mechanism with a distinct signature identifiable with conscious states, the scientific payoff *could* be enormous. The direct strategy, therefore, is worth a good shot.

The downside, of course, is that the mechanism might be experimentally very difficult to identify until neuroscience is *much* further along, since the signature may not be obvious to the naive observer. Our current misconceptions about the phenomena to be explained, or about the brain, may lead us to misinterpret the data even if the mechanism with its distinct signature exists to be identified. Or there may be other unforeseeable pitfalls to bedevil the approach. In short, all the usual problems besetting any ambitious scientific project beset us here.

In recent years, the direct approach has become more clearly articulated and more experimentally attractive, in part occasioned by new techniques that made it possible to investigate closely related functions such as attention and working memory.

Francis Crick, probably more than anyone else, has a sure-footed scientific sense of what the direct approach would need to succeed. He has drawn attention to the value of using low-level and systems-level data to narrow the search space of plausible hypotheses, and of constantly prowling that search space to provoke one's scientific imagination to come up with testable hypotheses. Crick has consistently recognized and defended the value of getting *some* sort of structural bead on the neuroanatomy subserving conscious states, not because he thought such data would solve the problems in one grand sweep, but because he realized it would give us a thread, which, when pulled, might begin to unravel the problem. He argued that experiments probing such a mechanism could make a plausible assumption, which I henceforth refer to as Crick's assumption:

Crick's assumption   There must be brain differences in the following two conditions: (1) a stimulus is presented and the subject *is* aware of it, and (2) a stimulus is presented and the subject is *not* aware of it.[5]

With the right experiments, it should be possible to find what is different about the brain in these two conditions.

Within this lean framework, the next step is to find an experimental paradigm where psychology and neuroscience can hold hands across the divide; in other words, to find a psychological phenomenon that fits Crick's assumption and *probe* the corresponding neurobiological system to try to identify the neural differences between being aware and not being aware of the stimulus. This would give us a lead into the neural correlate of consciousness and hence into the mechanism. Fortunately, a property of the visual system known as *binocular rivalry* presents just the opportunity needed to proceed on Crick's assumption.[6]

What is binocular rivalry?

Suppose that you are looking at a computer monitor through special box with a division down the middle, so each eye sees only its half of the screen. If the two eyes are presented with the *same* stimulus, say a face, then what you see is one face. If, however, each eye gets different inputs—the left eye gets a face, and the right eye gets a sunburst pattern—then something quite surprising

Stimuli

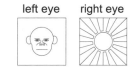

Subject's perception

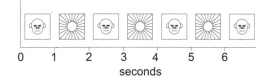

Figure 4.3 Bistable perception resulting from binocular rivalry. If different stimuli are presented to each eye, after a few moments of confusion, the brain settles down to perceiving the stimuli in an alternating sequence, where the perception of any given stimulus lasts only about 1 second. (Courtesy of P. M. Churchland.)

happens. After a few seconds, you perceive *alternating* stimuli: first sunburst, then face, then sunburst, then face. The perception is *bistable*, favoring neither one over the other, but switching back and forth between the two stimuli (figure 4.3). The reversal happens about once every 1–5 seconds, though the rate can be as long as once every 10 seconds. Many different stimuli give bistable perceptual effects, including horizontal bars shown to one eye and vertical bars to the other. So long as the stimuli are not too big or too small, the effect is striking, robust, and quite unambiguous.[7]

For the purposes of Crick's assumption, this setup is appealing: the opposing stimuli (e.g., the face and sunburst pattern) are *always* present, but the subject is *perceptually aware* of each only in alternating periods. Consider, for example, the face. It is *always* present, but now I am aware of the face, now I am aware of the sunburst pattern. Consequently, we can ask, What is the difference in the brain between those occasions when you *are* aware of the face and those when you are *not*?

Precisely *why* binocular rivalry exists is a question we leave aside for now, as there are various speculations but no definitive answer. It is fairly certain, however, that it is not a retinal or thalamic effect, but an effect of cortical processing. The most convincing hypothesis, favored by Leopold and Logothetis, is that binocular rivalry results from a system-level randomness that

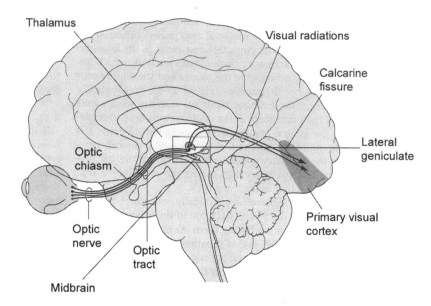

Figure 4.4   A diagram of human brain from the medial aspect showing the projections from the retina to the lateral geniculate nucleus of the thalamus and midbrain (superior colliculus and pretectum), and from the thalamus to cortical area V1 of the cerebral cortex. (Based on Kandel, Schwartz, and Jessell 2000.)

typifies exploratory behavior in general and whose function is to ensure that the brain does not get stuck in one perceptual hypothesis.[8]

On the neurobiological side, what is experimentally convenient about binocular rivalry is that in the visual system, cortical area STS (superior temporal sulcus) is known to contain individual neurons that respond preferentially to faces. This "tuning" of neurons, as it is called, is something that can be exploited by the experimentalist in the binocular rivalry setup (figures 4.4 to 4.6). This means that the cellular responses during presentation of rival stimuli can be recorded and monitored.

Area STS was identified, and its tuned neurons characterized, using single-neuron recording techniques in the monkey. This technique involves inserting a microelectrode into the cortex and recording the action potentials in the axon of a single neuron (figure 4.7).[9] On the basis of lesion data and fMRI studies, we know that human brains also have areas that are especially responsive to faces. Although such macrolevel data are extremely important, it has to be balanced by microlevel data from the single neuron. By and large, looking for single neurons whose activity correlates with conscious perception is something

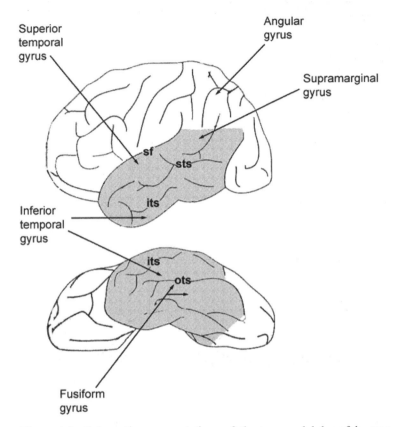

Figure 4.5 Schematic representations of the temporal lobe of human brain (shaded areas). The upper panel shows a side view (lateral aspect), and the lower panel shows the underside (ventral aspect). There are three general regions on the lateral surface of the temporal lobe: the superior temporal gyrus, the middle temporal gyrus, and the inferior temporal gyrus, which extends around to the ventral aspect of the temporal lobe. The ventral aspect includes the fusiform gyrus, also referred to as the occipitotemporal gyrus, and the parahippocampal gyrus, also referred to as the lingual gyrus. Abbreviations: its, inferior temporal sulcus; ots, occipitotemporal sulcus; sf, Sylvian fissure; sts, superior temporal sulcus. (Based on Rodman 1998.)

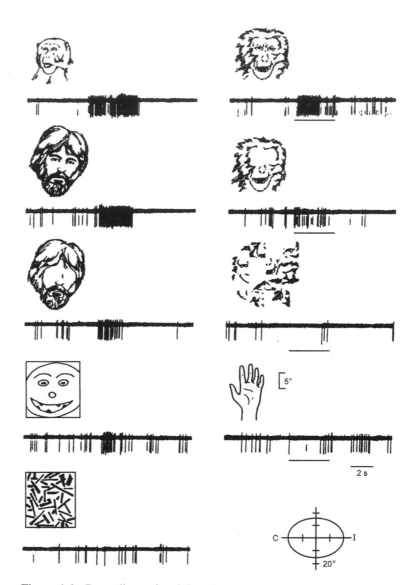

Figure 4.6 Recordings of activity of a cell with a large receptive field in the superior temporal gyrus as pictures of faces, degraded faces, or nonfaces are visually presented to a monkey. The cell responds most vigorously to faces, human or monkey or baboon. Activity is diminished if the eyes are removed or if the face's features are all present but jumbled. It responds better to a cartoon face than to the jumbled features or a nonface. When the monkey is shown a hand or a meaningless pattern, the cell response drops to its base firing rate. (From Bruce et al. 1981.)

Intracellular recording by mircoelectrode

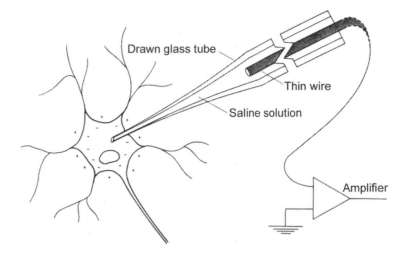

Figure 4.7 An idealized experiment for measuring the potential difference across a cell membrane. The electrode is a fine glass capillary with a tip no more than .1 micrometer in diameter, filled with a saline solution.

that must be done in monkeys. Nevertheless, by using an existing medical opportunity, Kreiman, Fried and Koch (2002) were able to repeat the Logothetis experiment in fourteen human surgical patients. Each had intractable epilepsy. To localize the seizure onset focus before surgery, eight depth electrodes were implanted in the medial temporal lobe of each patient. Recordings from these electrodes during bistable perception showed that about two thirds of the visually selective cells tracked the percept; none tracked the perceptually suppressed stimulus. Macaque monkeys are a good substitute for humans in the binocular-rivalry experiment because human and monkey brains are structurally very similar, and in particular, their visual systems are organizationally and structurally very similar. There is nevertheless a residual problem in using monkeys instead of humans, which is that humans can verbally answer "face" when they see a face, but the monkey cannot.

The tactic for overcoming this human/monkey difference is to train the monkey to respond by pressing a button with its left or right hand to indicate whether it sees a face or a sunburst. Monkeys are first trained in a standard (nonrivalrous) paradigm in which there is a correct answer and they are rewarded accordingly. That is the only way we have, so far, to let the monkey know what behavior we want. Once trained, monkeys are presented with rivalrous stimuli (face to one eye, sunburst to the other) to see how they respond. It is reassuring that monkeys' response behavior matches that of humans: it indicates an alternation in perception of the face versus the sunburst at about once per second.

A specific and significant doubt remains, nonetheless. Although monkeys may indeed be visually aware, they may not be using visual awareness to solve *this* problem. We know from human psychophysics that subjects can perform well above chance on a visual identification task even though they *report* that they are merely guessing their answers rather than judging on the basis of a conscious perception.

What adds fuel to this doubt is that the learning curves of the monkeys look like the learning curves of *operant conditioned* rats. In other words, we cannot assume that the experimenter's intent suddenly dawned on the monkey and it thought to itself, "Oh I get it. When I see *faces* I press *this* button, and when I see sunbursts I press *that* one!" and with that insight its performance jumps to nearly perfect. In fact, the monkeys show gradual improvement over days and even weeks rather than an abrupt improvement indicative of insight. The learning curves mean that the behavior of the animals is consistent with the *possibility* that connectivity is strengthened between visual area STS and motor cortex without visual awareness being part of the loop after all.

It is highly desirable to find ways to determine empirically, with a decent degree of probability, whether the animal uses *conscious* visual perception to solve the problem. Flexibility in response might be such an indicator. For example, if the monkey uses awareness to solve problems in anything like the way humans do, then the monkey should be able quickly to learn a new motor action to respond to the very same stimulus. If it uses both the new and the original response, the two should agree. The monkey should also appear surprised if a particular trial is easy and it gets the answer wrong. This sort of flexibility is characteristic of human conscious perception, and it is the kind of thing that should be demonstrable if the monkey is using visual awareness in solving the problem. Although we must shelve this problem for now, it is essential to acknowledge the need for developing experimental procedures on animals that overcome these problems.[10]

Inspired by the empirical problems confronting the experimentalist, the a priori skeptic might tender a much more tenacious skepticism about animal awareness. For example, the skeptic might complain that the monkey can only exhibit *behavior*, whereas the human can actually *talk*. So, the objection continues, we have no reason to think that the monkey is aware *at all*, *ever*, under *any* conditions.[11] The objection presupposes that speech is really a *direct* indication of consciousness, whereas button pressing is not.

Notice, first, that speech too is *just behavior*—behavior that humans have learned to perform. Even if the monkey did show verbal behavior, the determined skeptic would *still* complain that we could not be certain that its speech involves awareness as human speech does. Bonobo chimpanzees such as Kanzi and Pambanisha do display some verbal behavior, but the a priori skeptic waves this off as "mere conditioning."[12] We are now venturing into Skepticism, with a capital "S."

A thoroughly general Skepticism takes the form "How do I know that *any person*, let alone *some monkey*, is ever conscious? Indeed, how do I know that anything other than I exists? And moreover, how do I know that *I* was conscious before *this* very moment?" Part of the trouble with *this* brand of skepticism is that *no* empirical controls could allay the doubt one whit, *in principle*. The Skeptic thus overplays his hand, with the consequence that general Skepticism is hard to take very seriously beyond a moment or two.

A Skeptic can insist that there is no decisive proof that one is not dreaming, or that the universe was not created five minutes ago complete with fossil record, memories, history books, crumbling Roman ruins, and so on. Indeed, *there is no* decisive proof of the impossibility of what was just sketched. Still, as a hypothesis about reality, it is a bit silly.[13] *Specific* doubts about a *specific* experiment are a very different matter, however, and they do indeed have to be answered, one and all. In the absence of identifiable reasons for thinking that *only* humans can be visually aware, the similarities in monkey and human brains suggest that it is reasonable for me *provisionally* to assume that the monkey has visual awareness qualitatively *not very different* from ours. This is not a dogmatic declaration that monkeys are indeed visually aware as we are, but it is a useful *working assumption*, one that can sustain some interesting experiments. Nonetheless, it could be false, and it could be *falsified* empirically.

The binocular rivalry experiments

The neural correlates of visual awareness in binocular rivalry were first experimentally probed by neuroscientists Nikos Logothetis and Jeffrey Schall in 1989. Logothetis and Schall were using upward-moving and downward-moving gratings as stimuli. Their monkeys had been trained in advanced to indicate what they saw by pressing specific buttons, and the recording of single cells was done in visual cortical area MT. More recently (1997), Scheinberg and Logothetis have used a face and a sunburst pattern, and recorded in STS. Henceforth I shall frame the discussion around the face/sunburst stimuli, and I shall say "The monkey *sees* the face" as shorthand for "The monkey presses the button indicating its learned response to face stimuli," and so forth.

Simplified, the results are as follows. Consider a set of neurons, $N_1, \ldots, N_5$, that were previously identified as responding preferentially to *faces*. (Suppose, for simplicity in this discussion, that faces are *always* present to the left eye, and sunbursts always to the right eye.) What do those neurons do when the monkey sees the *sunburst*? Some of them, perhaps N_1 and N_2, continue to respond, because of course the face is still present to the left eye, even if it is not consciously seen. Other face neurons, perhaps N_3 and N_4, do not respond. Now for the critical result: when and only when the monkey indicates that it *does see* the face, N_3 and N_4 respond (and as always, N_1, N_2 respond so long as the face is present) (figure 4.8).

Here is why this is interesting. Some neurons seem to be driven by the external stimulus; that is, they respond to the stimulus regardless of whether the monkey consciously perceives it. Others seem to respond only when the monkey sees—*consciously sees*—the stimulus. More exactly, the distribution of responses in STS was this: about 90 percent of the face neurons fire when and only when the monkey indicates it sees a face; the remainder always fire so long as the face is present on the monitor.

Can we say that the responsivity of the neurons in the 90 percent pool is *correlated with visual perception* (visual awareness)? Yes, but we need to go carefully here. Over a fairly generous time scale, "correlated with" could include events that are not identical with the state of perceptual awareness but are part of the causal sequence. More exactly, the data do not exclude the possibility that the responses of STS neurons are actually the causal antecedents—or possibly causal sequelae—of neural activity that *is* the awareness. In other words, we cannot simply conclude that this subset of STS neurons is the seat of visual awareness of faces. Progress has been made, but we do not want to overstate our conclusions.[14]

Although the binocular-rivalry experiments are a little complicated, they are important because they illustrate something that will surprise convention-bound philosophers. With the right experiment, you *can* make progress, even at the level of the single neuron, in investigating the neural causes or neural correlates of visual awareness. It shows, contra the naysayers, that headway, albeit only a little, is possible. Moreover, image data, using fMRI on humans, is consistent with the single-neuron results.[15] With further experiments, this beginning allows us to push on into territory that will be fruitful.

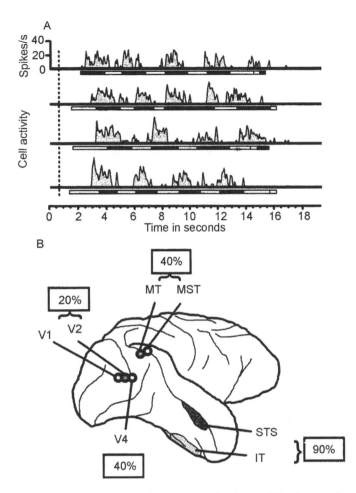

Figure 4.8 The neuronal responses of a face cell in the monkey brain during bistable perception. In the experiment, a monkey is trained to hold down one lever, e.g., the right-hand lever, when it sees a face, and to hold down the other lever when it sees a sunburst pattern. (A) The four horizontal graphs represent four observation periods, and the dashed vertical line indicates the onset of a rivalrous presentation (e.g., face and sunburst pattern). The animal's behavioral response is shown below the line, the shaded area representing the period during which animal holds down the appropriate lever. The cell response is shown above the line. The high rate of activity of the face cell begins just before, and ends just before, the period during which the animal holds down the face lever. The period of high activity (between 0 and 50 spikes/second) lasts for about 1 second. (B) The brain areas that contained the cells whose activity correlated with the monkey's subjective perception when responding to stimuli known to drive cells in that area. The greater the synaptic distance of the cortical area from the retina, the greater the percentage of cells driven by the subjective perception. Abbreviations: IT, inferior temporal; MT, middle temporal; MST, medial superior temporal sulcus; STS, superior temporal sulcus; V1, striate cortex; V2, V4, extrastriate cortex. (From Leopold and Logothetis 1999.)

Other experiments, similarly motivated, link up with the Logothetis results. Here is one strategy. To get a visual perception called "the waterfall illusion," you stare at a waterfall for several minutes. When you look away at a *still* surface, such as a gray blanket, you see upward motion, a kind of reverse, and illusory, waterfall. Roger Tootell used this phenomenon to run an experiment that complements the Logothetis and Schall experiment. The focus here will be on the neural correlates of conscious perception of upward motion induced in the *absence* of an externally present upward stimulus. Tootell used the non-invasive scanning technique fMRI to determine what cortical visual area showed greater activity when a human subject consciously perceives the waterfall illusion. He found, not unexpectedly, that motion-sensitive areas such as MT show increased activity with the onset of perception of the waterfall illusion. In this experiment too, it remains unknown whether MT neurons are actually neural correlates of consciousness, or whether they are just an element in the causal antecedents or consequences thereof.[16]

Hallucinations in human subjects present a different possibility for exploring what happens in the brain when a visual experience is present but the stimulus is *not*. Recently this has been elegantly pursued using fMRI by a group in London led by Ffytche.[17] Patients who suffer eye damage, for example as a result of detachment of the retina or glaucoma, lack normal vision. In some cases, these patients periodically experience highly vivid visual effects, though they are perfectly normal neuropsychiatrically. The character of the hallucinations varies from subject to subject, and unlike visual imagery, the visual objects appear to be in the outside world, and neither their appearance nor the nature of the visual image is under voluntary control.

One subject saw cartoonlike faces; another saw colored, shiny shapes rather like "futuristic cars." In the fMRI scanner, subjects signaled the onset of their visual hallucinations, and the scan data were analyzed. The data showed association of hallucinations with activity in the ventral visual regions, but with little activity in early visual cortex (V1). More specifically, if a subject hallucinated in color, an area independently identified as important in color processing was more active than if the hallucination was in black and white. Face hallucinations were associated with cortical subareas independently known to be involved with face processing, including the inferior temporal region (figure 4.9).

What do the Ffytche data mean? On their own, they do not solve the mystery, of course, but they are at least consistent with the data from binocular rivalry and from the waterfall illusion. These converging data suggest that a subset of neurons in visual cortical areas may support conscious visual perception.

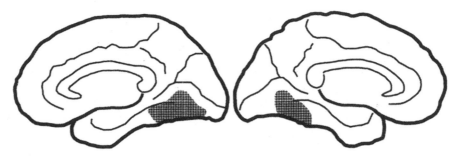

Figure 4.9 Bilateral lesions in the shaded region cause propopagnosia (loss of the capacity to identify individual faces). (Courtesy of Hanna Damasio.)

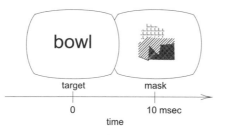

Figure 4.10 Visual masking. As the subject views the monitor, a word is presented, followed about 10 msec later by a noisy jumble—the mask. In these conditions, the subject sees only the mask, not the word.

Another experimental approach, also using fMRI, involves comparing brain activity during presentation of stimuli that are not consciously perceived and during presentation of stimuli that *are* consciously perceived. The experiments exploit an earlier behavioral result by Anthony Marcel, in which he showed that nonperceived stimuli had a quantifiable effect on subject's task performance. More specifically, Marcel flashed a word for about 10 msec., then immediately followed the word with a masking stimulus (a noisy visual stimulus flashed in the same location as the stimulus). The presentation of the mask somehow interferes with normal visual processing and the flashed item is not seen (figure 4.10). Subsequently, subjects were given a lexical-decision task, in which a string of letters was presented and the subject's task was to specify whether the string was or was not a word. Marcel showed that the subject's performance, measured in reaction time, was better for those words that had been presented in the *masked* condition than for words never presented. Moreover, processing of the flashed stimulus went beyond the mere physical shape of the stimulus because the effect was case-insensitive. (i.e., "BIRD" versus "bird"). This elegant experiment demonstrated a level of *semantic* processing even when subjects reported no conscious perception of the stimulus.

Dehaene and colleagues used the Marcel paradigm and recorded activity in normal subjects using fMRI in the masked and the visible conditions.[18] They showed that even in the masked condition, there is activity in both the fusiform gyrus and the precentral gyrus, areas that independent experiments indicate are active during conscious *reading* (see again fig. 4.9). In the condition where the stimulus was seen and not masked, the activity in the fusiform gyrus appeared to be about twelve times as strong as in the masked condition, and there was additional activity in the dorsolateral prefrontal cortex. The data suggest that the difference in brain activity in the two conditions is owed to conscious awareness of the stimuli.

Clever as the experiment is and important though the data are, several cautions are in order. First, the areas showing increased activity involve hundreds of millions of neurons, so the data are giving us a very general portrait, not detailed information about specific neurons or neuron-types and their role in awareness. Second, the data are consistent with the possibility that the greater activity in the nonmasked trial is caused by activation of a large range of neural networks whose stored information is associated with the flashed word. The mask may have associations too, but many fewer than a word. In the masked case, activation of networks associated with the word is probably interrupted by the mask, whereas the mask, being junk, provokes few associations. As the authors rightly note, the effects of the mask appear to start very early in the visual system, and propagate to higher levels. If the greater activity seen in the nonmasked case reflects greater numbers of activated associations, these associations might well be entirely nonconscious. They might be caused by a conscious representation, or by whatever it is that causes the conscious representation. Consequently, we cannot be sure that the greater range of activation in the unmasked case corresponds to conscious activity per se.[19]

Loops and conscious experience

An idea that has long been central to the approach of neuroscientist Gerald Edelman[20] is that loops (also referred to as *re-entrant pathways* and as *back projections*) are essential circuitry in the production of conscious awareness.[21] The idea is that some neurons carry signals from more peripheral to more central regions, such as from V1 to V2, while others convey more highly processed signals in the reverse direction, for example from V2 to V1. At an anatomical level, it is a general rule of cortical organization that forward-projecting neurons are matched by an equal or greater number of back-projecting neurons. Back-projecting neurons are a feature of brain organization generally, and in some instances, such as the pathway from V1 to the lateral geniculate nucleus (LGN) of the thalamus, back-projecting neurons are more numerous by a factor of ten than the forward-projecting neurons. Anatomically, then, the equipment is known to exist.

Why do Edelman and others think back projections have some particular role in consciousness? Part of the rationale for this point is that perception *always* involves classification; conscious seeing is *seeing as*.[22] Normally, one *sees* a fearful human face as fearful, rather than simply as a face followed by the explicit inference, "Aha, the eyes are especially wide open, etc., so this face is showing fear." In fact, most of us instantly recognize a fearful face but cannot articulate precisely what configuration of facial features is required for a face to show fear (figure 4.11). So we could not say what an *explicit inference* could use for *premises*, anyhow. Smells are often imbued with a *hedonic* dimension of meaning. The smell of rotten meat, for example, is disgusting to humans, whereas to vultures, it is appealing. Separating *in experience* the pure odor of rotten meat from the anhedonic nastiness of the smell is impossible.

Integrating hedonic components, emotional significance, associated cognitive representations, and so forth, with features of perception detected by the sensory systems almost certainly relies on loops—pathways projecting a signal back from structures such as the amygdala and hypothalamus (which have powerful roles in emotions and drives) to the sensory systems themselves, and pathways from so-called *higher areas* of cortex (e.g., prefrontal regions) to *lower areas* (e.g., V1). That we directly perceive a face with its fearful expression implies that information about the emotion must be routed back to the visual system at some level. A purely feedforward neural network cannot achieve this kind of integration.

Artificial neural network (ANN) research indicates that many of the consciousness-related functions—STM, attention, sensory perception, meaning— are handled most powerfully and efficiently by networks with recurrent projections. The range of functions that back projections perform has not been precisely demonstrated in real neural networks, and there are serious technical difficulties to be overcome before back-projection physiology can get very far. Nevertheless, the fact that back projections in ANNs render those systems vastly more powerful, and more powerful *in the ways relevant to consciousness-related functions*, is highly suggestive.[23]

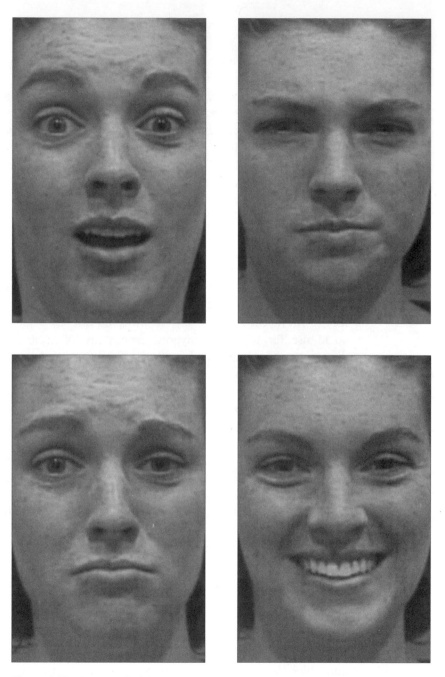

Figure 4.11 Human facial expressions of four emotions: fear, anger, sadness, and happiness. (Faces courtesy of Dailey, Cottrell, and Reilly. Copyright 2001 California Facial Expressions Database [CAFE].)

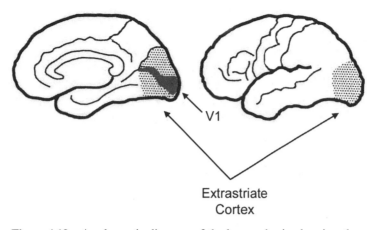

Extrastriate
Cortex

Figure 4.12 A schematic diagram of the human brain showing the position of V1. On the left is the medial view; on the right is the lateral view. In the visual cortex, V1 is located in the calcarine sulcus in the medial aspect, shown in dark shading. The extra striate cortex is shown with dotted shading. (Courtesy of Hanna Damasio.)

   Experimental evidence is beginning to come in to support this idea. For example, Pascual-Leone and Walsh exploited the fact that transcranial magnetic stimulation (TMS) of cortical visual area V1 will cause the subject to experience small flashes of light, while stimulation of cortical visual area MT will produce flashes of light that move.[24] The anatomical fact of importance is that there are back projections from MT to V1. (In fact the back projections typical of cortical organization are also seen in the brainstem and spinal cord, as well as in structures such as the hypothalamus. They are essentially everywhere.) So here is their experiment: stimulate MT in a manner normally adequate to produce moving flashes of light, and also stimulate V1, but at an intensity so low that it does not cause perception of lights, but high enough to interfere with the normal effect of back-projected signals from MT. If back-projected signals from MT are necessary to see moving flashes, then in this condition, no moving flashes will be seen. These are indeed the results. Subjects see flashes, but not moving flashes.
   As always, optimism must be tempered with skeptical questions. One major question concerns what exactly is the effect of TMS at the neuronal level, how focal the stimulation really is, and how far the effect spreads, cortically and subcortically. A further problem arises from the nature of human brain anatomy. In the macaque monkey, V1 is on the dorsal surface of the brain. In human brains, V1 is on the *medial* surface of the occipital lobe (figure 4.12).

Consequently, if you aim to stimulate V1 with TMS, you will also stimulate the dorsal regions, and activity in the pathways from the incidentally stimulated areas can be predicted to affect both V1 and V2. The worry is that the incidentally stimulated areas confound the results.

In any case, even if back projections are *necessary* for consciousness, we know that they are not *sufficient*. Back projections function in phylogenetically older parts of the brain, such as the spinal cord; some are active when subjects are under anesthesia, in a deep sleep, or in a coma. If a subset of cortical back projections are indeed subserving awareness of visual stimuli, it will be important to determine which axons they are and what precisely is the nature of their signals.

Theorizing and narrowing the hypothesis space

In addition to designing experiments to identify the neural correlates of consciousness, pulling together data bearing on the conditions for visual experience and isolating structural and functional constraints can help narrow the hypothesis space. Especially in the early stages of the problem, this is a very useful strategy, particularly because some of the concepts needed to articulate a good hypothesis undoubtedly need to be invented as the search space narrows ever more.

Loops are likely to be one structural constraint on the substrate for consciousness. As Francis Crick and Christof Koch suggest, other constraints that emerge from the experimental literature include the following:[25]

- The neurons whose collective activity constitutes being aware of something are distributed spatially. Transiently, they form a "coalition" that lasts for the duration of the awareness of a particular perception, such as visual awareness of Lincoln's face. Individual neurons can be elements in different coalitions as a function of the percepts. For example, a particular neuron might be part of a coalition that constitutes being aware of Lincoln's face, but it also might be part of a coalition that constitutes being aware of a human hand, or a coalition for a dog face.

- Neurons in the coalition whose activity constitutes a perceptual awareness probably need to reach a threshold in order for the coalition's activity to constitute perceptual awareness.

- Normally, though perhaps not necessarily, a coalition emerges as a consequence of synchrony of firing in neuron populations that project to the coalition members. This synchrony of firing is part of the causal conditions for reaching the threshold.

- When neurons involved in perceptual awareness do fire above that threshold, they continue firing for a short but sustained period of time (e.g., longer than 100 milliseconds but not as long as a minute).

- Attention probably up-regulates the activity of the relevant neurons, getting them closer to their threshold.

- In awareness of a certain visual phenomenon, say the face of Lincoln, some neurons will be activated as part of the cognitive background, while some will be activated as essential to the experience itself. These latter neurons Crick and Koch call "essential nodes," to distinguish them from neurons that contribute to the cognitive background. Included in the cognitive background are the *expectation* that the face is the front of the head, and various nonconscious, *tacit beliefs*, e.g., that if Lincoln had been born in Australia, he would not have been president of the United States. The cognitive background includes also various *associations* and *inferential* connections, for example, the association with the civil war, and the capacity to infer from "Lincoln was president of the United States in 1864," the statement that "Lincoln is not now president of the United States."

- At any given moment there is probably a competition between various essential-node neurons for which neurons will fire at the threshold and hence which representation will be conscious. Thus, if I am paying close attention to events on television, I may not hear the lawnmower running next door. This implies that the essential-node neurons in the auditory system will have lost out in the competition to those in the visual system representing the events on the television.

Ideally, the items in this list will jell to form a kind of prototheory of neural mechanisms supporting perceptual awareness. In the role of prototheory, the list may provoke experiments to confirm or disconfirm any one of its items, and thus move us closer to understanding the nature of consciousness. Having some sort of theoretical scaffolding is a clear improvement over groping haphazardly. Even if none of the items on the list turns out to be part of the explanation of consciousness, the exercise is valuable, because it orients us toward thinking of the problem of consciousness in terms of *mechanisms*, that is, in terms of causal organization. Identifying neural correlates is one thing, and likely a useful thing, but the goal we ultimately want to reach is identifying causal mechanisms so as to understand *how* consciousness occurs.

A methodological question about neural correlates

In the foregoing experiments, there was evidence of neural activity correlated with conscious awareness. Nevertheless, I expressed caution concerning what such correlational evidence signifies. The major reason has already been stated: finding correlations between neural activity and a subject's reports of perceptual awareness is *consistent* with any of the following: (1) the neural activity is a background condition for perceptual awareness, (2) the neural activity is part of the cause, (3) the neural activity is part of the sequelae of the awareness, (4) the neural activity parallels, but plays no direct role in, perceptual awareness, and (5) the neural activity is what perceptual awareness can be *identified* with (the *identificand*).

Ultimately, if we want to be able to explain the nature of consciousness in neural terms, what we seek is the *identification* of some class of neural activity with perceptual awareness. That is, we want our data to justify interpretation (5). As is evident, however, correlational data per se do not rule out all alternatives except (5). That some event x is a correlate of some phenomenon y does tell you a *little*, such as that you *may* be on the right path for finding the *identificand*. For similar reasons, that some event z fails to correlate with some phenomenon y suggests that you may be on the wrong path. This is not the whole pudding, nor is it nothing, and one has to start somewhere.

Determining that two phenomena are systematically correlated requires testing under a wide range of conditions. It is not enough, for example, to get fMRI data showing that in awake subjects, a specific cortical visual area is highly active whenever the subject reports visual awareness of an object. We want also to know whether there is activity in that brain region when the subject is not conscious. For example, it is essential to know whether the brain of a subject in a coma or in a persistent vegetative state or under anesthesia shows activity in that brain region when a visual stimulus is presented. This is not idle skepticism. Activity in various cortical areas is known to occur in response to an external stimulus in precisely these unusual conditions. A patient in a persistent vegetative state, for example, exhibits no signs of awareness, and in particular, no behavioral sign of awareness when shown a familiar person. Nevertheless, when the subject was shown familiar faces, the so-called "face area" of the cortex showed a pattern of increased activity similar to that of the normal subject.[26] As Damasio correctly notes, such data are powerful clues that neurons in the visual cortex may not be the generators of visual conscious experience. Rather, their activities are representations that the subject might be aware of *if* he were conscious. So until the tough cases have been excluded by experiment, no conclusion can be drawn from correlations in the relatively easy cases.

There is, however, the deeper problem touched on earlier; it is the problem of knowing what you are looking at. It is reasonable to hope that there is a class of neural activity correlated *always* and *only* with perceptual awareness, and that such activity is *identifiable* as conscious awareness. Nonetheless, even if there is such a class of activity, knowing that *this* measured activity belongs to *that class* may be discoverable only very indirectly. In other words, we might be looking straight at an instance of the class without in the slightest recognizing that it is an instance. This will happen if, as is very likely, the physical substrate does not have a property that is salient to the naive observer, but is recognizable only through the lens of a more comprehensive *theory* of brain function.

An analogy may make this point clearer. In the nineteenth century, the nature of light was a profound mystery. Suppose, to be fanciful, that nineteenth-century physicists address the mystery by seeking the microstructural correlates of light. They hope that there is a particular class of microstructural phenomena that is *always* and *only* correlated with light, and that such activity, or something connected to it, is *identifiable* as light. The rough idea is to look for the "defining property"—the *identificand*, as we may refer to it.

Since those of us living now have the benefit of post-Maxwellian physics, we know that the defining property is characterized abstractly and nonobservationally by the theory of electromagnetic radiation. That is, Maxwell realized that the equations characterizing light matched perfectly the equations characterizing radio waves, x-rays, and other electromagnetic phenomena. He rightly concluded that light just *is* yet another form of electromagnetic radiation. Observable properties give no hint of this, but the match of deep, unobservable properties gave the game away.

Here is the question: could our imagined pre-Maxwellian correlation hunters notice, even if they looked closely, that radio waves and light share that same deep property? Probably not, since, until they understand a good deal more about electromagnetic radiation, they lack the conceptual resources to see what *counts as the same property*. This is because they do not yet have the slightest inkling that light *is* electromagnetic radiation, or that x-rays, gamma rays, etc., even exist (see plate 1, following p. 186).

Or think of the problem this way: How would *you* know, independently of Lavosier's work on oxygen, that rusting, metabolizing, and burning are the same microphysical process, but that sunlight and lightning are *not*? What property would you look at? And if you did by luck make a guess that the first three phenomena share a microstructural property, how would you test your idea?

This is *not* to say that looking for the neural correlates of consciousness is futile. On the contrary, at this very early stage of the neurobiological investigation of consciousness, it is undoubtedly wise to give it the best shot possible. My point is that it is also wise to recognize the pitfalls and to appreciate that they are not merely technological, but derive also from the absence of a firmly planted *theoretical* framework for understanding how the brain works.[27]

The experiments discussed in this section, and others with a similar general conceptual slant, are important because they have opened doors. From the vantage point of 1980, when such experiments were barely conceivable, they look downright spectacular. At the very least, they inspire researchers to invent better and better experimental designs. It should be noted, however, that the examples in this section do share a certain conceptual slant that is open to criticism. All are focused mainly on the *cerebral cortex*, and all are drawn from the *visual system*. This narrowing of the focus can be valuable, especially when different experimental strategies unearth complementary results, as those discussed above do to some extent. Focusing narrowly allows us to probe deeply, if not broadly, and that can be rewarding.

Nevertheless, for all we can tell now, it could turn out that other modalities play a role in consciousness that is more straightforward and less complicated than the role of vision. Possibly, exploration of olfactory or somatosensory processing will reveal principles obscured thus far. More seriously, it could turn out that it is not *cortical* neurons—or not cortical neurons *alone*—whose activity is identifiable with awareness, but rather, the activity of various *noncortical* neurons in the brainstem, thalamus, hypothalamus, and so forth.[28] It is common knowledge that subcortical activity does figure in the causal antecedents. Whether some subcortical activity is more than that, however, is a possibility we shall explore in section 1.4.

1.4   The Indirect Approach

Attention, short-term memory, autobiographical memory, self-representation, perception, imagery, thought, meaning, being awake, self-referencing—*all* seem to be connected in some way with being conscious of something. The indirect approach proposes that once we understand the neurobiological mechanisms of each of these diverse functions and the relations between them, the story of consciousness will more or less come together on its own. That is, once we have a more substantial *theory of brain function in general*, we will have the means to develop a theory of the conditions under which these functions involve conscious awareness. In this respect, therefore, the approach is *indirect*. The strategy favors continuing to investigate, both neurobiologically and behaviorally, these diverse brain functions and how they connect with each other. Because its success depends on understanding most of the functions of the brain, this strategy may take longer to bear fruit than the more direct route.

Is consciousness identifiable with some *one* of these functions, with, say, being awake? Is consciousness anything over and above being awake? Consciousness is not the same as being awake, since you can be awake but still not be conscious of your saccadic eye movements or of things you are not attending to (such as tongue movement) or of masked or subthreshold stimuli. Moreover, we seem to be conscious of our dreams, even though we are asleep while we dream.

Is consciousness identifiable with paying *attention*?[29] Probably not, though the two may indeed be very closely linked. There is more than one attention system, and in both, shifts in attention can precede awareness. This implies that consciousness cannot just *be* attention. In "bottom-up" attention, a subject can normally orient to a moving object nonconsciously detected in peripheral vision. Reading text provides another well-studied example where attention and visual awareness do not coincide.[30] In reading, the eyes do not smoothly traverse the text, but jump from chunk to chunk (a chunk is about 17 characters in length). Remarkably, the fovea typically lands on the most informative part of the chunk, such as on the word "cantaloupe" rather than on the word "the" (figure 4.13). This shows that eye movements are not a lock-step operation, but are sensitive to specific features of the stimulus. How is this achieved? At each eye-movement fixation, the subject reads the text on which the eye is focused. The foveated text is what the reader is aware of. During this fixation period, attention shifts to the right,[31] and via peripheral vision, the next suitable foveation site is selected. Then the eyes shift, and one is aware of the next chunk of text.

There are other examples where a brain appears to devote attentional resources to something the subject is not aware of. For example, failure to suppress noise and irrelevant information messes up performance in tennis and speech making and problem solving. If, however, you consciously and

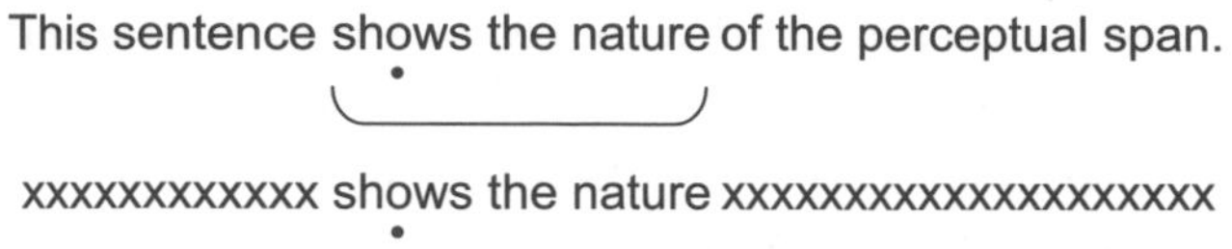

This sentence shows the nature of the perceptual span.

xxxxxxxxxxxx shows the nature xxxxxxxxxxxxxxxxxxxx

Figure 4.13   The attentional (perceptual) span is the zone from which useful information can be extracted on a given fixation. The fixation point is indicated by a bullet. The zone in words ("shows the nature") displays the width of the attentional span. Notice that the span is asymmetric. The maximum perceptual span is 2 to 3 characters to the left (the beginning of the current word) and about 15 characters to the right (2 words beyond the current word). Regions comprised of *x*s flank the subject's attentional span. During a gaze shift in reading, the next 17 *x*s are replaced by words. In this reading experiment, subjects remain unaware that *x*s flank the attentional span and are replaced with words during a gaze shift. (Courtesy of John Henderson.)

purposefully pay attention to irrelevant information in order to suppress it, you really mess up. So if suppression is an aspect of an attentional mechanism, it is presumably a nonconscious aspect. One might counter that such suppression does not involve *attention*, because attention, at least for the "top-down" system, is, by definition, conscious. This move should be avoided. In the absence of independent supporting evidence, it is circular.

The more important point, perhaps, is that we still have a lot to learn about the phenomena that we refer to as "attention." It does appear, for example, that different neurotransmitter systems are associated with distinct aspects of attention: noradrenalin with alerting, acetylcholine with orienting, and dopamine with suppressing conflicting information. In fact, it is still unclear what computational tasks attention is supposed to perform.

Consciousness as global workspace

An important corollary of the indirect approach is that to be productive, research should target the contrast between the *roles* of conscious representations and nonconscious representations in the cognitive economy as a whole.[32] Greater flexibility in perception, planning, imagining, reasoning, motor control, and, in the human case at least, for *reporting* what you experience has been touted as the obvious distinctive difference made by consciousness in the organism's behavior. If you are not conscious of a touch or a pain, for example, then you cannot report that you have it, and if the nonconscious representation plays any role in motor behavior, it will be a more reflexive than considered role.

How might this flexibility owed to conscious representation be explained in terms of brain functions? The suggestion is that conscious representations are more *broadly accessible* in the brain than are nonconscious representations. Therefore, the flexibility of cognitive function could be explained in terms of information distribution. So if we could understand how information is more broadly accessible, we might make progress in understanding the neurobiology of conscious representations. Dennett has cast the idea in even stronger terms, namely, that wide accessibility per se *constitutes* consciousness. As he asserts, "Global accessibility *is* consciousness."[33]

This general concept of accessibility sketched by Dennett was elaborated with more empirical detail by Baars, who proposed the *global-workspace model* of consciousness.[34] Simplified, Baars's thought that a state is a conscious state when its neural information is globally accessible, that is, available for use in such diverse functions as perceptual categorization, motor control, planning, decision making, and recollection of long-term memories. His seminal metaphor is that of a conventional bulletin board, where information can be posted, making it accessible to others who can, on a need-to-know basis, access and read the bulletin board. Readers can also post their own things on the bulletin board. Some information is not broadcast (the nonconscious signals). His suggestion was that the neurons mediating consciousness are, in their *informational* aspects, like a bulletin board; that is, certain neural networks are connected so as to have what amounts to a shared workspace.

Baars understood very well that the workspace metaphor was only a metaphor, and that it must be cashed out eventually in neuronal terms, that is, in terms of real circuits, real neurons, and real activity. He speculated that the reticular formation, a finger-like structure in the brainstem known to be essential in orienting and arousal, was the crucial part of the anatomy for determining what information got onto the bulletin board at any given time. The thalamus, with its vast cortical projections, he suggested, is the mechanism for bulletin-board broadcasting. Although these very general speculations shift the discussion a little closer to testability, a difficult part of the task is to specify what "global access" means in neuronal terms, and to do so without surreptitiously defining "global access" as "conscious access," and hence getting stuck with circularity. Why is this difficult?

Brains, as we have seen, are composed of elements that send and receive signals carrying information relevant to behavior. Another way of putting this same point, but viewed from the receiving rather than the sending perspective, is to say that brains are in the access business. Access, in varying degrees of breadth, is ubiquitous in nervous systems. But what does "access" mean, neurobiologically?

To a first approximation, we can say that a neuron *b* has access to the information carried by the activity of a neuron *a* if the activity in *a* causes activity in *b* and this causal link constitutes a transfer of information from *a* to *b*. This is just a different way of saying that neuron *a* sends information to neuron *b*. We could, so far as I can tell, drop talk of access and state the hypothesis solely in terms of sending and receiving information. Granting that we do not yet understand how precisely[35] to characterize the nature of information in nervous systems, we can provisionally use this rough-hewn notion. On this basis, therefore, we can say that information in retinal ganglion cells, for example, is accessible to neurons in the thalamus but not to neurons in the spinal cord. And we can say that neurons in the motor cortex make motor commands accessible to neurons in the red nucleus, the cerebellum, the basal ganglia, and the spinal cord.

If "access" is the name of the brain game in general, how do we specify in neuronal terms what *global* access is in a way that makes it the key to consciousness? "Global" in this context does not, of course, literally mean global, because given the nature of brain connectivity, the information does not in fact go everywhere. The key idea must be that the information is made accessible *very broadly*. In the recent discussion of the workspace approach, the term is tied to anatomical properties: there are specific long-distance neurons (long-axon neurons) in the parietal cortex, cingulate cortex, dorsolateral prefrontal cortex, and superior temporal cortex that allegedly are the workspace neurons (figure 4.14). The idea is that increased activity of these long-axon neurons makes information available to selected populations of neurons, for example, in the visual system. Before getting on the bandwagon, let us, in normal critical fashion, give the hypothesis a long, hard look.

First, it is unclear whether the shifting neuronal population whose activity allegedly constitutes awareness is the sending population (workspace neurons) or the receiving population or both the sending and receiving populations.

Second, broad accessibility, if anatomically defined in terms of long-axon neurons, or long-axon neurons with unusually high numbers of neurons in the projective field, is certainly not unique to the areas cited. For example, it typifies many neurons in motor and premotor cortex, as well as neurons in the thalamus, amygdala, brainstem, and, well, just about everywhere (figure 4.15). So defining the workspace neurons by means of these specific structural criteria is less than satisfactory.

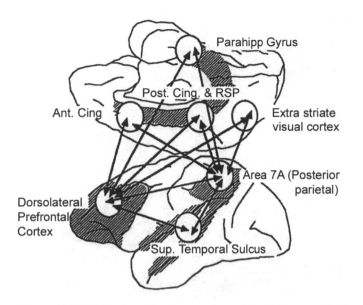

Figure 4.14 This schematic diagram is used by Dehaene and Naccache (2001) to illustrate some of the connections between the parietal cortex and the prefrontal cortex in the monkey brain that subserve "global access." The upper panel presents the medial view (inverted), and the lower panel the lateral view. The cross-hatched areas receive projections from the medial pulvinar nucleus of the thalamus, which receives projections from a variety of areas, including visual cortical area V1 and the superior colliculus. Not shown are the many subcortical connections from the dorsolateral prefrontal and posterior parietal cortical areas to striatum, claustrum, thalamus, and reticular formation. (Based on Goldman-Rakic 1988.)

Can the workspace population be defined by a combination of structural and functional criteria? Perhaps the functional criteria can be sketched out by working backwards from functions made more flexible or deliberate or intelligent by conscious representations. For example, planning or deliberating or trying to perform a task is greatly hampered if a person is in a coma or in a persistent vegetative state or asleep or given subthreshold stimuli. Accordingly, one could hypothesize that the global-access neurons are those active during tasks that involve attention, effort, or deliberation. On this supposition, a great deal of effort has gone into determining which brain areas are implicated in the performance of certain tasks that demand attention, working memory, or conscious perception, with the aim of identifying as workspace neurons those involved in all these functions. Lesions studies, along with fMRI, EEG, and

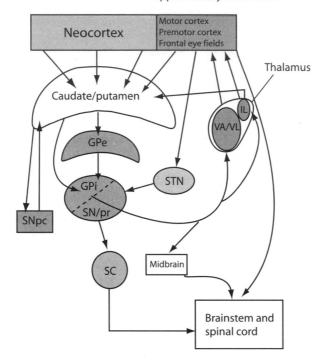

Figure 4.15 A schematic drawing of some of the pathways between cortical areas and neuronal structures mediating motor functions. Abbreviations: Gpe, globus pallidus pars externa; Gpi, globus pallidus pars interna; IL, intralaminar thalamic nuclei; SC, superior colliculus; SNpc, substantia nigra pars compacta; SNpr, substantia nigra pars reticulata; STN, subthalamic nucleus; VA/VL, ventral anterior and ventral lateral nuclei of the thalamus. (Based on Zigmond et al. 1999.)

single-cell studies in monkeys, have been cited as implicating the particular class of neuronal connections specified in figure 4.14.

So far as so good, but let us test the approach not by selecting favorable evidence from the available data pool, but by deliberately searching for counterexamples. That is, let us see whether there are circuits that qualify under the structural and functional criteria, but which even the proponents of the hypothesis would not want to consider as workspace neurons.

As one possible counterexample, consider again eye movements. The question is this: do eye-movement neurons in the frontal eye fields qualify as workspace neurons? If *they* do, then what *doesn't*? If they do not, why are they excluded? First, eye-movement signals are widely distributed, which means they are widely accessible. The neurons in the frontal eye fields project to the pons, prefrontal cortex, parietal cortex, and basal ganglia, requiring long axons. Hence they satisfy the structural criteria. Moreover, the pathways go to and from some of the same areas as those cited in the global workspace hypothesis. Second, activity in these neurons does enhance the ability to see, make decisions, learn skills, etc. Eye-movement information is important in making head movements, postural adjustments, whole-body movements, and, if you can make them, ear and nose movements. As noted earlier, patients in a coma or persistent vegetative state are greatly compromised in their behavioral flexibility, but they are also compromised in their visual scanning, even if the eyes are mechanically opened. So the functional criteria are satisfied. Apparently, given the criteria on offer, therefore, frontal eye-field neurons should qualify as workspace neurons.

The problem is that we seem not to be conscious of eye-movement decisions. By and large, we do not consciously deliberate about our incessant eye movements, and we are generally unaware of them. With the possible exception of rare visits to the optometrist, I have no experience of eye-movement decisions. The logic so far invites the conclusion that normal eye movements constitute a counterexample to the workspace criteria for "consciousness neurons." Although it may be possible to shore up the criteria in a scientifically principled way, it is far from obvious how to achieve that.

Unfortunately, putting the global-workspace hypothesis under scrutiny makes it less, rather than a more, comprehensible in neuronal terms. This is especially disappointing when we recall that according to Dennett's promising assessment of the workspace hypothesis, global access just *is* consciousness. Dennett's own story of global access is, of course, complicated by his conviction that the consciousness we humans have is not shared by animals, because they do not have language and cannot talk to themselves.[36]

Moreover, of the features that do make the hypothesis appealing, two are worrisome. First, much of its appeal derives from our familiarity with bulletin boards, workspaces, accessibility of websites, and so forth, in the *nonneuronal* world. We understand these things in their literal contexts. It would be convenient if the metaphor were true of the brain without too much patching and doctoring. But is it? Invaluable as metaphors are, they can seduce us into believing we understand more than we truly do. In the hypothesis at hand, trucking in the workspace metaphor tends to obscure the fact that it is very unclear what "global access" means in neurobiological terms.

Second, the allure of the metaphor invites us to celebrate the data that fit and ignore the data that are awkward. The problem with seeking confirming data is that just about any theory, false or true, wacky or ingenious, is consistent with lots of data.[37] This was the case with the caloric theory of heat, the Ptolemaic theory of the heavens, the grassy-knoll theory of the assassination of President Kennedy, and just about all of alien abduction stories. As Karl Popper famously insisted, it is easy to get data that fit; what counts for the believability of a theory, however, is passing a tough test. Finding that some data do satisfyingly fit the hypothesis, we are duty bound to wade into hostile territory and see whether the hypothesis can survive the really tough tests.[38]

With the critical flags now hoisted, I should add that the hypothesis does look robust enough to merit testing, and that is more than can be said about many hypotheses regarding the physical basis of consciousness. The heartening thing about the global-workspace hypothesis is that it has its feet solidly in the empirical mud. In the coming years it will be essential to confront the hypothesis with potentially falsifying tests, as well as to assemble supporting data. Notwithstanding Dennett's argument that it makes no sense to talk about animal consciousness, animals experiments will continue to be extremely important. Like all investigations concerning cognitive function, this hypothesis needs to be given time to develop closer ties with basic neurobiology.

Self, subjectivity, and consciousness

Antonio Damasio's attack on the problem is launched at the systems level rather than the neuronal level. His motivating insight is that the capacity for consciousness is the outcome of high-level *self-representational* capacities.[39] For the conceptual backdrop to this idea, recall the discussion in chapter 3 (pp. 70–90) stressing that inner regulation and sensorimotor coordination are the basic platform for the evolutionary development of cognition. Thus nervous systems have integrative organizations for ranking *goals*, making behavioral *decisions*, and evaluating relevant *perceptual* signals in the context of specific behavioral plans. We used the notion of an internal model—specifically the *Grush emulator*—to conceptualize self-representational capacities that deploy an inner representation of the body in relation to its environment.

What, according to Damasio, is the connection between consciousness and self-representation? Roughly, the idea is this: Under evolutionary pressure, the sophistication of the simple integrative internal models increased, consistent with the organism's need for staying alive and maintaining niche-suitable coherence in behavior.[40] At some stage, new circuitry enabled a neuronal population to represent the *internal model* itself. It could represent some items in the model (themselves representations) as standing in relation to representations of states of the body. That is, the circuitry could represent certain of the organism's current perceptual and emotional states *as* states of itself, it could categorize some representations as being *of* objects external to the body, and, most important, it could represent the relation between them.[41]

Thus if I step on a cactus, a certain class of neural events is represented as inner (e.g., my pain), while others are represented as being of the outer world (e.g., the visual representation of the cactus). The relation between them is also represented, inasmuch as the brain sees the external thing (the cactus) as the source of the inner state (the pain), and represents control over its own body to avoid contact with the cactus as a way of avoiding pain. The properties recognized visually (green, spiny) are seen as properties of the cactus, whereas the properties of the pain are categorized as belonging to me. For convenience, we can call such representations of relationships between representations *metarepresentations*, since they are higher-order representations that are *about* lower-order representations. This richer neural architecture enables second-order evaluative structures and second-order planning and predictive structure.

Why would metalevel representational categorization constitute an change favored in the competition for survival? To a first approximation, because it permits richer comparison, evaluation, and learning. With the envisioned metarepresentational capacity, I can emulate myself in various conditions and evaluate my options. I can envision myself as feeling hungry and hunting a rabbit on one option, as finding a mate under another option, as portaging my canoe under another option.[42] Moreover, I can sequence my self-representations in my plans so as to maximize my goal achievements. Those organisms whose brains happen to excel in the coherencing and integration business have a better chance at reproductive success than those whose brains coherence poorly. The metarepresentational upgrade endows the organism with a greater range of capacities to manipulate its body image in problem solving, developing impulse control, making long-term plans, and drawing upon relevant stored knowledge. In short, it makes the organism smarter.

Why should this metarepresentational integration constitute the basis for the capacity for *consciousness*? After all, computers can have metarepresentations without being conscious. As I understand him, Damasio answers thus. First, banish the intuition that when you become conscious of something, a pain for example, a little light in effect shines on the pain, making it conscious. If that metaphor creeps into your understanding, you are headed for mysticism. Needless to say, being aware of a pain is neurobiologically different from not being aware of it, but that difference is neither literally nor metaphorically having the nonphysical flashlight of the soul shining down upon the pain. Whatever the difference is, it is likely a difference identifiable at the systems level and constituted by specific activities of widely distributed neuronal populations.

Second, metarepresentations per se do not yield consciousness. The metarepresentational capacities serving consciousness must involve self-attribution ("This pain is mine"), self-representation (having a point of view), self-control ("I will wait to eat"), and the recognition of the relations between inner and outer things ("I can eat *that*" or "*That* thing can hurt me").

Third, with the metaintegrative operations referred to, conscious experiences just turn out to be items in the integrated schema. The hypothesis is therefore reductionistic in the sense that it identifies consciousness of a pain, for example, with a representation in the metarepresentational schema. That is, consciousness of pain is just what you get when the representation of the relevant somatosensory signal is metarepresented as standing in the "belongs to" relation to the self-representation. According to the hypothesis, the identification is just a biological fact about the brain, just as it is a physical fact that light *is* electromagnetic radiation or a neurobiological fact that an epileptic seizure is synchronous firing of large populations of excitatory neurons.

Whence the *qualitative* differences between experiences, such as the difference between the pain of a burn and the sound of a mosquito or the smell of skunk? On this approach, these differences are the wholly natural consequence of representing signals as having different sources (e.g., retina versus olfactory epithelium) or as having different significance for the organism (e.g., safe versus dangerous) or as having different action-relevant categorizations (e.g., spider versus grizzly) or the like. Exactly how these qualitative differences depend on these factors should be sorted out as neuroscience proceeds.

Other questions need to be considered. We have conscious experience of only some among a range of internal signals. For example, one can be conscious of bladder distension, but not of one's blood pressure. What determines which among the variety of internal signals are signals included in the high-level integration that enables one to experience them? This has to be answered in the context of evolutionary biology and of what would and would not be favored by natural selection. Consequently, the answer will depend on whether the type of state in question is one where it made sense for Mother Nature to permit the organism behavioral control and options. What, then, about blood pressure?

Maintaining the appropriate blood pressure is a constant priority of the nervous system, never to be put behind eating or sex or satisfying one's curiosity. Not surprisingly, therefore, it is automatically regulated by the autonomic nervous system, not relegated to cognitive functions that may be unreliable on occasion or unregulated during sleep. Modern medicine aside, there are no behavioral options for getting blood pressure to its appropriate values, as there are behavioral strategies for finding a safe place to rest or finding water. These kinds of considerations explain why representation of blood pressure is not included in the metalevel integration that gives rise to representations of an experience as "mine," and why, therefore, there was no survival advantage in having wiring to support conscious awareness of changes in blood pressure. Similar observations can be made about peristaltic movements of the stomach and intestines.

Among the kinds of states of which we can be conscious, what determines which ones we are in fact aware of at any given point in time? The answers here will derive from the wider neurocomputational theory of how the brain achieves its various integrative feats—how its sets and resets priorities, how attention can be directed top-down but can be overridden by important bottom-up signals, and so on. Given the envisioned metalevel representational and integrative capacity, what the organism *currently* is aware of is a function of how its integrative architecture has determined what it should *now* watch and listen for, what it should *now* do, what memories are *now* relevant to current goal-planning functions, what behavioral options are *now* viable, and so on. That is, the coordinated operation of neurocognitive functions—attention, short-term memory, long-term memory, perception, emotion, choice, and imagination—will result in the organism's being aware of some states but not others.

Since nothing like a full-fledged theory of the nature of integration is on the table, it is not surprising that the details needed to explain how and when signals are consciously represented as "my experiences" are out of reach. Is Damasio's hypothesis therefore too fragmentary and sketchy to evaluate, let alone bank on? Or is there evidence suggesting it is on the right track? There is some evidence, and while a full discussion of that evidence would be too lengthy, perhaps a first-pass answer and a list of references will constitute a beginning.[43]

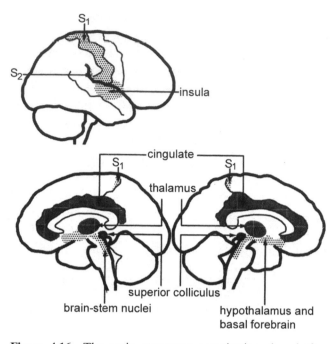

Figure 4.16 The main structures constituting the platform for self-representation, according to Damasio's hypothesis. (Courtesy of Hanna Damasio.)

In addressing the testability issue, Damasio highlights evidence indicating the special importance to consciousness of the following: nuclei in the brainstem tegmentum, the cingulate cortices and the parietal cortices directly behind them, the hypothalamus, and the intralaminar nuclei of the thalamus. Small lesions to the brainstem tegmentum, hypothalamus, posterior cingulate, or the intralaminar nuclei result in coma or persistent vegetative state (figure 4.16). Damage to cingulate cortices, especially in the posterior sector and the adjoining parietal cortices, also compromise consciousness. By contrast, surprisingly large segments of frontal or sensory or motor cortex can be removed without loss of consciousness, though, of course, other deficits will appear.

In a very difficult but revealing study using positron emission tomography (PET), Fiset and colleagues gave normal volunteers the drug propofol, an anesthetic widely used in medical practice to induce general anesthesia.[44] Propofol is an experimentally promising drug because there is a precise and known relationship between concentration and level of sedation. Very tiny changes in concentration correlate with differences between mild sedation, deep sedation, and unconsciousness, the latter defined as unresponsiveness to verbal commands. Fiset and colleagues found that the brainstem nuclei, and consequently the thalamic structures to which they project, were preferentially affected by propofol. Other regions cited by Damasio as part of the self-representational substructure, including the posterior cingulate cortex, also showed changes correlated with propofol concentrations sufficient for unconsciousness.

Brainstem structures are also known to mediate attentional functions, along with levels of arousal, and to control the shifts in state from being asleep, to dreaming, to being awake. Additionally, there is a convergence of input to the brainstem signaling the states of the vestibular system, musculoskeletal frame, viscera, and internal milieu (see chapter 3, figure 3.3). Drawing on anatomical and physiological data, Damasio notes that specific small regions (nuclei) in the brainstem contain integrated information about current activity and recent changes relevant to the organism's state and its goals. Depending on this state-of-the-critter report, modulation of cortical activity is caused by other brainstem nuclei. At the systems level, this to-ing and fro-ing between state-of-the-critter profiles and cortical modulation means that attention is paid to some things and not others, that some things are learned, that some relevant things are actively remembered, and that some choices are favored over others as the organism moves about its environment making its living.

Obviously, hordes of details remain to be worked out by neuroscience and psychology even if this hypothesis is more or less in the right neck of the woods. For starters, we would like to understand exactly how specific brainstem structures regulate shifts in attention, exactly how internal models are organized, updated, interconnected, and modified. As with other hypotheses herein entertained, Damasio's hypothesis too must confront potentially falsifying tests.

Progress in neuroscience and the indirect approach

In the last several decades, progress on all aspects of brain function has been truly impressive. No meaningful summary of this progress is possible in a few pages. In subsequent sections, however, I shall make specific use of relevant neuroscientific developments in the course of analyzing and responding to those who think that neuroscience, in principle, can never, *ever*, lead us to a deeper understanding of conscious experience. In later chapters on representation and knowledge, I shall again draw upon relevant developments.

Impressive progress notwithstanding, it is also true that neuroscience as a field is still young and still groping for its general, "exoskeletal" explanatory principles. This probably means we are especially prone to losing the forest for the trees, particularly when experimental research is vigorous—more prone than, for example, scientists in molecular biology or cell biology. To a first approximation, those fields enjoy the benefits of having established the general principles governing their target phenomena.

So far, the same cannot truly be said for neuroscience. Although there are indeed fruitful ideas of a highly general sort, and although the rise of computational modeling has helped enormously in conceptualizing the problem of how macroeffects emerge from microphenomena, the fact remains that neuroscience has not achieved the explanatory maturity of, for example, cell biology. The reasons for the relative immaturity are not surprising. They include the truly staggering complexity of the system under study and the monumentally difficult problems confronting the development of reliable, revealing experimental techniques. They also include *conceptual lacunae*. As noted earlier, we do not yet really understand what the notion of *information* should mean in a biological or psychological context. Moreover, we do not yet fully understand how neurons code information, whatever information *is*. These issues will be discussed a little more in chapter 7. I mention them now to balance my genuine optimism for future discoveries regarding consciousness on both the direct and the indirect routes. Like many neuroscientists, I view the pioneering aspects of neuroscience as part of what makes the field so very exciting. Virtually nothing is humdrum, so much is open territory, and surprises are an almost daily affair.

1.5   Concluding Remarks

The main aim of section 1 has been to see what happens if we consider consciousness as a natural phenomenon that can be investigated scientifically as well as introspectively. We saw that there are different strategies, driven by different hunches and directed by differences in scientific feel for the problem. Progress is evident in many investigations, though techniques for safely investigating the brains of humans at the micronetwork level remain to be developed. In the next section, I canvas a range of reservations about any and every neurobiological approach to understanding consciousness.

2   Dualism and the Arguments against Neuroscientific Progress

2.1   Life and Conscious Experience

At this stage of our knowledge, none of the functions—attention, short-term memory, being awake, perceiving, imagining—can plausibly be equated with consciousness, but we are learning more about consciousness, bit by little bit, as scientific progress is made on each of the topics. In this respect, the virtues of the indirect approach to consciousness may be analogous to the virtues of the indirect approach to the problem of *what it is to be alive.* Just as identifying a micro-organizational correlate to being alive was not the winning strategy for the problem of life, so perhaps, by analogy, trying to identify a micro-organization correlate of consciousness *may* not be the winning strategy for the problem of awareness. But is the analogy between the problem of being alive and the problem of consciousness a *useful* analogy? Let's consider how it might be useful.

What is it for something to be alive? The fundamental answer is now available in college biology courses. Modern cell biology, molecular biology, physiology, and evolutionary biology have discovered so much that a *comprehensive,* if *not complete,* story can now be told. To be alive, cells need a cytoplasm containing structures such as mitochondria, to produce energy. They need the means of replication, such as DNA, along with microtubules to orchestrate cell division. They need protein-manufacturing apparatus, and so need ribosomes, enzymes, mRNA, tRNA, and DNA. They need specialized membranes, such as bilipid layers with specialized protein channels to admit certain molecules into the cell under specific conditions and to keep others out under certain conditions. They need endoplasmic reticulum for metabolic processes, lysosomes for digestion, and Golgi apparatus for sorting, finishing, and shipping cell products. The biochemistry segment of the course would talk about water, carbon compounds, amino acids, and proteins. The physiology segment of the course would discuss how tissues like muscle, and organs like kidneys, function. At the end of the course, one would have, at least in outline, the scientific account of what it is for something to be alive.

A biology professor winding down the course at the end of the year, might hear this complaint: "I now understand all *that,* but you still have not explained to us what *life itself* is." The reply is, roughly, that life is *all that.* You understand what is it for something to be alive when you understand the physical processes of metabolism, replication, protein building, and so forth. Once you know all that, there is no other phenomenon—*livingness itself*—to be explained. Certainly, there are many questions still unanswered concerning how cells work, but these are questions such as "How does a transmembrane protein get inserted?" not questions such as "How does the *life force* get into the cell?"

Unconvinced, someone might persist, noting that textbook explanations really involve the interactions of *dead stuff*—ribosomes, microtubules, etc.—but what he wants to know is what *living* (being alive) itself is, what the *essence* of life is. Surely, it may be contested, being alive cannot emerge from mere dead stuff, no matter how it is arranged and organized.

The assumption behind this persistent question was a seriously debated hypothesis in the not very distant past. By 1920, however, the assumption was already seriously behind the scientific times. The assumption, known as vitalism, is that things are alive because they are infused with the "life force" or "vital spirit" or "urge." Vitalists are convinced that being alive cannot be a function of the dynamics and organization of dead molecules. Even as late as 1955, a few scientists still clung to the conviction that a nonphysical "urge" transforms a cell from a dead organization to a living organization.

Nevertheless, what modern biology has discovered is there is no vital spirit over and above a complex—*really* complex—organization of physical properties. The urge intuition takes a beating when the details of metabolism, protein production, membrane functions, and replication are understood. When you see how it all comes together, you see that no vital spirit is needed in the explanation. This is an example where *the nonexistence of something is established as highly probable, not through a single experiment demonstrating its nonexistence, but through acceptance of an explanatorily powerful framework that has no place for it.* The same thing happened to "impetus" as Newton's physics became accepted and, as we saw in chapter 2, to "caloric fluid." This is not to say that the nonexistence of caloric fluid or vital spirit has been absolutely *proved*, but because these concepts play no explanatory role whatever in science, they are deemed to be outdated theoretical curiosities.

Those who pursue the scientific approach to consciousness believe that developments analogous to those in the biology of "life" will allow us to understand consciousness. That is, we are beginning to understand the neurobiology of sleep, dreaming, attention, perception, emotions, drives, moods, autobiographical memory, perceptual imagery, motor control, motor imagery, and self-representation. We are beginning to understand the neurobiology of what happens under various anesthetics, in a coma, in subthreshold perception, and in hallucinatory states. With more complete explanations of all, the nature of conscious phenomena should be understood, at least in a *general* way. Lots of detailed questions will remain, of course, but science is like that. What the research program envisions is that this understanding is an empirical possibility, not an empirical certainty.

If, having understood all those functions, someone were to persist, "But what about consciousness itself. Consciousness cannot come out of nonconscious physical stuff, no matter what its dynamics and organization," we shall have to respond more or less as we do now with the vitalists. We go back through the relevant science all over again. If the objection under consideration assumes that consciousness cannot be a brain function *because* consciousness is a soulish thing, science may be up against dogmatism, as it was with vitalism circa 1950.

Dualism, as we know from discussion in chapters 2 and 3, is not likely to be falsified by a single experiment or two showing the nonexistence of the soul. Rather, dualism is rendered improbable because the explanatory framework of psychology and neuroscience, though incomplete, and embedded within the larger framework of physics, chemistry, and evolutionary biology, is *much* more powerful than any dualist competitor. This could change, but so far the empirical evidence does not point that way.[45] As things stands, the concept of a nonphysical soul looks increasingly like an outdated theoretical curiosity.

Even granting that dualism is essentially moribund, a number of philosophers and scientists wish to argue that consciousness cannot *ever* be understood in terms of brain function. Even if dualism is false, they claim, neurobiological research on consciousness is a waste of time, and neurophilosophy is a snare and delusion. Although a host of such arguments exist, I shall analyze only those generally regarded as the strongest, the most widely held, or the most appealing.

2.2 Nine Naysaying Arguments[46]

A common argument consists in stressing what we *do not know*, and using this as a premise for concluding what we *cannot* know. Colin McGinn, for example, says that the problem of how the brain could generate consciousness is "miraculous, eerie, even faintly comic."[47] Finding the problem difficult, he concludes, "This is the kind of causal nexus we are precluded from ever understanding, given the way we have to form our concepts and develop our theories." He thinks that for us to understand the nature of consciousness is like a mouse understanding calculus. McGinn is by no means alone here. A number of contemporary thinkers believe they can already tell that the question is unanswerable—not just now, not just given what we know so far, but unanswerable *ever*. Zeno Vendler chides the ambitions of neuroscience by saying that it is obvious from the nature of sensation, that our sensing selves "are in principle beyond what science can explain."[48] That we are trying to unravel the mystery is, in Vendler's view, a consequence of the overweening assumption that there are no questions science cannot answer. How can we respond to McGinn, Vendler, and other naysayers?

In each of the following subsections, I shall briefly entertain one naysaying objection and try to assess its cogency.[49]

I cannot imagine *how science could explain awareness!*

This is one of the most popular naysaying arguments, advanced frequently by philosophers and sometimes by scientists. What can be said in response?

In general, what substantive conclusions can be drawn when science has not advanced very far on a problem? Not much. One of the basic skills philosophers teach in logic is how to recognize and diagnose the range of nonformal fallacies that lurk under ostensibly appealing arguments: what it is to beg the question, what a non sequitur is, and so on. A prominent item in the fallacy roster is *argumentum ad ignorantiam*—argument from ignorance. The canonical version of this fallacy uses ignorance as the key premise from which a substantive conclusion is drawn. The canonical version looks like this:

We really do not understand much about a phenomenon *p*. (Science is largely ignorant about the nature of *p*.)
Therefore, we do know that

· *p* can never be explained, or

· nothing science could ever discover would deepen our understanding of *p*, or

· *p* can never be explained in terms of properties of kind *s*.

In its canonical version, the argument is obviously a fallacy: none of the proffered conclusions follow, not even a little. Surrounded with rhetorical flourishes, brow furrowing, and hand wringing, however, versions of this argument can hornswoggle the unwary.

From the fact that we do not know something, nothing very interesting follows—we just don't know. Nevertheless, the temptation to suspect that our ignorance is telling us something positive, something deep, something meta-physical or even radical, is ever-present. Perhaps we like to put our ignorance in a positive light, supposing that but for the awesome complexity of the phenomenon, we (smart as we are) *would* have knowledge. But there can be many reasons for not knowing, and the specialness of the phenomenon is, quite regularly, not the most significant reason. I am currently ignorant of what caused an unusual rapping noise in the woods last night. Can I conclude it must be something special, something unimaginable, something *alien, other-worldly*? Evidently not. For all I can tell now, it might merely have been a raccoon gnawing on the compost bin. Lack of evidence for something is just that: lack of evidence. It is not positive evidence for something else, let alone something of a spooky sort. That conclusion is not very thrilling, perhaps, but when ignorance is a premise, that is about all you can grind out of it.

Moreover, the mysteriousness of a problematic phenomenon is *not a fact about the phenomenon*. It is merely an epistemological fact about *us*. It is a fact about where we are in current science. It is a fact is about what we currently do and do not understand, about what, using the rest of our understanding, we can and cannot imagine. It is not a property of the problem itself.

It is sometimes assumed that there can be a valid transition from "We cannot *now* explain" to "We can *never* explain" if we have the help of a subsidiary premise, namely, "I cannot *imagine* how we could ever explain." But the subsidiary premise does not help, and this transition remains a straight-up application of argument from ignorance. Adding, "I cannot imagine explaining *p*" merely adds a psychological fact about the speaker, from which, again, nothing significant follows about the nature of the phenomenon in question.

Vitalists, we noted earlier, argued that life could be explained only by invoking a nonphysical kind of thing, a vital spirit; living things have it, dead things do not. A favored argument for vitalism ran as follows: I cannot *imagine* how you could get living things out of dead molecules. Out of bits of proteins, fats, sugars how could life itself emerge? It seemed obvious from the sheer mysteriousness of life that the problem could have no solution in biology or chemistry. We know now, of course, that this was all a shortsighted mistake.

Neuroscience is very much in its infancy. So if someone or other cannot imagine a certain kind of explanation of some brain phenomenon, it is not terribly significant. Aristotle could not imagine how a complex organism could come from a fertilized egg. Given early science (300 B.C.), it is no surprise that he could not imagine what it took many scientists hundreds of years to discover. I cannot imagine how ravens can solve a multistep problem in one trial, or how an organism integrates visual signals across time, or how the brain manages thermoregulation. But this is a (not very interesting) *psychological* fact about *me*. One could, of course, use various rhetorical devices to make it seem like an interesting fact about oneself, perhaps by emphasizing that it is a really, *really* hard problem, but if we are going to be sensible about this, it is clear that one's inability to imagine how thermoregulation works is, at bottom, pretty boring.

The "I cannot imagine" gambit suffers in another way. Being able to imagine an explanation for *p* is a highly open-ended and under-specified business. Given the poverty of delimiting conditions of the operation, you can pretty much rig the conclusion to go whichever way your heart desires. Logically, however, that flexibility is the kiss of death.

Suppose that someone claims that he *can* imagine the mechanisms for sensorimotor integration in the human brain but *cannot* imagine the mechanisms for consciousness. What exactly does this difference in imaginability amount to? Can he imagine the former in detail? No, because the details are not known. What, precisely, can he imagine? Suppose he answers that in a very general way he imagines that sensory neurons interact with interneurons that interact with motor neurons, and via these interactions, sensorimotor integration is achieved. Now if *that* is all it takes to be able to imagine, one might as well say that one *can* imagine the mechanisms underlying consciousness. Thus, "the interneurons do it." The point is this: if you want to contrast being *able* to imagine brain mechanisms for attention, short-term memory, planning, etc., with being *unable* to imagine mechanisms for consciousness, you have to do more that say that you can imagine neurons doing one but cannot imagine neurons doing the other. Otherwise, you simply beg the question.

There could be zombies

This time the attack on neurobiological strategies derives from a so-called "thought experiment," which roughly goes as follows. (1) We can imagine a person, like us in all the aforementioned capacities (attention, short-term memory, verbal capacity, etc.), but lacking the *experience* of pain and the *experience* of seeing blue. That is, he would lack *qualia* (pronounce kwa-lee-a), i.e., the *qualitative* aspect of conscious experience, such as feeling pain or feeling dizzy, seeing colors, hearing a C-minor chord. This person would be *exactly* like us, save that he would be a *zombie*. He would even say things that we do, such as "I have a funny feeling in my tummy" as the airplane suddenly descends and, on a fine summer afternoon, "The sky is very blue today." The next premise of the argument says this: (2) If the scenario is *conceivable*, it is *logically possible*. The conclusion says, (3) Since a zombie is logically possible, then whatever consciousness is, it is *explanatorily independent* of brain activities. That is, even a complete explanation of every aspect of the human brain will not explain consciousness. This is because a true explanation *must* foreclose the logical possibility of there being a zombie. (Something akin to this was argued by Saul Kripke in the 1970s, by Joseph Levine in the 1980s, and again by David Chalmers in the 1990s.)

To most of us, this argument is puzzling, because many things are logically possible but not empirically possible, such as a 2-ton mouse or a spider that can play the flute. Why should we suppose that the logical possibility of a zombie tells us anything interesting about what research could be successful? After all, what neurophilosophy is really interested in is the actual empirical world and how it works. The reply depends on the pivotal claim about the standards for an explanation, namely, that *a proper explanation must foreclose logical possibilities*.

Assuming that this is the pivotal claim here, we need to recognize how absurdly strong a claim it is. Not only does it rule out explaining consciousness in terms of brain function, but it also rules out explaining consciousness in terms of *soul function* or *spooky-stuff function* or *quantum gravity* or *anything else* you might think of. So strong is the demand it places on successful explanation that no scientific explanation of any phenomenon has ever met it, or ever could meet it.

As we saw from the discussion in chapter 1, section 3, explanatory reductions require that a new theory successfully reconstruct most of the features of the reduced phenomenon, as antecedently understood. But this falls far short of any logical entailments from the former to the latter such that *previously conceived possibilities* are now *logically impossible*. Good explanations rule out *empirical* possibilities, not logical possibilities. Historically speaking, no scientific reduction/integration has ever met such an absurdly strong requirement.

A further problem with *all* such "conceivability" arguments is that they want to draw an interesting conclusion about the nature of how things *really* are. *Nothing* interesting follows, however, from the fact that some particular human is, or is not, able to imagine something. That something *seems* possible does not thereby guarantee it *is* a genuine possibility in any interesting sense, so why should we think that the zombie idea *is* genuinely possible? To insist on its possibility on grounds that the premises are grammatical is to *confuse a real possibility with mere grammaticality*.

For the sake of argument, I have played along with the underlying assumption that we understand quite well the scope and limits of the domain of the logically possible. Nevertheless, this assumption is deeply flawed. Quine demonstrated in 1960 that such an assumption is actually just a bit of philosophical self-deception. A few hand-picked examples of what is and is not logically possible seem straightforward enough, but outside of these, all is fantasy, or group-think, or depends on self-serving definition. Not surprisingly, the especially controversial cases are those where philosophers want logical possibility to give them some real metaphysical leverage. And the argument at hand is very much a case in point. Standing back a bit, one does find something unconvincing in the idea that the conveniently elastic and philosophically concocted notion of logical possibility should dictate to neurobiology what it can and cannot discover—ever.

To see from a different perspective why the argument gets messed up, run an analogous zombie argument with respect to life. It says that we can imagine a planet where "deadbies" are things composed of cells with membranes, nuclei with DNA, the usual organelles, and so forth. Deadbies reproduce, digest, respire, metabolize, manufacture proteins, grow, and so forth, just as organisms on Earth do. Unlike us, however, deadbies are not *really* alive. This is a logical possibility. So life is *explanatorily independent* of biology.

Here too the premises are *possible* in the very weak sense that they are grammatical, but so far as we know, they do not state a *real* possibility. Here is another feeble thought experiment: imagine a planet where the velocity of molecules in a gas increases, but lo and behold, its temperature does not. Does this tell us that temperature is *explanatorily independent* of mean molecular kinetic energy? Certainly not. What does this tell us about the *actual* relation between mean molecule kinetic energy and temperature in a gas? Not a single thing.

I take the zombie argument to be a demonstration of the feebleness of the class of thought experiments that are factually isolated from the relevant science but nonetheless hope to draw a scientifically relevant conclusion.[50]

The problem is too hard

This objection is also very common, and is often advanced along with sundry other objections, both those discussed above and some from those given below. How valuable is it?

Can we tell how hard a problem is when we do not have a whole lot of science on the subject? To fill out the point, consider several lessons from the history of science. Before the turn of the twentieth century, people regarded as trivial the problem of explaining the precession of the perihelion of Mercury, that is, the fact that the elliptical orbit of Mercury constantly but slowly advances in the plane of its orbit. This movement was an annoying deviation from what Newton's Laws predict, but the problem was expected ultimately to sort itself out as more data came in. Essentially, it looked like an easy problem.

With the advantage of hindsight, we can see that the assessment was quite wrong: it took the Einsteinian revolution in physics to solve the problem of the precession of the perihelion of Mercury. By contrast, the composition of the stars was thought to be a *really* hard problem. How could a sample ever be obtained? As soon as you try to get close enough to take a sample, you burn. But with the advent of spectral analysis, that turned out to be a readily solvable problem. When heated to incandescence, the elements turn out to have a kind of fingerprint, easily seen when light emitted from a source is passed through a prism.

Consider now a biological example. Before 1953, many people believed, on rather good grounds actually, that to address the copying problem (transmission of traits from parents to offspring), we would first have to solve the problem of how proteins fold, i.e., how a string of amino acids bends and twists so that it ends up having a highly specific shape unique to that protein. The copying problem was deemed a much harder problem than the problem of how a string of amino acids takes on the correct shape, and many scientists believed it was foolhardy to attack the copying problem directly. This was partly because it was generally believed that it would take something as complex as a protein to be the carrier of hereditary information. DNA, a mere acid, was considered too simple to qualify as a candidate.

As we all know now, the key to the copying problem lay in the base-pairing of DNA, and the copying problem was solved first. Humbling it is to realize that the problem of protein folding (secondary and tertiary folding) is *still* not solved.

What is the point of these stories? They illustrate the fallacy in arguments from ignorance. From the vantage point of ignorance, it is often very difficult to tell which problem will turn out to be more tractable than some other, and whether we have even conceptualized the problem in the best way. Consequently, our judgments about relative difficulty or ultimate tractability should be appropriately qualified and tentative. Guesswork has a useful place, of course, but it is best to distinguish between blind guesswork and educated guesswork, and between guesswork and confirmed fact. The philosophical lesson is this: when not much is known about a topic, don't take terribly seriously someone else's heartfelt conviction about what problems are scientifically tractable. Learn the science, do the science, and see what happens.

How can I know what **you** *experience?*[51]

This worry takes several closely related forms, the oldest and most familiar of which is the so-called "inverted spectrum problem." The general worry is that the facts of anyone's phenomenal experience are always underdetermined by *any and all physical* facts, including all neurophysiological facts, that we might come to know about that person. (By "*p* is underdetermined by *q*," philosophers mean that *p* cannot be strictly *deduced* from *q*; *q* may provide evidence for *p*, but not absolutely conclusive evidence.) Accordingly, the argument concludes, phenomenal facts must be distinct and independent facts in their own right, a class of facts that can never be explained in purely physical terms. This general argument finds specific expression in the following thought experiment.

Consider the possibility that you and I share the same range of visual color experiences, but in all those cases where I have the subjective experience of red (as when I look at a ripe tomato in broad daylight), you have the subjective experience of green, the experience that I get when I look at the lawn. Suppose, moreover, that these divergent color experiences are systematic: when I look at the rainbowlike spectrum projected by a prism, I see red on the left-hand side, fading progressively into orange, yellow, green, and blue as I look to the right, but in that same objective situation, you see blue on the left-hand side, fading progressively to green, yellow, orange, and red as you look to the right. In short, your internal spectrum of color experiences is mapped onto the external world in a fashion that is exactly the inverse of my own. But this internal difference is hidden by the fact that we apply our shared color *terms* to external objects in all of the same ways.

This, let us suppose, is entirely conceivable. But, continues the antiphysicalist argument, this possible inversion of our respective color qualia stubbornly *remains* perfectly conceivable no matter how much we might know about each others' brains, and no matter how similar we might be in our physical behavior, our physical constitution, and our internal neural activities. Our brains could be identical, and yet our conscious experiences could still diverge. The physical facts, apparently, do not "logically fix" the phenomenal facts, and so the phenomenal facts must be some kind of facts above and beyond the merely physical facts. Therefore, concludes the argument, we must look beyond the physical sciences for any explanation of phenomenal experiences. They evidently constitute a realm of nonphysical facts.

Is this argument compelling? To answer that, we must closely examine its logic. First, this argument too relies on what is and is not alleged to be imaginable/conceivable in order to generate support for its conclusion. The *key* premise asserts, "Our brains could be *identical* in every respect, but our qualia could *differ*." Not surprisingly, the "could" is the "could" of conceivability, not the "could" of "actually could." As noted in analysis of the zombie argument, that something is logically possible implies absolutely nothing about empirical or real possibility.[52]

If the key premise collapses, the argument collapses. Is perhaps the premise that our brains could be *identical* in every respect but our qualia could *differ* just *obviously* true, and hence not in need of any defense? Not at all. Given the weight of available empirical evidence showing that differences in conscious experience do in fact involve differences in brain activity, the premise cannot be sold as obviously true. For example, we know that if you decrease the activity in the neurons projecting from a decayed tooth to the brainstem, the pain disappears. If nothing is done, the pain persists. Direct stimulation of the hand area of the somatosensory cortex during surgery produces changes in sensations in the hand. We entirely lack any examples where we know the brain remains *exactly* the same but the conscious experience changes. If there is a causal relationship between neuronal activity and conscious experience, as there certainly seems to be, then the *falsity* of the key premise is exactly what one would predict.

Can the premise be defended by claiming that in the actual world there are known examples where brains are *identical* in every respect and our qualia do differ? That strategy would indeed begin to add real substance to the argument. Yet it is never adopted, for the simple reason that there are no examples, there is no factual evidence to bring to bear.

A distinct line of defense of the key premise asserts that the premise is true because qualitative experiences are *nonphysical properties*. Consequently, it is alleged, our brains could be *identical* in every respect but our qualia could *differ*. The weakness in this defense is that it invokes dualism, which, on independent grounds, appears to be highly improbable. Nevertheless, in a spirit

Table 4.1 Key premise: our brains could be absolutely identical but our qualia could differ

Brief defense of the key premise	Brief criticism of the defense
It is conceivable.	So what?
It is empirically well supported.	Show us the data.
Dualism is true.	Dualism is improbable.
The conclusion is true, so the premise must be true.	Circular arguments are worthless.
By definition, qualia are independent of brain states.	Circular arguments are worthless.

of thoroughness, we shall explore this possibility in much greater detail below (pp. 182–192).

A last ditch effort consists in defending the key premise on grounds that conscious experiences are not identifiable with any property of the nervous system. This move is ineffective because this very claim is what the argument is supposed to *show*, not what the argument gets to *assume*. If you defend the key premise by appeal to the very conclusion your argument is supposed to establish, the argument is utterly worthless—it simply runs in a circle. The illusion of progress can be conjured, however, especially if the defense of the key premise is left implicit and hence hidden from inspection. Incidentally, a variant on the circular argument consists in *defining* qualia as psychological states that are not identifiable with any pattern of neuronal activity. This is no better than simply arguing by restating the conclusion as a premise.

In sum, here is the logical fix the argument finds itself in. It cannot just help itself to the key premise "Our brains could be *identical* in every respect but our qualia could *differ*" on grounds that is it obviously true. The defense of the key premise can, jointly or severally, take five forms (see table 4.1). Succinct criticism of these defenses are given in table 4.1.

The inverted-spectrum argument gets into trouble not because it envisages perceptual differences between subjects that are difficult to detect. The argument gets into trouble because it wants to crank out a very strong conclusion about the *nature of things* from essentially no facts; i.e., it wants to establish an a priori truth. It needs to persuade us that qualitative differences in experience are *undetectable*; not just undetectable given only behavioral data, but undetectable no matter what facts—behavioral, anatomical, physiological—are available.

Given the utter poverty of its cohort of defenses, dualism actually emerges as the strongest argument against a neurophysiological explanation of consciousness. At least the dualist has the option of launching an empirical argument for dualism. The empirically sensitive dualist will want to argue that if the facts prevent us from discovering whether one subject's color experiences are inverted with respect to those of another, then these facts constitute evidence in favor of dualism. In the next section, therefore, we shall take a closer look at the empirical possibility that one person's color experience might be systematically different from that of another, and whether we could indeed discover that this was so from the psychology and neuroscience of the visual system.

What happens if we get more empirical?

First, the argument, as stated above, betrays a much-too-simple conception of our actual color experiences.[53] The monochromatic linear spectrum produced by a prism presents only a small percentage of the visual color qualia enjoyed by normal human perceivers. That spectrum is missing brown, for example, and pink, and chartreuse, and sky blue, and jade green, and black and white too, for that matter. Indeed, it has been known for some time that the space of human color qualia is not one-dimensional, or even two-dimensional, but is fully three-dimensional. The Munsell color solid (plates 3 and 4) displays the structure of that fairly complex space. Notice that every color discriminable by humans occupies a unique place within that space, a place fixed by the unique family of similarity and dissimilarity relations that it bears to all of the other colors that surround it, both near and far. Two distinct colors could not exchange their respective positions without thereby fouling up many of the similarity relations that structure the original space.

Notice also that the overall shape of this space is nonuniform. For whatever reasons, tying *equal distances* in this space to *equal increments of color discriminability* yields the decidedly nonspherical phenomenal space of plates 3 and 4. Most notably, yellow bulges out from the central axis and up towards the white pole, and at lower brightness levels, it fades to being indiscriminable from dark gray more swiftly than any other color. (In fact, this is roughly how Munsell pieced together his original model of our color space in the first place—by asking people to judge relative similarities and just barely discriminable color differences over a large sample of colored chips.) Additional experiments have shown that we can make finer discriminations among diverse external stimuli within the greenish, yellowish, and orangeish regions of our color space than we can in the blueish regions.

If we are going to perform a color-inversion thought experiment, then we need to imagine something a little more complex than the one-dimensional spectrum flip usually suggested. Specifically, we need to imagine that the subject of the proposed inversion has his phenomenal color solid either rotated (180°, say) or mirror-inverted relative to its normal family of causal connections to external stimuli—thus, the yellow part of his color space gets activated when he looks at the sky, the blue part of his color space gets activated when he looks at bananas, and so forth—*while all of the internal similarity relations of his three-dimensional color space remain exactly the same* (just as in the original thought experiment). Is there anything impossible or inconceivable about this scenario?

Not a thing. Such an inversion is perfectly conceivable. But we should notice that it would be behaviorally (that is, physically) *detectable* in short order. In comparison with normal humans, the inversion subject would be able to make more and finer discriminations than we can among external objects that we describe as various shades of blue, and he would suffer a relative discriminatory deficit among objects that we describe as various shades of red, yellow, orange, and green. (There are probably good evolutionary reasons why normal subjects make finer discriminations among the greens, for example, than among the blues. Birds, with a fourth cone type sensitive to wavelengths in the ultraviolet range, will make finer discriminations among the blues than *we* do.) Moreover, the inversion subject would locate the familiar color *boundaries* in different places. Some external objects that have different shades of the same color, according to us, will fall into entirely different color classes, according to him.

This follows from the refined and more accurate assumptions of our updated thought experiment, as specified at the top of this page. The inversion subject's objective perceptual capacities would be systematically different as well, in ways clearly predicted by the thought experiment, once it is properly performed. Evidently, it is *not true*, even on present scientific knowledge, let alone on all possible future knowledge, *that our color qualia could be differently connected to the external world without any physical or behavioral divergences to herald that phenomenal inversion.* The idea that our color qualia could be inverted, completely independently of any objectively detectable effects, had a superficial plausibility only because of our ignorance of the nonuniform structure of human phenomenal color space and the diversity in our discriminatory capacities, across the colors, that experiments have revealed. Repair that ignorance, as we have done, and the dualist must take his thought experiment back to the drawing board. That, you may be sure, the creative dualist will do.

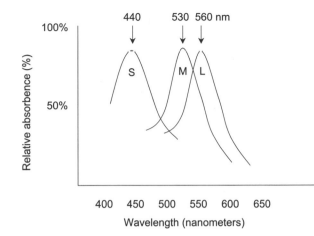

Figure 4.17 The neural-response curves for the three types of cones. Cones for short (S), medium (M), and long (L) wavelengths provide overlapping but differential responses to light of different wavelengths. These curves are defined by the absorption spectra of the three pigments found in normal cones.

Connecting qualia and neuronal organization

But let us put the dualist aside for a moment, and ask the independently interesting questions, Why does human phenomenal color space have three dimensions? Why *those* three dimensions in particular? And why does it have the nonuniform shape that it does? What gives rise to the curious phenomenal arrangement of plate 3 in the first place?

Apparently, the shape of phenomenal color space arises quite naturally and inevitably from the physical organization and response profiles of the various neurons in the brain's visual pathways. The fundamentals of the story, according to vision researchers, are surprisingly simple and elegant. The story begins with the three types of light-sensitive *cone* cells scattered across the human retina. Unlike the *rod* cells, with which they are mixed, each cone type is preferentially sensitive to its own narrow band of wavelengths, as illustrated in figure 4.17 and plate 2. This allows the retina to do a crude *spectral analysis* of the mixture of various wavelengths entering the eye.

But this is only the first stage of color vision. The crucial stage is the next one. The cone cells in the retina make a set of excitatory and inhibitory synaptic connections, via the optic nerve, to a subsequent population of neurons in the lateral geniculate nucleus (LGN), as illustrated schematically in figure 4.18.

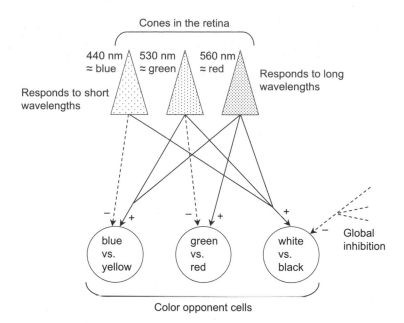

Figure 4.18   A simplified diagram of neural circuits in opponent-process theory. Opponent responses are derived from the outputs of three classes of cones. Excitatory connections (+) are shown by solid lines, and inhibitory connections (−) are shown by broken lines.

That LGN population is also divided into three distinct kinds of cells, but their response properties are quite different from the cones that project to them. As you can see, the middle cell—labeled "green vs. red"—is the site of a constant tug-of-war between the excitatory signals received from the M-cones (roughly, the green part of the spectrum) and the inhibitory signals received from the L-cones (roughly, the red part of the spectrum). Its resulting activity is thus an ongoing measure of the relative *balance or ratio* of medium wavelengths over long wavelengths currently hitting the relevant part of the retina. (Notice, by the way, that the M- and L-cone curves in figure 4.17 and plate 2 overlap to a substantial degree. This means that our green-versus-red tug-of-war cell will be hypersensitive to small shifts, up or down, in the wavelength of monochromatic light in the spectral regions immediately to the right and left of the crossover point of the two curves.)

Similarly, the left-most cell—labeled "blue vs. yellow"—is the site of a tug-of-war between the excitatory signals from the S-cones (roughly, the blue part

ELECTROMAGNETIC SPECTRUM

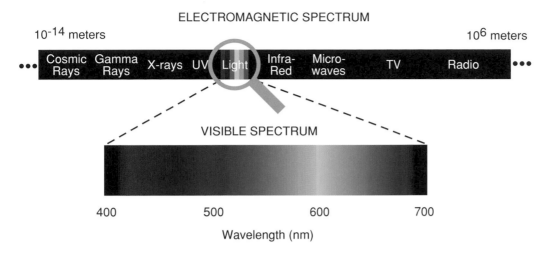

10^{-14} meters

10^6 meters

| Cosmic Rays | Gamma Rays | X-rays | UV | Light | Infra-Red | Micro-waves | TV | Radio |

VISIBLE SPECTRUM

400   500   600   700

Wavelength (nm)

Plate 1 The electromagnetic spectrum. Radiant energy is characterized by its wavelength, which varies continuously from very small to very large. Visible light occupies the limited range from 400 to 700 nanometers (10^{-9} meters). It is the only form of electromagnetic radiation that people sense directly. (From Palmer 1999.)

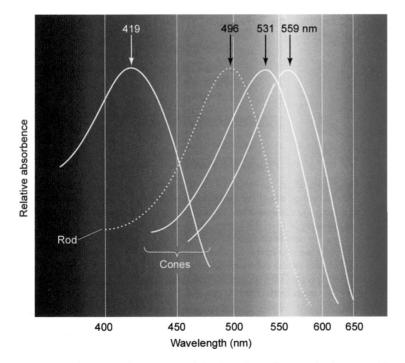

Plate 2 The absorption spectra of the four photopigments in the normal human retina. There are three types of cones, distinguished by three types of photopigments sensitive to light at distinct wavelengths. The sensitivity curve for rhodopsin, the photopigment in the rods, is also shown.

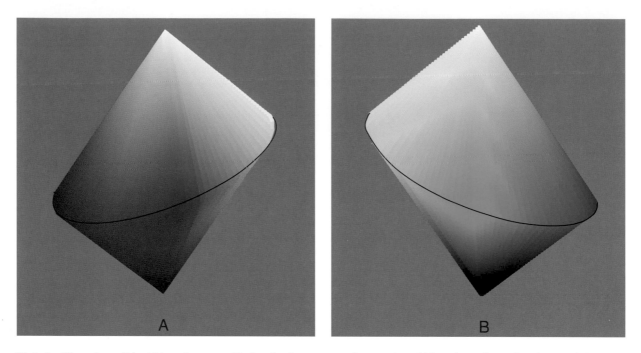

Plate 3   The color solid within color space. Each color is represented as a point within a three-dimensional space defined by the dimensions of hue, saturation, and lightness. This figure shows the outer surface of the color solid separately for the red side (A) and the green side (B). (From Palmer 1999.)

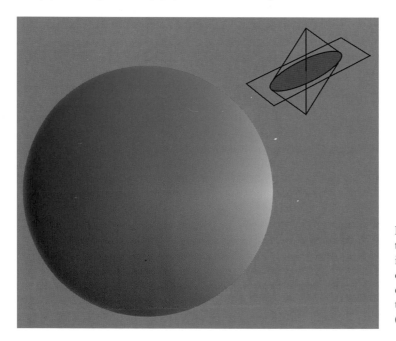

Plate 4   The color circle. This oblique section through the color solid shows the color circle, including the most saturated colors around its outer edge. Neutral gray is at the center, and the colors at various intermediate levels of saturation are located at intermediate positions. (From Palmer 1999.)

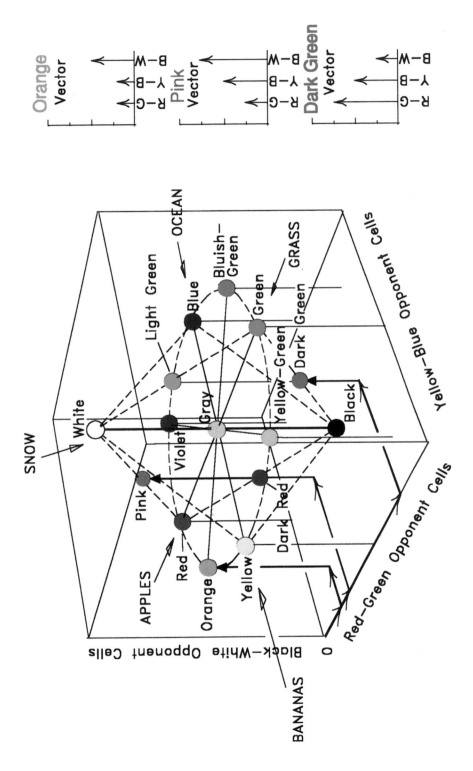

Plate 5 The vector space of opponent-cell coding, with some standard causal connections that it bears to the external world. Gray is roughly in the center of the space, white is at the top middle, and black at the bottom middle. The baseline activity for opponent cells is located midway along the opponent-cell axis. Sample vectors—for orange, pink, and dark green—are displayed as histograms at the side. These vectors are traced within the color space proper. Note the isomorphism with the phenomenological color space shown in plates 3 and 4, both in its internal relations and its external connections. (From P. M. Churchland and P. S. Churchland 1997.)

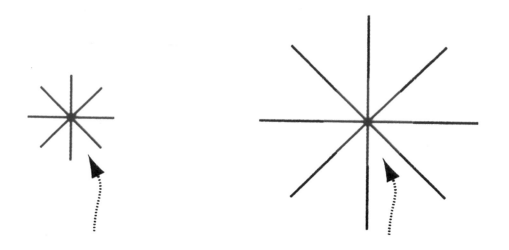

Plate 6   The left object is a set of intersecting red lines. The right object is made by attaching black lines to the tips of the red lines in the left object. Now, however, you see a definite red tint in the space where the arrow points in the right figure, but not where the arrow points in the left figure. A photometer indicates that the light in each case is identical. (From Hoffman 1998.)

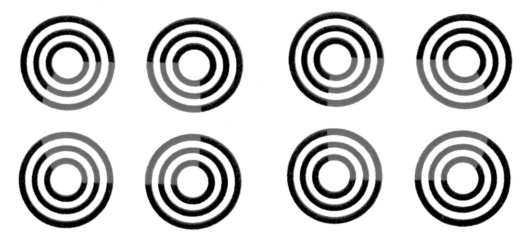

Plate 7   This is a stereoptic display. The two sets of four circles can be fused to make a single set by crossing your eyes slightly. In each set, the blue color is confined to lines on the segments of the circles, yet it appears to fill the intervening space to make a single semitransparent blue tissue spread across each of the circles. When the two sets are fused, the semitransparent blue tissue has clear boundaries and appears to curve out well in front of the black circles. (From Hoffman 1998.)

of the spectrum) and the inhibitory signals from both of the L- and M-cones (very roughly, the yellow part of the spectrum). Its activity reflects the balance of wavelengths from the shorter end of the spectrum over wavelengths from the medium and longer end. (Notice in figure 4.17 and plate 2, however, that in this case there is almost no crossover of the relevant curves. So our system will display no hypersensitive discriminations within this area of the spectrum.)

Finally, the right-most cell—labeled "white vs. black"—is the site of a tug-of-war between excitatory signals from all three types of retinal cones (the L, M, and, to a lesser degree, the S cells) versus inhibitory signals averaged over the stimulus-levels reaching the retinal surface as a whole. The activity of that cell is thus a measure of how much *brighter or darker* is its local portion of the retina, compared to the brightness levels hitting the retina as a whole.

These three types of LGN cells—called "color opponent cells" for reasons that are obvious from the diagram—constitute a most interesting arena for the coding of information about the character of the light hitting any spot on the retina. The simultaneous activity levels of all three cell types constitute a three-dimensional comparative analysis of the peculiar wavelength structure of the light hitting any part of the retina to which they are connected. Not to waste words, this analysis constitutes the brain's initial representation of external color. In fact, we can graphically represent any particular neural representation of this sort as a single point in a three-dimensional space, a space whose three axes correspond to the possible activity levels of each of the three types of color-opponent cells, as in plate 5.

When we do that, something quite arresting emerges. The range of *possible* coding triplets—that is, the range of simultaneous activation-level patterns possible across the three kinds of color-opponent cells—does not include the entire volume of the three-dimensional cube portrayed in plate 5. The available range is constrained to an irregular central subvolume of that cube, as illustrated. This is because the three cell types have activation levels that are *not entirely independent* of each other, as can be seen from the wiring diagram of figure 4.18. The several corners of the coding cube are thus "off limits" to the trio of color-opponent cells.

More specifically, when one calculates what the actual *shape* of that interior volume will have to be (from the details of figure 4.17 and plate 5, from the relative numbers and influence of the three cone types, and from the specific overlap of their wavelength response profiles), that interior volume turns out to have the same shape, and to have its various parts associated with the *same* colors, as the original Munsell solid of plate 3. Most obviously, the yellow portion bulges out and up towards the white pole, and in and down towards the black pole. Moreover, equal increments of discriminability within the green, yellow, and orange regions of that neuronal activation space correspond to finer increments of external wavelength than do equal increments within the blue region, just as we found in our own discriminatory capacities.

To a first approximation, and at a rather abstract level, the mapping means we are looking at *the neuronal basis for our phenomenal color space*. The general characteristics of the neuronal basis for the existence, dimensionality, global shape, and chromatic orientation of our internal space for color qualia, as experimentally mapped out by Munsell and subsequent generations of visual psychologists, are discernible. In this *very general sense*, it is mildly tempting to hypothesize that we can discern the basic principles governing color qualia.

It is tempting to say this because, as you have just seen, the various possible coding triplets stand to each other in all of the same similarity/proximity relations that our color qualia stand to each other, and they stand in all of the same causal relations to stimulus objects in the external world, and they stand in all of the same causal relations to subsequent internal cognitive activities, such as believing or saying that the lawn is green. Now, in general, in science, if explanatory power is greatly enhanced by making a cross-level identification, such as between light and electromagnetic radiation, or between temperature and mean molecular kinetic energy, then the identification looks like a reasonable bet.

In the case at hand, if we *hypothesize* that phenomenal color qualia are *identical with* coding triplets across our opponent cells, then the *systematic parallels in their causal and relational properties* are *explicable* rather than *coincidental*. The point is, the causal and relational properties displayed by qualia and by coding triplets will be systematically the same if the qualia and the coding triplets are *themselves* one and the same thing, in the same way that temperature and mean molecular kinetic energy, light and electromagnetic waves, and water and H_2O are one and the same thing.[54]

Is it possible that during inattention to color or even under anesthesia, perhaps, the coding triplets might be active, but no color qualities are experienced? Well, we do not know, but this is something we could find out. Additionally, it is safe to assume that there are many other events that must be taking place elsewhere, for example in the brainstem. To be a little more accurate, therefore, we should restate this *very provisional* hypothesis to say that the coding triplets are one component of a set of components that are *jointly sufficient* for color experience, and that there are a host of background conditions, many of which remain to be discovered.

So, yes, the hypothesis is undoubtedly too simple to be correct. Nevertheless, my point is to emphasize the significance of the *fit* between the antecedently determined qualia profile and the neuronal-coding triplet profile. I should mention too that a range of other color perceptual phenomena, such as various color illusions, afterimages, and the various forms of color blindness, are also plausibly explained within this framework.[55] This expanding range of explanatory success lends credence to the reductive promise of the general approach; i.e., we have here the same sorts of evidential grounds and explanatory opportunities that standardly motivate reductive claims throughout science. And to that degree, we can get a grip on why materialism seems more plausible than dualism. For example, the task of the dualist's original thought experiment—to invert the qualia without changing anything physical or behavioral—is now one step harder yet to imagine. If the inversion is to preserve the metric of similarity and discriminability relations that structure our phenomenal qualia, then it will require wholesale changes in the synaptic connections that project to our various color-opponent cells, and/or major changes in the profile or location of the normal response profiles of our three cone-cell populations. It is these features of our nervous system, as we saw, that give rise to that nonuniform metric in the first place.

An inversion is still possible, to be sure, but if it were imposed, it would show up not just in the subject's color-discrimination behaviors (as we saw before); it would also show up in the form of *changed behavior in his cones* and/or massive physical adjustments to the *wiring* that connects his retinal cone cells to his LGN opponent-cells. Evidently, as our understanding of the brain's coding activities gradually expands, the claim that qualia might be inverted among us, without *any* behavioral or physical differences among us, looks less and less plausible.

The dualist tries again

"Still," the Dualist might say, "it remains *conceivable*. We need only invert as well the *metric of the similarity/discriminability* relations, *in addition* to inverting the causal map of color qualia onto the external world, and the inversion will then require no synaptic adjustments and it will lead to no differences in discriminatory behavior."

That is strictly true, although changing the global metric of the space of possible qualia raises the issue of whether we have thereby made a significant change in the nature of the qualia themselves. If every color in the original space now bears a *different* set of similarity and dissimilarity relations to every other color in the original space, are we still talking about the same family of colors that we started with? It is not clear that we are. But let us not insist on this point. Who are we to insist that *any one* of the features we have been discussing is *essential* to the nature of color qualia, and could not *conceivably* be switched around without compromising their identity? In the absence of any *settled* scientific understanding of what qualia really *are*, any such insistence would be premature and prejudicial. It is the job of unfolding research, in the fullness of time, to provide us with authoritative grounds for claims about the essential versus the accidental features of our color qualia.

The dualist is hoist by his own petard

But if this is a lesson we materialists must learn to swallow, it is a lesson *no less obligatory for the dualist*. And for him it has an unwelcome edge to it, for the dualist's thought experiment, in all of its versions, depends on a preferential fixing of "how they present themselves to introspective judgment" as the *essential* feature of color qualia, while downgrading all other features of color qualia (and, as we saw, there are quite a few of them) as inessential contingencies, invertible without penalty at the drop of a thought experiment. But this very insistence is also premature and prejudicial, however much it may reflect the uncritical convictions of untutored common sense. The dualist *has no more right to that premise* than the functionalist has to "functional role" as *the* essential feature of color qualia, or the reductionist has to "family of similarity relations" as their essential feature. To insist on any one of these, *before* our science on the matter is completed, is to do science by *fiat* instead of by conceptual exploration and empirical evaluation.

Two points will drive this lesson home. The first is that the dualist himself can be victimized by an alternate instance of his own strategy, as follows.

Intrinsic-character-as-judged-by-introspection cannot be the defining feature of phenomenal qualia, since I can quite easily imagine that half the population suffers from "phenomenal judgment inversion syndrome," an undetectable malady whereby the faculty of judgment makes systematically inverted, and systematically *mistaken*, judgments about the identity of the phenomenal qualia had by the subject. Our judgmental take on our qualia, therefore, can hardly be definitive of their true nature. Accordingly, we shall have to dig even deeper still to find the identifying essence of color qualia. (See pp. 118–123.)

Though I am disinclined to defend this argument, its mere existence is instructive. Conceivability, it seems, is a two-edged sword.

To this it may be replied, perhaps in exasperation, "But qualia are *by definition* those things whose appearance *is* the reality!" As an observation about common usage, this claim may be strictly correct. But so were the following historical claims, famously uttered and with equal exasperation. "But atoms are by *definition* those things that cannot be split! (The Greek word "a-tom" means not cuttable.) So you can forget about subatomic particles." Or equally fatuously, "But the Earth (*terra firma*) is by *definition* that-which-does-not-move! So you can forget about its revolving around the Sun."

These remarks illustrate the second major point. As Quine first argued, and many others have underscored since, *the meaning of words is not independent of beliefs about what those words apply to*, and also, *no claim is immune to revision or rejection in the face of sufficiently compelling new science*. If science discovers, as it did, that the Earth does in fact move, there is no point in trying to counteract the evidence by saying, "But by 'Earth' I mean, in part, the thing-that-does-not-move." This strategy is futile, for the plain and simple reason that whether the Earth moves or does not move depends on the *facts* of the matter. It does not depend on an existing dictionary entry plus human resolve to protect the dictionary from revision. In the present context, this means that the ultimate nature of phenomenal color qualia is something to be determined by empirical research, and not by preemptive linguistic analyses and thought experiments based on them. Thought experiments can be useful exploratory devices, but they have no authority in dictating empirical facts.

So who is right?

None of this entails that the dualist hypothesis about the ultimate nature of color qualia is false. Despite the emptiness of the inverted-spectrum thought experiment as an *argument* for the truth of dualism, color qualia might still be a metaphysically basic feature of *some* nonphysical sort. What, then, will decide this issue?

The issue will be decided by the comparative virtues of the explanatory theories produced by both parties to the debate. You have seen, for what it is worth, what the physical sciences currently have to offer in the way of explaining human color experience: the opponent-cell activation-space theory of human color coding. You have seen some of the evidence for it and some of its explanatory prowess. Though far from proven, it plainly has at least some virtues. We can reopen the discussion when the dualist produces a competing explanatory theory (a competing explanation of the shape of the Munsell color solid, for example), a theory with *comparable specificity, supporting evidence, and explanatory power*. In the end, the issue is scientific, and competing theories must be decided on their respective scientific merits. That is the ultimate lesson of this section.

Doesn't neuroscience leave something out?

Before moving on, it is useful to address one residual worry about the ability of any purely physical theory—such as the one just examined—to account for the qualitative character of our internal phenomenal experience. After all, knowing the theory of neural coding across various color-opponent cells doesn't tell me how to recognize, in *introspection*, a visual sensation as a sensation of red. And so, hasn't it thereby left something out? After all, I could be color blind, and thus phenomenally ignorant of that domain of experience. But learning the neuronal theory just outlined wouldn't help me one bit to repair that phenomenal ignorance.[56]

This last sentence is entirely true. To have the perceptual skill of discriminating and recognizing colors requires more than just knowledge of the theory of how our color-discriminating system works: it requires that the theory also be *true of* oneself. It requires that *one actually possess a functioning instance of the neuronal system that the theory describes*. A color-blind person doesn't have that system, and so he is doomed to be phenomenally ignorant where colors are concerned. Learning the theory of that missing system will be no help on that score.

But this doesn't mean there is anything inadequate about the *theory*, especially when that theory gives a detailed explanation of what *produces* the various forms of color blindness (the lack of one or more retinal-cone types, which leads to the partial or total loss of information reaching the several types of color-opponent cells), and especially when the theory tells you what to do to *repair* that discriminatory/representational deficit (namely, artificially induce the genetic expression of the missing cone type(s), and induce the growth of their missing synaptic connections with the LGN color-opponent cells).

The residual worry about leaving something out thus involves the confused expectation that having-a-certain-cognitive-skill (namely, being able to have and discriminate color qualia) should *result from* knowing-a-certain-theory (namely, the color-opponent-cell theory). But the two are quite different things, and simply knowing the latter (the theory) won't give you the former (the skill). However, if the theory at issue is *true of* you—if you actually *have* the neuronal system that the theory describes—then you will certainly have the skill at issue. You will be able to discriminate colors by spontaneous internal reaction to their intrinsic qualitative natures. That ability is what needed an explanation in the first place. And an explanation of that ability is precisely what the color-opponent theory provides.

It is ridiculous to expect a reduction from the behavioral level directly to the neuronal level

This observation is sometimes used to support the conclusion that consciousness cannot be explained neurobiologically. The conclusion, however, just does not follow, and hence the argument is a non sequitur. Here is why.

Nervous systems appear to have many levels of organization, ranging in spatial scale from molecules such as serotonin, to dendritic spines, neurons, small networks, large networks, brain areas, and integrated systems (see again figure 1.1). Although it remains to be empirically determined what exactly are the functionally significant levels, it is unlikely that explanations of macro-effects such as face recognition will be explained directly in terms of the most microlevel. More likely, high-level network effects will be the outcome of smaller networks, and those effects in turn of the participating neurons and their interconnections, and those in turn of the properties of protein channels, neuromodulators, and neurotransmitters, and so forth. Emerging from efforts to understand these levels are a range of *midlevel concepts* applicable to mid-level neuronal organization and computation.

One misconception about the reductionist strategy interprets it as seeking a *direct* explanatory bridge between the highest level and the very lowest levels. This idea of "explanation-in-a-single-bound" does indeed stretch credulity, but neuroscientists are not remotely tempted by it. In contrast, the direct and indirect approaches predict that reductive explanations will proceed stepwise from highest to lowest, both agreeing, of course, that the research should proceed at all levels simultaneously. As more of the brain's organizational midlevels and their functions becomes known, a vocabulary suitable to those levels and functions will certainly develop.

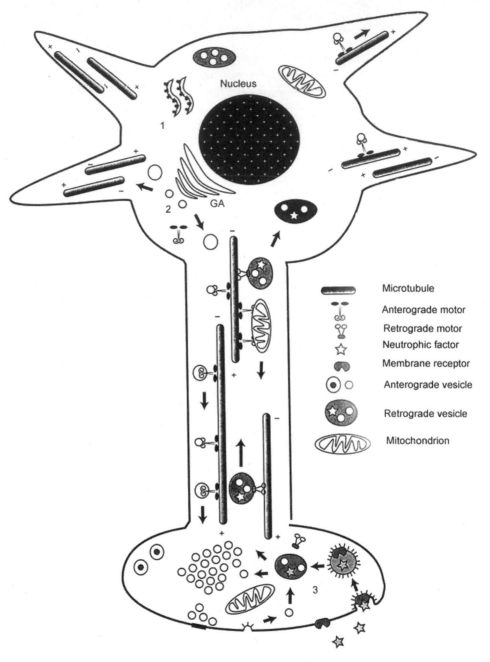

Nucleus

1

2

GA

Microtubule

Anterograde motor

Retrograde motor

Neutrophic factor

Membrane receptor

Anterograde vesicle

Retrograde vesicle

Mitochondrion

3

Figure 4.19 This schematic diagram of a neuron and some of its organelles shows the position of long (100 μm) microtubules in the axon and the shorter microtubules in the dendrites. Axonal microtubules are oriented with the same polarity; dendritic microtubules have mixed polarity. The microtubules have a diameter of about 14 nm. Notice

Consciousness is not a neural effect but a subatomic effect

Roger Penrose, a Cambridge mathematician, and Stuart Hameroff, an Arizona researcher on anesthesics, also harbor reservations about explaining awareness neurobiologically, but are moved by rather different reasons (Penrose and Hameroff 1995). They believe the dynamic properties at the level of neurons and networks to be incapable of generating consciousness, regardless of the complexity. For Penrose and Hameroff, the key to consciousness lies in quantum events in tiny protein structures—microtubules—within neurons. Microtubules are in fact found in *all* cells. They have a number of functions, including mediating cell division. In neurons, they are used for the transport of proteins up and down the axon and the dendrites. So our question is this: why do Penrose and Hameroff believe that a subatomic phenomenon holds the secret? And second, why do they find microtubules a particularly likely structure to mediate consciousness? I shall very briefly sketch their answers to these questions.

The answer to the first question is that Penrose believes the nature of mathematical understanding transcends the kind of computation that could conceivably by done by neurons and networks. As a demonstration of neuronal inadequacy, Penrose cites the Gödel Incompleteness Result, which concerns limitations to theorem-provability in axiom systems for arithmetic. What is needed to transcend these limitations, according to Penrose, are unique operations at the quantum level. Quantum gravity, were it to exist, could, he believes, do the trick. Granting that no adequate theory of quantum gravity exists, Penrose and Hameroff argue that microtubules are about the right size to support the envisioned quantum events, and they have the right sort of sensitivity to anesthetics to suggest that they do sustain consciousness (figure 4.19).

The details of Penrose and Hameroff's theory are highly technical, drawing on mathematics, physics, biochemistry, and neuroscience. Before investing time

that the microtubules do not extend into the synaptic end bulb of the axon. Neurotransmitter is synthesized in the cell body by the endoplasmic reticulum (1), packaged by the Golgi apparatus (2), and transported down the axon or the dendrites by protein motors on the microtubule. The speed of anterograde transport is 100–400 mm per day. Vesicle proteins not sorted for reuse at the synpase are packaged into larger vesicles for transport back to the soma for recycling. Neurotrophic factors collected from intracellular space are also transported back to the cell body. The speed of retrograde transport is about 50–200 mm per day. (3) Mitochondria are the site of the cell's energy production. (Based on Zigmond et al. 1999.)

in mastering the details, most people want a measure of the theory's "figures of merit," as an engineer might put it.[57] Specifically, is there any hard evidence in support of the theory, is the theory testable, and if true, would the theory give a clear and cogent explanation of what it is supposed to explain? After all, there is no dearth of crackpot theories on every topic, from consciousness to sun spots. Making theories divulge their figures of merit is a minimal condition for further investment.

First, a brief interlude to glimpse the positive views Penrose has concerning the question of how humans understand mathematics. In 1989 he suggested as unblushing a Platonic solution as Plato himself proposed circa 400 B.C.: "Mathematical ideas have an existence of their own, and inhabit an ideal Platonic world, which is accessible via the intellect only. When one "sees" a mathematical truth, one's consciousness breaks through into this world of ideas, and makes direct contact with it. . . . Mathematicians communicate . . . by each one having *a direct route to truth*" (1989, 428; Penrose's italics).

As a solution to questions in the epistemology of mathematics, Platonism is not remotely satisfactory. Given what we now know in biology, psychology, physics, and chemistry, the Platonic story of mathematical understanding is as much a fairy tale as the claim that Eve was created from Adam's rib. Far better to admit that we have no satisfactory solution than to adopt a "And God said Lo" solution.

Let us return now to evaluating the quantum-gravity-microtubule theory of conscious experience. The figures of merit are not encouraging. First, mathematical logicians generally disagree with Penrose on what the Gödel result implies for brain function. Additionally, the link between conscious experiences such as smelling cinnamon and the Gödel result is obscure, at best.[58]

Now, is there any significant evidential link between microtubules and awareness? Hameroff believes that microtubules are affected by hydrophobic anesthetics in a way that causes loss of consciousness. But there is no evidence that loss of consciousness under anesthesia depends on the envisaged changes in the microtubules, and only indirect evidence that anesthetics do in fact—as opposed to "could conceivably"—have *any* effect on microtubules. On the other hand, plenty of evidence points to proteins in the neuron membrane as the principal locus of action of hydrophobic anesthetics.[59]

Is there any hard evidence that the subatomic effect they cite, namely quantum coherence, happens in microtubules? *Only that it might.* Would not the presence of cytoplasmic ions in the microtubule pore disrupt this effect? *They might not.* Surely the effects of quantum coherence would be swamped by the millivolt signaling activity in the neuronal membrane? *They might not be.* Can the existence of quantum coherence in microtubules be tested experimentally? *For technical reasons, experiments on microtubules are performed in a dish (in vitro), rather than in the animal.* If tests under these conditions failed to show quantum coherence, would that be significant? *No, because microtubules might behave differently in the animal, where we cannot test for these effects.* Does any of this, supposing it to be true, help us explain such things as recall of past events, filling in of the blindspot, hallucinations, and attentional effects on sensory awareness? *Somehow, it might.*

The want of directly relevant data is frustrating enough, but the explanatory vacuum is catastrophic. Pixie dust in the synapses is about as explanatorily powerful as quantum coherence in the microtubules. Without at least a blueprint, outline, prospectus, or *something* showing how, if true, the theory could explain the various phenomena of conscious experience, Penrose and Hameroff have little to tempt us. None of this shows that Penrose and Hameroff are definitely wrong, only that their theory needs work. Whether it is worth additional work depends on how one assesses the theory's figures of merit.

Science cannot solve all problems

Finally, consider Zeno Vendler's admonition: science cannot expect to solve all problems, answer all questions.[60] Let's agree with him—some questions may never be answered. What, we must inquire, is entailed by *this* problem—the problem of the neurobiology of consciousness? Absolutely nothing. Because significant progress has been made by neuroscience on many questions about the mind, it does look as though further progress is possible. We may at some point hit the wall, but so far, at least, no reason has emerged to indicate the wall has already been hit. What Vendler offers is not an argument, but off-the-shelf Faustian rhetoric.

2.3 Conclusions

The principal aim of this chapter has been to convey my sense of where things stand on the question of brain-based explanations for conscious phenomena. The chapter does not pretend to be a survey of all views, since there are an almost limitless number of those. Nor are all of them equally worth discussing. Of the theories I do discuss, some get better report cards than others. These judgments reflect my particular, and quite possibly mistaken, opinions concerning what is productive and important, what is logically compelling or a logical shell game.

The main philosophical argument submitted for uncompromised dissection concerns the "inverted spectrum" argument. In my experience, this particular problem is an unparalleled quagmire. Most of us are curious enough to want to get into it. We vaguely sense that there is *something* to it, though exactly what remains a bit foggy. We are reasonably confident that we can get to the crux of it and come away with a clearer understanding. In the end, however, we tend to find ourselves in an unholy jam, wondering how we got in the jam and how we can avoid embarrassing ourselves further. My goal was to lay bare the entire structure of the argument, following the various lines to their end, however tangled the path. If this works, readers should be able to identify the logical strengths or fallacies, and determine precisely what significance, if any, the argument has for neuroscientific attacks on the problems of conscious phenomena.

In addition to the inverted-spectrum argument, I considered a range of other philosophical arguments allegedly demonstrating the futility of looking to neuroscience for answers to questions about the nature of consciousness. Though each of the skeptical arguments considered boasts a considerable following, and for that reason alone must be dissected carefully, none is convincing once examined. Nor do they *collectively* create a credible skepticism even if *individually* they do not. That they are flawed does not, of course, show that neuroscience will in fact be successful in expanding our understanding of consciousness. It shows only that the skeptics' conclusions regarding the mere *possibility* are unconvincing. The most convincing answer to skepticism is, of course, explanatory progress in neuroscience.

Suggested Readings

Churchland, P. M. 1988. *Matter and Consciousness*. 2nd ed. Cambridge: MIT Press.

Churchland, P. M. 1995. *The Engine of Reason, The Seat of the Soul*. Cambridge: MIT Press.

Crick, F., and C. Koch. 2000. The unconscious homunculus. In T. Metzinger, ed., *Neural Correlates of Consciousness*, pp. 103–110. Cambridge: MIT Press.

Damasio, A. R. 1999. *The Feeling of What Happens*. New York: Harcourt Brace.

Dennett, D. C. 1991. *Consciousness Explained*. Boston: Little Brown.

Hobson, J. A. 1999. *Consciousness*. New York: Scientific American Library.

Llinás, R. 2001. *I of the Vortex*. Cambridge: MIT Press.

Metzinger, T. 2003. *Being No One: The Self-Model Theory of Subjectivity*. Cambridge: MIT Press.

Palmer, S. E. 1999. *Vision Science: Photons to Phenomenology*. Cambridge: MIT Press. See especially chapter 13.

Parvizi, J., and A. R. Damasio. 2001. Consciousness and the brainstem. *Cognition* 79: 135–159.

Walsh, V., and A. Cowey. 2000. Transcranial magnetic stimulation and cognitive neuroscience. *Nature Reviews: Neuroscience* 1: 73–80.

Websites

BioMedNet Magazine: http://news.bmn.com/magazine

Comparative Mammalian Brain Collections: http://brainmuseum.org

Encyclopedia of Life Sciences: http://www.els.net

Higher Order Visual Areas: http://www.med.uwo.ca/physiology/courses/sensesweb/L3HigherVisual/l3v23.swf

The MIT Encyclopedia of the Cognitive Sciences: http://cognet.mit.edu/MITECS

5   Free Will

1   Introduction[1]

Much of human social life depends on the expectation that agents have control over their actions and are responsible for their choices. In daily life it is commonly assumed that it is sensible to punish and reward behavior so long as the person was in control and chose knowingly and intentionally. Without the assumptions of agent control and responsibility, human social commerce is hardly conceivable. As member of a social species, we recognize cooperation, loyalty, honesty, and helping as prominent features of the social environment. We react with hostility when group members disappoint certain socially significant expectations. Inflicting disutilities (e.g., shunning, pinching) on the socially erring and rewarding civic virtue help restore the standards.

In other social species too, social unreliability, such as a failure to reciprocate grooming or food sharing, provoke a reaction likely to cost the erring agent. In social mammals, at least, mechanisms for keeping the social order seem to be part of what evolution has bequeathed to our brain circuitry. The stability of the social-expectation baseline is sufficiently important to survival that individuals are prepared to incur some cost in enforcing those expectations. Anyone with dogs can observe the complex but general phenomenon of maintaining social stability in dog interactions. Mature dogs will teach pups what is unacceptable conduct, and typically dogs test newly encountered dogs, making it clear what territory is theirs and what person they will defend. Just as anubis baboons learn that tasty scorpions are to be found under rocks but cannot just be picked up, so they learn that failure to reciprocate grooming when it is duly expected may incur a slap. As discussed in chapter 3, much of our behavior is

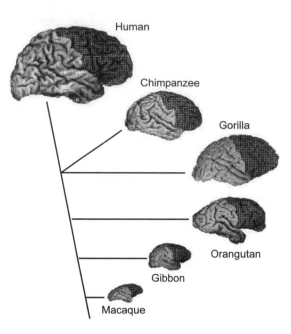

Figure 5.1   The frontal cortex (shaded) of six primates. The evolutionary relationships among the species are indicated by the connecting lines. Although the human brain is absolutely larger than the brains of the other primates, the proportion of frontal cortex is roughly the same across species. Frontal cortex has an important role in planning, impulse control, socialization, and the organization of behavior. (From Semendeferi et al. 2002.)

guided by expectations of specific consequences of events, not only in the physical world, and but also in the social world (figure 5.1).

If the reward and punishment system is to be effective in shaping social behavior, the actions for which the agent is rewarded or punished must be under the agent's control. The important question, therefore, is this: What is it, for us or baboons or chimpanzees, to have control over our behavior? Are we ever *really* responsible for our choices and decisions? Will neuroscientific understanding of the neuronal mechanisms for decision making change how we think about these fundamental features of social commerce? These are the places where issues about free will bump up against practical reality and our developing understanding of what is fair, what is reasonable, and what is effective in maintaining civil society.

2   Are We Responsible and in Control If Our Choices and Actions Are Caused?

One tradition bases the conditions for free will and control on a contrast between being *caused* to do something and *not* being so caused. For example, if someone falls on me and I hit you, then my hitting you was caused by the falling body; I did not choose to hit you. I am not responsible, therefore, for hitting you. Were you to punish me for hitting you, it would not help me avoid such events in the future. Examples emanating from this prototype have been extended to the broader idea that for *any* choice to be free, it must be absolutely *un*caused. That is, it is suggested that I make a free choice when, without any prior cause and without any prior constraints, I make a decision that results in an action. Examples allegedly illustrating freely chosen actions are Eisenhower's decision to send troops into Little Rock to enforce school desegregation, or my decision to go to the coffee shop for a cappuccino. This *contracausal* construal of free choice is known as libertarianism.[2] Is it plausible? That is, are the paradigm cases of free choices actually *uncaused* choices?

As Hume demonstrated in 1739,[3] the answer is *no*. Hume argued that our free choices and decisions are in fact caused by other events in the mind: desires, beliefs, preferences, feelings, and so forth. Thus Eisenhower's decision was the outcome of his beliefs about the situation and his desire to ensure that the federal school-integration law was not flouted. His decision did not suddenly spring uncaused into existence without preceding beliefs, thoughts, hopes, and worries. I went to get a cappuccino because I usually have one about this time in the afternoon, I wanted to have one, and I knew I had enough money to pay for it, and so on. Save for these causal antecedents, albeit *cognitive* causal antecedents, I would not have gone for coffee. By contrast, suppose that without any antecedent causes, I suddenly enter a saloon, ask for a glass of vodka, and gulp it down. I had no antecedent desire for vodka, no habit of going to a saloon anytime, let alone in the afternoon, and the behavior would be considered utterly at odds with my cognitive state and temperament. Is *this* the paradigm of free choice? Is *this* prototypically responsible behavior? Surely not.

Reflecting on these sorts of possibilities, Hume made the deeper and more penetrating observation that an agent's choices are not considered freely made *unless* they are caused by his desires, intentions, and so forth. Randomness, pure chance, and utter unpredictability are not preconditions for attribution of responsible choice. Hume puts the matter with memorable compactness:

"Where [actions] proceed not from some cause in the characters and disposition of the person, who perform'd them, they infix not themselves upon him, and can neither redound to his honor if good, nor infamy, if evil."[4]

Logic reveals, Hume argued, that responsible choice is actually *inconsistent* with libertarianism (uncaused choice). Someone may choose to climb onto his roof because he does not want the rain to come into his house, he wants to fix the loose shingles that allowed the rain in, and he believes that he needs to get up on the roof to do that. His desires, intentions, and beliefs are part of the causal antecedents resulting in his choice, even though he may not be introspectively aware of them *as* causes. If, without any determining desires and beliefs, he simply went up onto the roof—*for no reason*, as it were—his sanity and hence his self-control would be seriously in doubt.

More generally, a choice undetermined by anything the agent believes, intends, or desires is the kind of thing we consider *out* of the agent's control, and is not the sort of thing for which we hold someone responsible. Furthermore, desires or beliefs that are uncaused (if that is physically possible), rather than caused by other stable features of the person's character and temperament, likewise fail to be conditions for responsible choice. If a desire suddenly and without antecedent connection to my other desires or my general character were to spring into my mind—say, the serious desire to become a seamstress— I would suspect that someone must be "messing with my mind." The brain presumably has no mechanism for introspectively recognizing a desire to fix the roof *as* a cause, just as it has no way of detecting in introspection that growth hormone has been released or that blood pressure is at 110/85. A desire, nevertheless, is most certainly a cause.

Neither Hume's argument that choices are internally caused nor his argument that libertarianism is absurd have ever been convincingly refuted. Notice, moreover, that his arguments hold regardless of whether the mind is a separate *Cartesian substance* or a pattern of activity of the physical brain. And they hold regardless of whether the etiologically relevant states are conscious or unconscious.

In fact, moreover, the brain does indeed appear to be a causal machine. So far, there is no evidence at all that some neuronal events happen without any cause. True enough, neuroscience is still in its early stages, and we cannot absolutely rule out the possibility that evidence will be forthcoming at some later stage. Given the data, however, the odds are against it. Importantly, even were uncaused neuronal events to be discovered, it is a further, substantial matter to show that precisely *those* events constitute choice. They might, for all we can know, have to do with features of growth-hormone release or variations in the sleep/wake cycle.

Though all events in the brain may be caused, this does not imply that actions are predictable. Causality and unpredictability are entirely compatible. Causation concerns conditions that bring about an event, whereas predictability concerns what we *know* about such conditions. When an event occurs in a complex system, we may know that the event is causally governed, even though on any given occasion we may not know exactly what conditions actually obtain, and hence are unable to predict precisely the nature of the event. Nevertheless, despite our inability to make precise predictions, we can often make useful general predictions. Thus I might be able to predict that a dollar bill dropped from the top of the Eiffel Tower will fall to the ground in less than two minutes, but I will be unable to predict exactly the fluttering pattern and its precise downward trajectory. Those subtle changes in movement will depend on moment-by-moment changes in air currents, and these changes will occur much faster than I can take relevant measurements and do the relevant computations, even if I were lucky enough to have very powerful computational equipment. Every movement of the dollar bill is, nonetheless, caused.

Similarly, brain events relevant to decisions and choices are probably all caused events, but this does not imply that I can predict with any great precision what you will say if I ask you for directions from UCSD to the Salk Institute. I can predict roughly what you will say, however, if I know that you are familiar with the area, that you are alert, paying attention, are not easily disoriented, and that you tend to be forthcoming when asked for directions. I can also predict with considerable confidence that given the opportunity, a human will go to sleep at night for at least a few hours, that he will want to eat and drink at some time during a 24-hour period, that he will not want to sit for very long naked on an iceberg, and so on. I can predict that a neonate will suckle, a puppy will chew shoes, and that most undergraduates will name carrots as the first vegetable that comes into their minds. But these are rough and general, not precise, predictions.

The brain is a dynamical system of enormous complexity. The human brain is calculated to have about 10^{12} neurons and about 10^{15} synapses. The time scale for neuronal events is in the millisecond range. If we assume that synaptic events and neuronal events are the only causally relevant events, then to a first approximation, this means that the human brain has about 10^{15} parameters that can vary over roughly 1–100 milliseconds. (This is a conservative estimate, since there are intraneuronal events, such as gene expression, that are also relevant.) These figures mean that it is not physically possible to take all the relevant measurements and perform all the relevant computations to grind out a precise prediction in real time. So predicting on a neuron-by-neuron or synapse-by-synapse basis is even less realistic than predicting the precise path and flutter of the dropped dollar bill. The logical point, therefore, is this: causality does not entail predictability, and *un*predictability does not entail noncausality. Put another way, causality and unpredictability are entirely consistent.[5]

As we reflect on what would have to be true for us to have free choice, we tend to be impressed by the fact that absolutely precise prediction of an agent's behavior is really impossible given the relevant variables and time scales. We nurture the hunch that if you cannot predict whether I will choose a green salad or a beet salad, or whether I will choose to say "Hi" or "Good morning," then my choices are really uncaused and therein lies my freedom to choose. The hunch may be the more compelling if it gets support from this tacit assumption: since "uncaused" implies "unpredictable," "unpredictable" implies "uncaused." As I have shown, however, this is quite mistaken. The implication goes only one way. "Unpredictable" does *not* imply "uncaused." Once the logic of the relation between causality and predictability are clarified, no logical rationale remains for deriving expectations of noncausality from facts of unpredictability.

Nonetheless, the idea that randomness in the physical world is somehow the key to what makes free choice free remains appealing to those inclined to believe that free choice must be uncaused choice. With the advent of quantum mechanics and the respectability of the idea of quantum indeterminacy, the suggestion that somehow or other quantum-level indeterminacy is the basis for a "solution" to the problem of free will remains attractive to some libertarians.[6] Stripped to essentials, the hypothesis claims that although an agent may have the relevant desires, beliefs, etc., he can still make a choice that is truly independent of *all* antecedent causal conditions. On this view, the agent, not the agent's brain or his desires or his emotions, freely chooses between cappuccino and latte, for example. It is at the moment of deciding that the indeterminacy or the noncausality or the break in the causal nexus—whatever one wants to call it—occurs. The subsequent choice is therefore absolutely free.

This is meant to be an empirical hypothesis, and as such, it needs to confront neurobiologically informed questions. For example, what exactly, in neural terms, is the *agent who chooses*? How does the idea of an agent who chooses fit with what we understand about self and self-representational capacities in the brain? Under exactly what conditions do the supposed noncaused events occur?

Does noncausal choice exist only when I am dithering or agonizing between two equally good—or perhaps equally bad—alternatives? What about when, in conversation, I use the word "firm" rather than the word "stubborn"? Does it exist with respect to the *generation* of desires? Why not? There are also questions from quantum physics, such as these: What is the mechanism of amplification of the nondeterministic events? Were quantum effects of the envisioned kind to exist, how could they fail to be swamped by thermal indeterminacy?

These are just the first snowballs in an avalanche of empirically informed questions. Part of their effect is to expose the flagrantly ad hoc character of the hypothesis. That is, it is based more on a desire to prop up a wobbling ideology than on factual matters. Rather than fully discussing its merits and flaws now, however, I shall defer a closer analysis of the hypothesis of a quantum-level origin for uncaused choice until further details of the neurobiology of decision making are on the table. That will allow us to see what bearing the neurobiological data have on the question of causality and choice in the brain, and hence will provide a richer context for evaluating the hypothesis of noncausal choice. We return to this hypothesis, and its critics, therefore, in section 6.

Provisionally, therefore, let us adopt the competing hypothesis, namely that Hume is essentially right and all choices and all behavior *are* caused, in one way or another. The absolutely crucial point, however, is that not all kinds of causes are consistent with free choice; not all kinds of causes are equal before the tribunal of responsibility. Some causes excuse us from culpability; others make us culpable because they are part of the story of voluntary action. The important question is what are the relevant differences among causes of behavior such that some kinds play a role in free choice and others play a role in forced choice. That is, are there systematic *brain-based* differences between voluntary and involuntary actions that will support the notion of agent responsibility? This is the crucial question, because we do hold people responsible for what we take to be *their* actions. When those actions are intentionally harmful to others, punishment, varying from social disapproval to execution, may be visited upon the agent. When, if ever, is it fair to hold an agent responsible? When, if ever, is punishment justified?

Many possibilities have been explored to explain how the notions of control and responsibility can make sense in the context of causation. These fall under the general rubric of "compatibilism," which means that our work-a-day notion of responsibility is, at bottom, *compatible* with the probable truth that the mind-brain is a causal machine. First we shall consider some obvious but unsuccessful attempts at squaring responsibility and causation, and then we shall raise the possibility that increased understanding of the brain will aid in piecing together a plausible account.

---

3   Caused Choice and Free Choice: Some Traditional Hypotheses

3.1   Voluntary Causes Are Internal Causes

Can we rely on the following rule? "You are responsible if the causes are internal, otherwise not." No, for several reasons. A patient with Huntington's disease makes nonpurposeful, jerky movements as a result of internal causes. But we do not hold the Huntington's patient responsible for his movements, since they are the outcome of a disease that causes destruction in the striatum. He has no control over his movements, they are not voluntary, and they are not consistent with his actual desires and intentions, which he cannot execute. A sleepwalker may unplug the phone or kick the dog. Here too the causes are internal, but the sleepwalker is not straightforwardly responsible. In a rather attenuated sense, the sleepwalker may *intend* his movements, though he is apparently unaware of his intentions.

3.2   Voluntary Causes Are Internal, They Involve the Agent's Intentions, and the Agent Must Be Aware of His Intention

This revision to the above strategy also fails. A patient with obsessive-compulsive disorder (OCD) may have an overwhelming urge to wash his hands. He wants and intends to wash his hands, and he is fully aware of his desire and intention. He knows that the desire is his desire; he knows that it is he who is washing his hands. Nevertheless, in patients with OCD, obsessive behavior such as hand washing or footstep counting is considered to be out of the agent's control. OCD patients often indicate that they wish to be rid of hand-washing or footstep-counting behavior, but cannot stop. Pharmacological interventions, such as Prozac, may enable the subject to have what we would all regard as normal, free choice about whether or not to wash his hands.

3.3   Voluntary Causes Feel Different from the Inside

Another strategy is to base the distinction between voluntary causes and forcing causes on *felt* differences in inner experience between those actions we choose to do and those over which we feel we have no control. Thus it allegedly feels different when we evince a cry as a startle response to a mouse leaping out of the compost heap and when we cry out to get someone's attention and help. Is introspection a reliable guide to responsibility? Can introspection—attentive, careful, knowledgeable introspection—distinguish those internal causes for which we are responsible from those for which we are not? (See also Crick 1994 and Wegner 2002.)

Probably not. There are undoubtedly many cases where introspection is no guide at all. Phobic patients, the OCD patients just mentioned, and patients with Tourette's syndrome are obvious examples that muddy the waters. In a patient with claustrophobia, the desire not to go into a cave feels as much *his* as his desire not to go rafting without a life jacket. He can even give reasons for both—it could be unsafe, avoidable injuries could happen, etc. His desire not to go into a cave may be very strong, but so may his desire to eat when hungry or sleep with his wife. So mere *strength* of desire will not suffice to distinguish actions for which the agent has diminished responsibility and those for which he is fully responsible.

The various kinds of addictions present a further range of difficulties. A smoker feels that the desire for a cigarette is indeed *his*. His reaching for a cigarette may feel every bit as free as reaching to turn on the television or scratching his nose. He might wish it were not his, but so far as the *feeling* itself is concerned, it is as much his as his desire to quit smoking. The increase in intensity of sexual interest and desire at puberty is surely the result of hormonal changes on the brain, not something over which one has much control. Yet all of that interest, inclination, and alteration of behavior *feels*—from the inside at any rate—entirely free.

More problematic perhaps, are the many examples from everyday life where one may suppose the decision was entirely one's own, only to discover that subtle manipulation of desires by others had in fact been the decisive factor. According to the fashion standards of the day, one finds certain clothes beautiful, others frumpy, and the choice of wardrobe seems, introspectively, as free as any choice. There is no escaping the fact, however, that what is in fashion has a huge effect on what we find beautiful, and this affects not only our choices of clothes, but also such things as aesthetic judgment regarding plumpness or slenderness of the female body. Baseball hats worn backwards have been in fashion for about ten years and are considered to look good, but from another perspective, most people look less attractive if wearing a baseball cap backwards.

Social psychologists have produced dozens of examples that further muddy the waters, but a simple one will convey the point. On a table in a shopping mall, experimenters place ten pairs of *identical* panty hose and asked shoppers to select a pair and then briefly explain their choice. Choosers referred to color, denier, sheerness, and so forth, as their rationales. In fact, there was a huge position effect: shoppers tended to pick the pantyhose in the right-most position on the table. None of them considered this to be a factor, none of them referred to it as a basis for choice, yet it clearly was so. The ten pairs of panty hose were, after all, *identical* to one another. Other examples of priming, subliminal perception, and emotional manipulation also suggest that we will not get very far with appeals to introspection to solve our problem about which behavior is in our control and which is not.

3.4   Could Have Done Otherwise

In a different attack on the problem, philosophers have explored the idea that if the choice was free, the agent *could have chosen otherwise*. That is, in some sense, the agent had the power to do something else.[7] Certainly, this idea does comport with conventional expectations about voluntary behavior, and to that extent, it is appealing. Lyndon Johnson, historians say, could have done otherwise regarding Vietnam. He could have decided to stop the war in Vietnam in 1965 when he correctly judged it to be unwinnable. I could have decided not to get coffee, and perhaps to have water instead. Nobody forced me or coerced me; the desire for coffee was mine. So far so good. The weakness in the strategy shows up when we ask further, "What exactly does 'could have done otherwise' mean?" If all behavior has antecedent causes, then "could have done otherwise" seems to boil down to *"would have done otherwise if antecedent conditions had been different."* Accepting that equivalence means the criterion is too *weak* to distinguish between the shouted insults of a Touretter, whose tics including such unpredicted and undirected outbursts as "idiot, idiot, idiot," and those of a member of parliament responding with "idiot, idiot, idiot" to another honorable member's proposal. In both cases, had the antecedent conditions been different, the results would have been different. Nevertheless, we hold the parliamentarian responsible, but not the Touretter. So the proposed criterion seems not so much wrong as unhelpful in revealing the nature of the difference between the causes of voluntary behavior and the causes of *non*voluntary behavior.

A further problem lurking here is circularity. Testing for whether an agent could have done otherwise seems to be exactly the same as testing whether the behavior was voluntary. Hence, specifying what counts as voluntary behavior by referring to the possibility that the agent might have done otherwise just goes around in a small circle. It does not seem to get us anywhere.

4 Toward a Neurobiology of Decision Making and Free Choice

4.1 Prototypes and Responsibility

In our legal as well as daily practice, we accept certain prototypical conditions as excusing a person from responsibility, but assume him responsible unless a definite exculpatory condition obtains. In other words, responsibility is the default condition; excuse from and mitigation of responsibility has to be positively established. The set of conditions regarded as exculpatory can be modified as we learn more about behavior and its etiology. A different but related issue concerns what to do with someone who harms others but has diminished responsibility.

Aristotle (384–322 B.C.), in his great work *The Nicomachean Ethics*, was an early exponent of the principle that one is responsible unless there are exculpating reasons. And wise the principle is, so wise that the core of this approach is still reflected in much of human practice, including current legal practice. In his systematic and profoundly sensible way, Aristotle pointed out that for an agent to be held responsible, it is necessary that the cause of an agent's behavior be internal to the agent, i.e., there must be intent. In addition, he characterized as "involuntary" actions produced by coercion and actions produced in certain kinds of ignorance. As Aristotle well knew, however, no simple rule demarcates cases here. Clearly, ignorance is not considered excusable when it may be fairly judged that the agent *should* have known. Additionally, in some cases of coercion, the agent is expected to resist the pressure, given the nature of the situation. A captured soldier is supposed to resist giving information to the enemy. As Aristotle illustrated in his own discussion of such complexities, we seem to deal with these cases by judging their similarity to uncontroversial and well-worn prototypes. This is perhaps why precedent law is so useful.[8]

Increasingly, it seems unlikely that there is a sharp distinction—brain-based or otherwise—between the voluntary and the involuntary, between being in control and being out of control, either in terms of behavioral conditions or in terms of the underlying neurobiology. This implies not that there is *no* distinction, but only that whatever the distinction, it is not sharp. That is, it is not like the distinction between having a valid California divers' license and *not* having a valid California drivers' license. It is rather more like categories with a prototype structure, e.g., "being a good sled dog," "being a navigable river," "being a fertile valley." These sorts of categories are useful even though we cannot specify necessary and sufficient conditions for membership in such categories, but teach them by citing prototypical instances, along with contrasting prototypical *non*instances.

Once we consider being in control in this light, we instantly recognize the degrees and nuances typical of freedom of choice. An agent's decision to change television channels may be more unconstrained than his decision to pay for his child's college tuition, which may be more unconstrained than his decision to marry his wife, which may be more unconstrained than his decision to turn off the alarm clock. Some desires or fears may be very powerful, others less so, and we may have more self-control in some circumstances than in others. Prolonged sleep deprivation makes it extremely hard to stay awake, even when the need to do so is great. Hormonal changes, for example in puberty, make certain behavior patterns highly likely, and in general, the neurochemical milieu has a powerful effect of the strength of desires, urges, drives, and feelings.

These considerations motivate thinking of control as coming in degrees, and hence as falling along a spectrum of possibilities. Toward opposite ends of the self-control spectrum are prototypical cases that contrast sufficiently in behavioral and internal features to provide a foundation for a basic, if somewhat rough-hewn and fuzzy-bordered, distinction between being in control and not, between freely choosing and not, between being responsible and not. Moreover, as we consider various points on the spectrum, it seems likely that there are in fact *many* parameters relevant to being in control. Consequently, we should upgrade the simple one-dimensional notion of a *spectrum* to a multidimensional notion of a *parameter space*, where the dimensions of the parameter space reflect the primary determinants of in-control behavior.

In our current state of knowledge, we do not know how to specify all the parameters or how to weight their significance. And the relations among the parameters are not likely to be linear. We can nevertheless make a start. We do know now that activity patterns in certain brain structures—including the anterior cingulate cortex, hypothalamus, insula, and ventromedial frontal cortex—are important. For example, large bilateral lesions to anterior cingulate abolish voluntary movement, though the patient remains aware of his surroundings.[9] One fortunate patient recovered some voluntary function after a

FUNCTIONAL SUBDIVISONS OF THE CINGULATE CORTEX

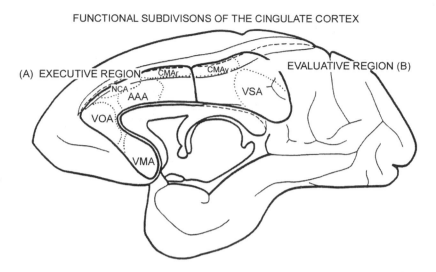

Figure 5.2 Functional division of the cingulate cortex of the rhesus-monkey brain. The executive region (A) and the evaluative region (B) are the two major divisions. Subdivisions in (A): visceromotor (VMA), vocalization (VOA), nociceptive (pain) (NCA), rostral cingulate motor (CMAr), and attention to action (AAA). Subdivisions in (B): ventral cingulate motor (CMAv) and visuospatial (VSA). (Based on Vogt, Finch, and Olson 1992.)

period of ininition. She also had good memories of her symptomatic episode, during which, she explained, "nothing mattered," and she said nothing because she "had nothing to say."[10] Smaller lesions to the anterior cingulate are associated with severe depression and anxiety (see figure 5.2).[11] If a lesion occurs in the middle area of the cingulate, patients may show loss of voluntary control over a hand. In the *alien-hand syndrome*, as this deficit is called, the hand behaves as though it has a will of its own. To the consternation of the patient, the hand may grab cookies or behave in socially inappropriate ways. One patient discovered he could regain some control over his misbehaving alien hand if he yelled at it, "Stop that!"

Imaging data implicate the anterior cingulate gyrus in the exercise of self-control over sexual arousal. In an fMRI study, male subjects were first exposed to erotic pictures and then were asked to inhibit their feelings of sexual arousal. Comparisons between the two conditions show that when subjects are responding normally to erotic pictures, limbic areas show increased activation. When subjects engage in inhibition of sexual arousal, this activation disappears, and the right anterior cingulate gyrus and the superior frontal gyrus become more highly activated.[12]

The anterior cingulate again emerges as a player in autism. One undisputed finding is that autistics have deficits in analyzing affective signals. Because limbic structures play a central role in affect, a leading hypothesis claims that autism results primarily from defective affective evaluation, owing to structural abnormalities in limbic system.[13] This hypothesis has been tested by comparing the microstructure of normal and autistic brains. Using whole-brain serial sections, researchers examined the brains of nine deceased autistic subjects. The only cortical structure to show abnormalities was the anterior cingulate gyrus, where the cells were smaller and the packing density greater. There were similar abnormalities in limbic subcortical structures, including the hypothalamus, amygdala, and mammillary bodies. Abnormalities in the cerebellum were also seen.[14]

Additionally, it is known that levels of neuromodulators, such as serotonin and dopamine, and of neurotransmitters, such as norepinephrine and acetylcholine, as well as of various hormones such as estrogen and testosterone, are highly pertinent parameters in the well-tuned decision-making neural organization. For example, obsessive-compulsive pathologies and depressive pathologies involving loss of motivation can be greatly modified by increasing serotonin levels (figure 5.3). It is also known that subjects with Klinefelter's syndrome (that is, those with XXY chromosomes) have poor long-term judgment and impulse control, even when they are cognitively capable. Yet the judgmental capacities of Klinefelter's subjects improve markedly when they are given constant administration of testosterone through a skin patch. Tourette's syndrome is much more controlled when patients are given serotonin agonists; the subjects simply do not feel the same desire to engage in their customary *ticcing* behavior. Since the anterior cingulate has been implicated in voluntary behavior, it is noteworthy that both the dopamine projections and the norepinephrine projections can influence activity in the anterior cingulate, and thus have an influence on executive and attentional functions (see figure 5.4).[15]

Appetite is a particularly promising parameter to consider in discovering the brain-based differences between being or not being in control. Gluttony allegedly is one of the seven deadly sins; overeating, we are repeatedly reminded, can be controlled by sheer will power. The discovery of the role of the protein leptin in eating, and in particular in over-eating, has provoked reconsideration of just how much freedom of choice to push back from the table the very obese actually have, and whether leptin-related interventions will give them greater control.[16]

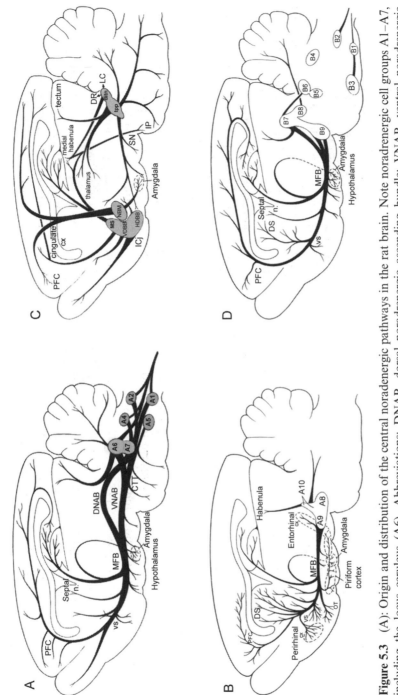

Figure 5.3 (A): Origin and distribution of the central noradenergic pathways in the rat brain. Note noradrenergic cell groups A1–A7, including the locus ceruleus (A6). Abbreviations: DNAB, dorsal noradrenergic ascending bundle; VNAB, ventral noradrenergic ascending bundle; CTT, central tegmental tract. (B): Origin and distribution of the central dopamine pathways. Note dopaminergic cell groups A8–A10. Abbreviation: OT, olfactory tubercle. (C): Origin and distribution of the central cholinergic pathways. Note rostral cell groups: nucleus basalis magnocellularis (NBM) (Meynert in primates), medial septum (MS), vertical limb nucleus of the diagonal band of Broca (VDBB), horizontal limb nucleus (HDBB). Abbreviations: Icj, islands of Calleja; SN, substantia nigra; IP, interpeduncular nucleus; dltn, dorsolateral tegmental nucleus; tpp, tegmental pedunculopontine nucleus; DR, dorsal raphe; LC, locus ceruleus. (D): Origin and distribution of the central serotoninergic pathways. Note cell groups in the raphe nucleus, B4–B9. Common abbreviations: MFB, medial forebrain bundle; PFC, prefrontal cortex; VS, ventral striatum; DS, dorsal striatum; cx, cortex. (From Robbins and Everitt 1995.)

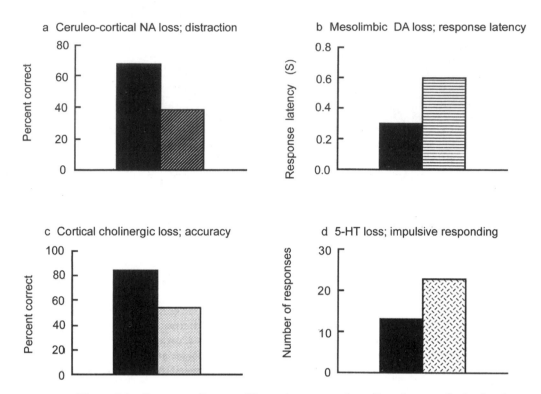

Figure 5.4   Summary diagrams illustrating contrasting effects in rats of selective damage to the noradrenergic (NA), dopaminergic (DA), cholinergic, and serotoninergic (5-HT) systems. A five-choice task was used. The diagrams highlight optimal conditions for exposing deficits in each condition. (a) The ceruleocortical NA system. No defict on the baseline, but accuracy reduced after distraction with white noise. (b) Mesolimbic DA depletion. Baseline speed and overall probability of responding are primarily affected. (c) Cortical cholinergic system. Baseline accuracy is impaired. (d) Serotoninergic depletion. No effects on accuracy, but impulsive responding is increased. The control groups are shown indicated by black bars. (From Robbins and Everitt 1995.)

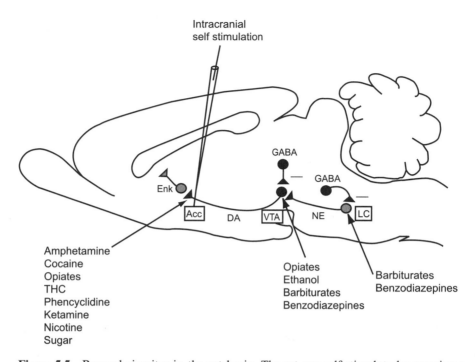

Figure 5.5 Reward circuitry in the rat brain. The rat can self-stimulate by pressing a bar that activates an electrode implanted in the region of the nucleus accumbens (Acc). Experiments show that specific drugs act on the Acc, the ventral tegmental area of the brainstem (VTA), and the locus ceruleus (LC). Abbreviations: DA, dopaminergic neurons; Enk, enkephalin- and other opiod-releasing neurons; GABA, GABA-ergic inhibitory interneurons; NE, norepinephrine-releasing neurons; THC, tetrahydrocannabinal. (Based on Gardner and Lowinson 1993.)

Leptin is a hormone released by fat cells. It acts on neurons in the hypothalamus that regulate feelings of hunger and satisfaction. Experiments on normal mice show that when the mouse has had an adequate meal, the leptin levels *increase*, and the mice leave the food for other pleasures. Some mice are different. They are obese, and they continue to eat even when their leptin levels rise. Genetic analysis shows that the receptor to which leptin binds can have a variety of mutations, and that the specific mutation predicts how overweight the animal is. For example, if the mouse has the *tu* mutation, it is somewhat tubby, relative to normals, and has *twice the leptin levels of normals*. If it has the *db* mutation, it is truly obese, and has ten times the leptin levels. There is something *very* different about the appetite regulation of the mutant animals (figure 5.5 shows the reward pathways).

If a person is born with the db mutation of the leptin-receptor gene, and if, in consequence, he feels as ravenous at the end of dinner as at the beginning, it seems inevitable that he will overeat. More precisely, it seems reasonable to assume that such a person will have less control over his eating behavior than a person with the standard version of the leptin receptor. He may have perfectly normal self-control when it comes to other matters, such as sex, alcohol, or gambling, but for food, his situation is markedly different because his leptin receptors in the hypothalamus are markedly different. The suggestion, therefore, is that the leptin receptor and its possible variations constitutes yet another component in the complex neurobiological profile of "in control" subjects, at least where food is concerned.

Many neural details remain to be uncovered, needless to say, but identifying the major neurochemical players is a profoundly important beginning. Beginnings such as these inspire the vision that neuroscience might ultimately be able specify a range of optimal values for the relevant parameters. When values fall within the optimal range, the agent's behavior is in his control. When values are suboptimal, the agent will be unable to control his behavior. In between, there may be gray areas where the agent is neither fully in control nor fully out of control (figures 5.6 and 5.7).[17]

Research from basic neuroscience as well as from lesion studies and scan studies will be needed to transform this speculative parameter space into a substantial, detailed, testable account of the features typical of in-control subjects. These properties may be quite abstract, for "in control" individuals may have different temperaments and different cognitive strategies.[18] As Aristotle might have put it, there are different ways to harmonize the soul. Nevertheless, the prediction is that some such general features probably are specifiable. It is relatively clear that dynamic-systems properties do distinguish between brains that perform well or poorly such tasks as walking. What I am proposing here is that more abstract skills, behaviorally characterized, such as being a successful shepherd dog or a competent lead sled dog, can also be specified in terms of dynamic-systems properties, dependent as they are on neural networks and neurochemical concentrations. My hunch is that human skills in planning, preparing, and cooperating, can likewise be specified. Not now, not next year, but in the fullness of time as neuroscience and experimental psychology develop and flourish.

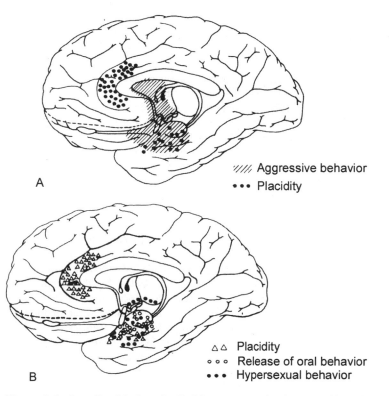

Figure 5.6 Localized lesions in limbic structures lead to specific behavioral changes. (A) Lesions resulting in increases in aggressive behavior and in placidity. (B) Lesions resulting in a release of oral behavior and in hypersexuality. (From Poeck 1969.)

In the next sections, we shall consider in more detail some of the evidence that speaks in favor of this general approach.

4.2 Are We More in Control and More Responsible When Emotions Play a Lesser Role and Reason Plays a Greater Role?

A view with deep historical roots assumes that in matters of practical decision, *reason* and *emotion* are in opposition. To be in control, on this view, is to be maximally rational and minimally emotional. To achieve rationality and self-control, one must maximally suppress emotions, feelings, and inclinations. In a metaphor sympathetic to this idea, Plato characterizes reason as a charioteer

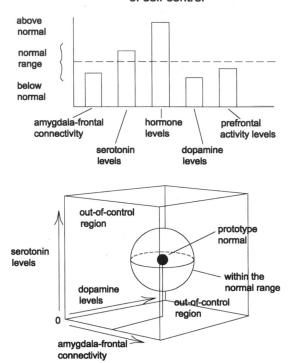

Figure 5.7 Some dimensions of control at the neural level. The top panel is a highly simplified representation of a subset of neural-level factors affecting self-control. The bottom panel is a parameter space in which the axes, drawn from the larger set of parameters, include leptin levels, amygdala-frontal connectivity, and serotonin levels. Values in the normal range would have to be determined experimentally. The parameter-space representation allows us to see that there are many ways of being normally in control, and many ways of being out of control, as a function of the values and interactions of many parameters. (Courtesy of P. M. Churchland.)

who is pulled along by the appetites and emotions, and who must beat them to avoid running amok.

Immanuel Kant is the philosopher best known for emphasizing on an opposition between reasons and emotions, and favoring the supremacy of reason. In his moral philosophy, Kant saw human agents as attaining virtue only as they succeed in downplaying feeling and inclination. He says, "The rule and direction for knowing how you go about [making a decision], without becoming unworthy of it, lies entirely in your reason. This amounts to saying that you don't learn this rule of conduct by experience or from other people's instruction; your own reason teaches and even tells you what to do."[19] The perfect moral agent, on Kant's view, is perfectly rational and entirely without emotion and feeling.[20] (Ronald de Sousa calls such an agent a "Kantian monster."[21])

The kinds of cases that inspire Kant's veneration of reason and his suspicion of the passions are the familiar heart-over-head blunders. In such cases, the impassioned do-gooder makes things worse, or one neglects long-term consequences while satisfying an immediate need. The fool does not look before he leaps. Othello, so overcome by jealousy that he failed to realize that he was being duped, kills Desdemona. In the grip of an overwhelming bitterness, Medea kills her children and herself. The moral failings of great tragedy are typically character flaws involving great emotions engulfing weak reason.

Understanding the consequences of a plan, both its long-term and short-term consequences, is obviously important, but is Kant right in assuming that feeling is the *enemy* of virtue, that moral education requires learning to disregard the bidding of inclination? Would we be more virtuous, or more educable morally, were we without passions, feelings, and inclinations?

Not according to David Hume. Hume asserted, "Reason alone can never be a motive to any action of the will; and secondly, it can never oppose passion in the direction of the will" (1739, 413). As he later explains, "'Tis from the prospect of pain or pleasure that the aversion or propensity arises towards any object: And these emotions extend themselves to the causes and effects of that object, as they are pointed out to us by reason and experience" (1888, 414). As Hume understands it, reason is responsible for delineating the various *consequences* of a plan, and thus reason and imagination work together to anticipate pitfalls and payoffs. But feelings, informed by experience, are generated by the mind-brain in response to anticipations, and incline an agent for or against a plan.

Common culture also finds something not quite right in the image of nonfeeling, nonemotional rationality. In the highly popular television series *Star*

Trek, three of the main characters are severally portrayed as typically hot-tempered, coldly reasonable, or moderate in all things. The pointy-eared semi-alien Mr. Spock lacks emotion. In trying circumstances, his head is cool and his approach is calm. He faces catastrophe and narrow escape with comparable equanimity. He is puzzled by humans' propensity to anger, fear, love, and sorrow, and correspondingly fails to predict the role of emotions in human affairs. Interestingly, Mr. Spock's cold reason sometimes results in bizarre decisions, even if they have a curious kind of "logic" to them.

By contrast, Dr. McCoy is found closer to the other end of the spectrum. Individual human suffering inspires him to risk much, ignore future costs, or fly off the handle, often to Mr. Spock's taciturn evaluation, "But that's illogical." The balance between reason and emotion is more nearly epitomized by the legendary Captain Kirk. By and large, his judgment is wise. He can make tough decisions when necessary; he can be merciful or courageous or angry when appropriate. He is more nearly Aristotle's ideal of someone who is wise in practical matters.

4.3   A Disconnection Effect: E.V.R.

Neuropsychological studies reveal a lot about the significance of feeling in wise decision making. Research by the Damasios and their colleagues on a number of patients with brain damage shows that when deliberation is cut off from feelings, decisions are likely to be impractical and disadvantageous in the long run. Thus S.M., whose amygdala has been destroyed, has no feelings of fear (see again figure 3.17). In complex circumstances, with no access to gut feelings of unease and fear, she is as likely as not to make a decision that normal people could easily foresee to be contrary to her interests.

In a rather more complex way, the point is dramatically illustrated by the remarkable patient E.V.R., who first came to the Damasios' lab at the University of Iowa College of Medicine more than a decade ago.[22] A brain tumor in the ventromedial region of E.V.R.'s frontal lobes had been surgically removed, leaving him with bilateral lesions. Following his surgery, E.V.R. enjoyed good recovery and seemed very normal, at least superficially. For example, he scored as well on standard IQ tests as he had before the surgery (about 140). He was knowledgeable, answered questions appropriately, and so far as mentation was concerned, seemed unscathed by his loss of brain tissue. E.V.R himself voiced no complaints. In his day-to-day life, however, a troubling picture began to emerge. Once a steady, resourceful, and efficient accountant, E.V.R. now made a mess of his tasks, came in late, failed to finish easy jobs, and so forth. Once a reliable and loving family man, he allowed his personal life to become a shambles. Because he scored well on IQ tests, E.V.R.'s problems seemed to his physician more likely to be psychiatric than neurological, and hence best treated with psychoanalysis. As we now know, the psychiatric diagnosis turned out to be quite wrong.

After studying E.V.R. for some time, the Damasios and their colleagues conjectured that his lapses in practical judgment had something to do with a disconnection between emotions and judgment. They repeatedly observed that although E.V.R. could state the correct answer to questions concerning what would be the best action to take (e.g., defer a small gratification now for a larger reward later), his own behavior often conflicted with his stated convictions (e.g., he would seize the small reward now, missing out on the large reward later).[23] When they tested whether E.V.R.'s emotional responses were in the normal range, they found intriguing abnormalities. For example, when shown horrifying or disgusting or erotic pictures, his galvanic skin response (GSR) was flat.[24] (Normals, in contrast, show a huge response while viewing such pictures.) Curiously, if asked to *say* what he saw in the pictures, E.V.R.'s emotional responses became somewhat more normal.

During the following years, new and more revealing tests were devised to probe more precisely the relation between reasoning logically and *acting* in accordance with reason. Antoine Bechara, working with the Damasios, developed a particularly revealing test. In this test, generally known as the Iowa Gambling Task, a subject is presented with four decks of cards and told only that his goal is to make as much profit as possible from an initial loan of money. Money can be made and lost as a function of turning over cards, one at a time, from any of the four decks. Subjects are not told how many cards can be played before the game ends (a series of 100) or what the payoffs are from any deck. One has to discover the winning strategy by trial and error. After a card is turned over, the subject is either rewarded with an amount of money or penalized and required to pay out money. Behind the scenes, the experimenter designates two decks, *C* and *D*, to be low-paying ($50) and to contain some moderate penalty cards; two other decks, *A* and *B*, pay large amounts ($100) but contain very high penalty cards. Things are rigged so that players incur a net loss if they play mostly *A* and *B*, but make a profit if they play mostly *C* and *D*. Subjects cannot calculate losses and gains exactly because there is too much mentally to keep track of (figure 5.8).

After about 15–20 trials, normal controls typically come to stick mainly with the low-paying/low-penalty decks (*C* and *D*) and duly make a tidy profit in the

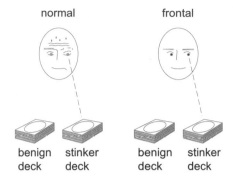

normal   frontal

benign   stinker   benign   stinker
deck   deck   deck   deck

Figure 5.8 The Iowa Gambling Task. Normal subjects begin to show autonomic-nervous-system reactions, such as perspiring, when they reach for the bad decks, but subjects with ventromedial frontal lesions do not. (Courtesy of P. M. Churchland.)

long run. In contrast, subjects with ventromedial frontal damage tend to end the game with a loss. They generally work the high-paying decks, despite the profit-eating penalty cards in those decks. Subjects with brain damage to regions other than ventromedial behave like controls. Yet the ventromedial patients had normal IQs.

As Bechara et al. note, even after repeated testing on the gambling task, as long as a month or as short as 24 hours later, E.V.R continued to play the losing decks heavily. When queried at the trial end, inevitably he correctly *reports* that *A* and *B* are losing decks and rues his strategy. To put it rather paradoxically, *rationally* E.V.R. does indeed know what the best long-run strategy is, but in exercising choice in actual situations, he goes for short-run gain, incurring long-run loss. To make matters more difficult for the Kantian ideal, his judgments of recency and frequency are flawless, his knowledge base and short-term memory are intact. Because E.V.R. can articulate well enough the future consequences of alternative actions, the problem cannot be lack of understanding of what might happen. That his "pure reasoning," displayed *verbally*, is at odds with his "practical decision making," displayed in *behavior*, suggests that the crux of the problem lies with E.V.R.'s lack of emotional responsivity to complex plans.[25]

Additional results came from a deeper analysis of skin conductance data taken by a galvanometer placed on the arm of each subject during the gambling task.[26] In the gambling task, neither controls nor frontal patients showed a skin response to card selections in the first few plays of the game (selections 1–10). By about the tenth selection, however, controls began to exhibit a skin response when they reached for the bad decks. When queried at this stage about how they were making their choices, controls (and frontal patients) said they had no idea whatever; they were just exploring. By about selection 20, controls continued to get a consistent skin response when starting to reach for the "bad" decks. In their verbal reports, controls said that they still did not know what was the best strategy, but that they had a feeling that maybe decks *A* and *B* were "funny." By selection 50, controls typically could articulate and follow the winning strategy. Frontal patients never did show a skin response in reaching for any deck. They remain free of any affective guidance. What is so striking is that for control subjects, choice was biased by feelings even before subjects were clearly aware of their feelings, and well before they could articulate the winning strategy. That many of our daily choices are likewise biased, without our being clearly aware of our feelings, seems likely.[27]

The significance of nonconscious biasing by emotion has implications for the economists' favored model of "rational choice." According to this model, the ideally rational (wise) agent begins deliberation by laying out all alternatives, calculating the expected utility for each alternative by multiplying the probability of each outcome by the value (goodies accruing) of each outcome. He ends by choosing the alternative with the highest expected utility score. In light of the data just considered, this model seems highly artificial, at least for the ongoing daily activity of actual humans. Perhaps it is roughly correct for a small range of somewhat artificial problems where the life-oriented computations that yield up the *relevant* options have already been performed. The point is that normally in the on-going business of life, the set of options we consciously consider is restricted by prior nonconscious, emotive-cognitive computation, i.e., restricted by the "dirty" computation that gives us a set of (mainly) relevant, sensible, and meaningful alternatives. This is a kind of computation about which we know very little. At any rate, the economists' model is unlikely to come even close to giving the whole story of rational choice, though it may be helpful once the set of reasonable alternatives is laid out.

On many occasions, one's brain seems to have things pretty well sorted out before conscious deliberation even begins. For example, in the grocery store I rarely bother to consider Delicious apples, since they are usually punky; I am not fond of eggplant, so I never pause over the eggplant bin. I never consider drinking a can of paint; I never ponder whether to make a fur bathing suit or porridge skis. I never consider beginning logic class with a demonstration of how to milk a cow. And so forth. All these are descriptions of options my brain *could* consciously entertain, but does not.

Subject A

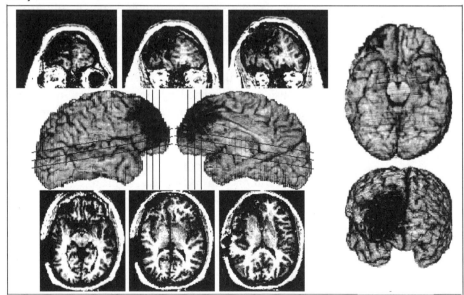

Subject B

One lesson taught us by E.V.R. and others with similar lesions (ventromedial frontal) is that whatever rationality in decision making *actually is*, independence from emotions is not its essence. When E.V.R. is confronted with a question ("Should I finish this job or watch the football game?" "Should I choose from deck *A* or from deck *C*?"), he is missing important emotional clues that something is foolish or unwise or problematic. Normally, neurons in the ventromedial frontal cortex project to and from areas such as the anterior cingulate cortex, amygdala, and hypothalamus, which contain neurons signaling body-state values. In patients with destruction of ventromedial cortex, the pathways are disrupted. Their frontal lobes, needed for a complex decision, have no access to information about the emotional valence of a complex situation, plan, or idea. Consequently, some of their behavior turns out to be foolish and unreasonable.[28] The point is not that patients like E.V.R. feel nothing at all. Rather, it is that in those situations requiring imaginative elaboration of the consequences of an option, feelings are not generated in response to the imagined scenario, because the ventromedial frontal region needed for integration of body-state representation and fancy scenario-spinning is disconnected from the gut feelings. In particular, the capacity to remember relevantly similar occasions with a recollection imbued with evaluative significance, is impaired.

An even more worrisome behavioral profile is seen when the prefrontal lesions occur early in development. Anderson and colleagues reported on two adults patients whose prefrontal lesions occurred before the age of 16 months.[29] Both scored normally on various intelligence tests, but both were severely impaired in their social behavior. In addition, they also showed defective social and moral reasoning, which suggests that the capacity to acquire moral understanding was itself diminished by the early lesions. Whereas E.V.R. and other late-onset lesion patients might do things that are socially inappropriate or foolish, they do understand and abide by moral rules (figure 5.9).

Figure 5.9 Neuroanatomical analysis. (a) A 3-D reconstructed brain of subject A. There was a cystic formation occupying the polar region of both frontal lobes. This cyst displaced and compressed prefrontal regions, especially in the anterior orbital sector, more so on the left than on the right. Additionally, there was structural damage in the right mesial orbital sector and the left polar cortices. (b) A 3-D reconstructed brain of subject B. There was extensive damage to the right frontal lobe, encompassing prefrontal cortices in the mesial, polar, and lateral sectors. Both the lateral half of the orbital gyri and the anterior sector of the cingulate gyrus were damaged. The cortex of the inferior frontal gyrus was intact, but the underlying white matter was damaged, especially in the anterior sector. (Reprinted from Anderson et al. 1999.)

4.4   Agents and Self-Representational Capacities

If the various emotions play an ongoing and indispensable role in formulating practically wise plans, both long-term and short-term, how does this fit into the framework for agency, self-representation, and consciousness developed in chapters 3 and 4? The answer is best laid out by referring once more to the Grush emulator. As discussed earlier, to a first approximation, the motivation for actions is anchored in the fundamental drives for food, sex, and survival. As plans develop, the imagination generates representations of plan sequelae. To these internally driven scenarios, as well as to perceptually driven representations, emotional responses are generated, via mediation of the brainstem structures, amygdala, and hypothalamus.[30] The central function of the emulator is to predict and evaluate consequences of proposed actions. As we saw, the emulator can be employed on-line in making immediate decisions and off-line for high-level decisions involving longer time scales. The various emotions have a central role in evaluating options and their consequences as threatening, rewarding, dangerous, risky, painful, satisfying, and so forth. If these affective states also represent the difference between threatening to *him* and threatening to *me*, then the states are, on Damasio's hypothesis, conscious feelings. In the context of acquired cognitive-cum-emotional understanding about the world, neuronal activity in these pathways calls forth certain memories, directs attention to certain perceptual and imaginative functions, and imbues certain perceptions with practical significance. In contrast to the computational mode of an iMAC or a PC, this is bio-computation, i.e., *dirty, me-relevant computation*.

The neural evaluation and assessment of options probably resembles less the clean, step-by-step execution of an algorithm than it does the rough-and-tumble jostling among puppies for access to the food supply. That is, the process whereby neural networks settle into the next decision probably involves a kind of competition, and the winning option moves ahead for assignment of detailed movements. To put it crudely in the familiar framework of folk psychology, a desire for immediate gratification can be outweighed by the fear of missing out on a more valuable good in the longer run; the pain of exercise can be endured for the sake of envisioned improvement in skiing performance; long and dreary hours in the lab are sustained by the glimmering possibility of satisfying one's curiosity. On those occasions when a weighty decision involves conscious deliberations, we are sometimes aware of the inner struggles, describing ourselves as having conflicting or ambivalent feelings. Some processes in decision-making take longer to resolve than others, and hence the wisdom in the advice to "sleep on" consequential decisions. Everyone knows that sleeping on a heavy decision tends to help us settle into the "decision minimum" we can best live with, though exactly how and why are not understood. Are these longer processes classically rational? Are they classically emotive? Probably they are not fittingly described by our existing vocabulary. They are the processes of a dynamical system settling into a stable attractor.

Introspection, as we know, is a highly limited and fallible guide to the dynamical aspects of these inner processes, and folk psychology is at best a crude interpretive filter in any case. Though introspection gives us some sense of the neural hurly-burly subserving choice, we have little conscious access to its neural nature. Nevertheless, good models of the interplay and competition among parameters, whatever exactly they are, will probably emerge in time.

According to conventional wisdom, *cognitive* factors are used to predict consequences, while *emotive* factors are used to evaluate the consequences, and the two are entirely separate functions. From the point of view of the brain, however, the situation is not that simple. The very formulation of certain general goals, such as going to college or starting a business, likely employs an inseparable alloy of cognitive-emotive elements. This is also true of more specific goals, such as taking the dogs to the beach or finding a babysitter. Scene segmentation and pattern recognition in perception are, save for unusual circumstances, shot through with affect and meaning. In momentous decision making, such as the decision to find the accused guilty or the decision to opt for doctor-assisted suicide, the competition alluded to is never a one-dimensional struggle between reason and emotion, but rather is a complex interplay between *this* cognitive-emotive consortium and *that* cognitive-emotive consortium. The decision to have a latte rather than a cappuccino is, relatively speaking, a completely trivial decision. Our choice really does not amount to a row of pins. Such trivial choices are not, however, the model for those life decisions which mark us as wise or foolish, as impulsive or measured, as lazy or ambitious. Consequently, in developing adequate models of decision making, we would do well not to make the latte-cappuccino choice the paradigm for choice generally.

5   Learning What's Reasonable and What's Not

Aristotle would have us add here the point that there is an important relation between self-control and habit formation. A substantial part of learning to cope with the world, defer gratification, show anger and compassion appropriately, and have courage when necessary involves acquiring appropriate *decision-making habits*. In the metaphor of dynamical systems, this is interpreted as contouring the terrain of the neuronal state space so that behaviorally appropriate trajectories are "well grooved" or strongly attractive. Clearly, we have much to learn about what this consists in, at both the behavioral and neuronal levels. We do know, however, that if an infant has damage in critical regions, such as the ventromedial frontal cortex or amygdala, then typical acquisition of the proper "Aristotelian" contours may be next to impossible, and more direct intervention may sometimes be necessary to achieve what normal children routinely achieve as they grow up.[31]

The characterization of a choice or an action as *rational* carries a strongly normative component; it is not sheerly descriptive. In contrast, consider describing an action as performed hurriedly, or with a hammer. Claiming that an action is rational normally carries the implication that the choice was conducive in some significant way to the agent's interests or well-being, or to those of kith and kin; that it properly took into account the consequences of the action, both long-term and short-term. Thus the evaluative component. Though a brief dictionary definition can capture some salient aspects of what it means to be rational and reasonable, it hardly does justice to the real complexity of the concept.

As children, we learn to evaluate actions as more or less rational by being exposed to prototypical examples of rational actions, as well as of foolish or unwise or irrational actions. Insofar as we learn by example, learning about rationality is like learning to recognize patterns in general, whether it be recognizing what is a dog, what is food, or when a person is afraid or embarrassed or weary.[32] As Paul Churchland has argued, we also learn ethical concepts such as fair and unfair, kind and unkind, by being shown prototypical cases and slowly learning to generalize to novel but relevantly similar situations.[33]

Peer and parental feedback fine-tune the pattern-recognition networks so that over time they come closely to resemble the standard upheld in the wider community. Nevertheless, as Socrates was fond of showing, articulating those standards is awesomely difficult, even when a person successfully uses the term "rational," case by case. Discriminating the reasonable from the unreasonable is a cognitive-emotive skill, like discriminating whether the river is now navigable by canoe, or whether and how attacking an enemy's position will succeed. Using prototype knowledge, we can see how Scott's skill in conducting his Antarctic exploration was pitiful, while Amundsen's was superb. Making the term "rational" precise in a way that fulfills the conditions for an algorithm is almost certainly impossible. Failures in programming computers to conform even roughly to common sense, or to understand what is relevant, are an indication of the nonalgorithmic, *skill-based* nature of rationality.

This is important, because most philosophers regard the evaluative dimension of ethical concepts to imply that their epistemology must be entirely different from that of descriptive concepts. What appears to be special about learning some concepts, such as rational, impractical, and fair, is that the basic wiring for feeling the appropriate emotion must be intact. That is, the prototypical situation of something's being impractical or shortsighted typically arouses unpleasant feelings of dismay and concern; the prospect of something's being dangerous arouses feelings of fear, and these feelings, along with perceptual features, are probably an integral part of what is learned in perceptual pattern recognition.

Frankly dangerous situations—crossing a busy street, encountering a grizzly with cubs—can likely be learned as dangerous without the relevant feelings. At least that is suggested by the Damasios' evidence from their patient S.M., who, as a result of amygdala destruction, has no feelings of fear. Although she can identify which *simple* situations are dangerous, this seems for her to be a purely cognitive, nonaffective judgment. Her recognition is poor, however, when she needs to detect menace or hostility or pathology in complex social or marketing situations, where no simple formula for identifying danger is available. As argued earlier, the appropriate feelings may be necessary for skilled application of a concept, if not for fairly routine applications. This is perhaps why the fictional Mr. Spock, lacking emotions, is plausibly poor at predicting what will provoke strong sympathy or dread or embarrassment in humans.

Stories, both time-honored ones and those passing as local gossip, provide a basic core of scenarios where children imagine and feel, if vicariously, the results of such choices as failing to prepare for future hard times (*The Ant and the Grasshopper*), failing to heed warnings (*The Boy Who Cried Wolf*), being conned by a smooth talker (*Jack and the Beanstalk*), vanity in appearance (*Narcissus*). As children, we can vividly feel and imagine the foolishness of trying to please everybody (*The Old Man and His Donkey*), of not caring to please anybody (Scrooge in Dickens's *A Christmas Carol*), and of pleasing the "wrong" people (*Pinocchio*). Many of the great and lasting stories, for example by Shakespeare, Ibsen, Tolstoy, Aristophanes, are rife with moral ambiguity, reflecting the fact that real life is filled with conflicting feelings and emotions. They remind us that simple foolishness is far easier to avoid than great tragedy.

Buridan's dithering ass was just silly.[34] Hamlet's ambivalence and hesitation was deeply tragic and all too human. In the great stories also is a reminder that our choices are always made amidst a deep and unavoidable ignorance of many of the details of the future, where coping with that very uncertainty is something about which one can be more or less wise. For all decisions save the trivial ones, there is no algorithm for making wise choices. Matters such as choosing a career or a mate, having children or not, moving to a new country or not, deciding the guilt or innocence of a person on trial, deciding whether to surrender or press on are usually complex constraint-satisfaction problems.

As we deliberate about a choice, we are guided by our reflection on past deeds, our recollection of pertinent stories, and our imagining the sequence of effects that would be brought about by choosing one option or another. Antonio Damasio calls the feelings generated in the imagining-deliberating context "secondary emotions" to indicate that they are a response not to external stimuli, but to internally generated representations and recollections.[35] As we learn and grow up, we come to associate certain feelings with certain types of situations, and this combination can be reactivated when a similar set of conditions arises. Recognition of a present situation as relevantly like a certain past case has, of course, a cognitive dimension, but it also evokes feelings that are similar to those evoked by the past case, and this is important in aiding the cortical network to relax into a solution concerning what to do next. This is the platform for one's neuroconscience.

6   Uncaused Choice Considered Again

Much of this chapter has focused on the emerging account of the neurobiology of decision making. The hypothesis on offer is that there are systematic neurobiological differences between being *in control* and being *out of control*, and that these differences can be characterized in terms of fuzzy-bordered subvolumes of the multidimensional parameter space. The in-control subvolume of the space may be relatively large, allowing for the fact that in-control humans have different habits, cognitive styles, emotional tone, and so forth. Similarly, the out-of-control subvolume may be very large, reflecting the fact that dysfunction to the reward system may yield an out-of-control profile that is very different from that of a dysfunctional anterior cingulate cortex, which in turn is different from that of a degenerating basal ganglia.

As noted in section 2, there are spirited defenses of a totally different hypothesis, namely that decisions made by in-control subjects are actually *uncaused* decisions, whereas decisions made by out-of-control subjects are *caused*. The most modern variation defends the idea that quantum indeterminacy is at the root, somehow, of uncaused choice. Though briefly introduced earlier, it is time now to reconsider the idea that real choice requires a break in causality milliseconds prior to the emergence of the brain state that constitutes the choice. An empirical hypothesis, it deserves to be weighed and evaluated as an empirical hypothesis and compared to the rather different picture of the brain discussed above.

Hume and his arguments aside, the credibility of the noncausal-choice hypothesis depends on whether it can mesh with what is known so far about neurons and nervous systems. Defenders of the hypothesis want it to be *consistent* with existing well-established neurobiological data, not openly to clash with the data. The hypothesis is that among the many details neuroscience has not yet discovered is this fact: for quantum mechanical reasons, voluntary choice is uncaused. Our task here is to ask whether, given what *is* well established neurobiologically, this appears to be a plausible hypothesis with promising research prospects. The hypothesis classifies a choice as voluntary if and only if it is uncaused. Caused choices, therefore, are deemed not free. As usual, we can begin by raising questions to which the hypothesis should have some noncontrived answers.

Why and how does a break in causality occur just for those particular brain events that supposedly are paradigm cases of choice? How does the brain work so that a simple behavior in conformity with good habit—routinely putting on my seat belt, for example—*is* caused, whereas choosing a latte rather than a cappuccino after dithering is *not* caused? What prevents these special noncausal events from occurring when a nicotine addict reaches for another cigarette or a child sucks its thumb or a highly trained but off-duty spy surveys his fellow passengers for assassins? If, as is entirely likely, the brain events constituting choice are distributed across many neurons, how is noncausality (quantum indeterminacy) orchestrated across the relevant population? If the brain events constituting choice are uncaused, what precisely are their relations to background desires, beliefs, habits, emotions, and so forth? Philosophical fantasies floated in abstraction from the tough and detailed constraints of the real world have an "in a single bound Jack was free" quality. Flippant answers to empirically informed questions are, of course, always possible: "It just works like that" or "Magic!" Unless the hypothesis can interdigitate with neurobiology and cognitive science to come up with nonfrivolous answers to these questions, however, it will continue to look nakedly ad hoc.

Before the hypothesis can be taken seriously, it will have to garner empirical confirmation and survive empirical tests. If uncaused choice is a quantum-level effect, as may be supposed, the aforementioned questions, as well as those raised in section 2, demand empirical answers. Under *exactly what conditions* do the supposed noncaused events occur? Does noncausal choice exist only when I am dithering or agonizing between two equally good—or perhaps equally bad—alternatives? How do quantum-level effects know (so to speak) when to occur and when not? Beyond the business of *decisions*, do quantum-level indeterminacies exist with respect to such processes as the generation of *desires*? Or *beliefs*? Why not? How is it they come into play with only some conscious decisions but not others? Does this break in causality occur at the synapse? If advocates of noncaused decision-making are serious, they will have to do more than wave the flag of quantum-level indeterminacy and claim that in a single bound choice is free. They will have to get into the business of empirical confirmation.

7   What Happens to the Concept of Responsibility?

We need now to return to the dominant background question motivating this chapter: if choices and decisions are caused, is anyone ever really responsible for his actions? One very general conclusion is provoked by the foregoing discussion. On the whole, social groups work best when individuals are presumed to be responsible agents. Consequently, as a matter of practical life, it is probably wisest to hold mature agents responsible for their behavior and for their habits. That is, it is probably in everyone's interest if we match up assignment of responsibility with being in control and adopt the default assumption that agents have control over their actions. Barring clear evidence that an agent's behavior was in the out-of-control subvolume of the parameter space, the agent is liable to punishment and praise for his actions. This is, of course, a highly complex and subtle issue, but the basic idea is that *feeling* the social consequences of one choices is a crucial part of socialization—of learning to be in the give-and-take of the group. It is part of acquiring the appropriate Aristotelean habits.[36] *Feeling* those consequences is necessary for contouring the parameter-space landscape in the appropriate way, and that means *feeling* the approval and disapproval meted out. Having social institutions that reinforce those feelings helps maintain civil life.

A child must learn about the physical world by interacting with it and bearing the consequences of his actions, or by watching others engage the world, or by hearing about how others engage the world. Similarly, learning about the social world involves direct or indirect cognitive-affective learning about the nature of the social consequences of a choice. This must, of course, be consistent with reasonably protecting the developing child, and also consistent with compassion, kindness, and understanding. In short, I do not want the simplicity of the general conclusion to mask the tremendous subtleties of child rearing. Nevertheless, if the only known way for "social decency" circuitry to develop requires that the subject generate the relevant feelings pursuant to social pattern recognition, then the responsibility assumption may be preferable to any version of a thorough-going assumption of nonresponsibility.

This leaves it open, of course, that under special circumstances agents should be excused from responsibility or be granted diminished responsibility. In general, the law courts are struggling, case by case, to make reasonable judgments about what those circumstances are, and no simple rule really works. Neuropsychological data are clearly relevant here, as for example in cases where the subject's brain shows an anatomical resemblance to the brain of E.V.R. or S.M. Quite as obviously, however, the data do *not* show that no one is ever really responsible, that no one is really deserving of punishment or praise. Nor do they show that when life is hard, one is entitled to avoid responsibility. To most of us, the "Twinkie defense" seems a travesty of justice, but so does ignoring someone's massive lesion in the ventromedial frontal cortex.

Is direct intervention in the circuitry morally acceptable? This too is a hugely complex and infinitely ramifying issue. My personal bias is twofold. First, in general, at any level, be it an ecosystem or immune system, intervening in biology always requires immense caution. When the target is the nervous system, then caution by another order of magnitude is warranted. Yet not taking action is still doing something, and *acts of omission can be every bit as consequential as acts of commission.*

Second, the movie *Clockwork Orange*, typically conjured up by the very idea of direct intervention by the criminal justice system, probably had a greater impact on our collective amygdaloid structures than it deserves to have. Certainly, some kinds of direct intervention are morally objectionable. So much is easy. But *all* kinds? Even pharmacological? Is it possible that some forms of nervous-system intervention might be more humane than lifelong incarceration or death? I do not wish to propose specific guidelines to allow or disallow any form of direct intervention. Nevertheless, given what we now understand about the role of emotion in reason, perhaps the time has come to give such guidelines a calm and thorough reconsideration. Approaching these questions with a careful Aristotelian determination to be as wise as possible may be preferable to giving free rein to unreflective self-righteousness. Ideological fervor, on the right or on the left, can often do greater harm than unhurried common sense.

8   Conclusions

I have considered three vintage philosophical theses in the context of new data from neuroscience: (1) feelings are an essential component of viable practical reasoning about what to do (David Hume), (2) moral agents come to be morally and practically wise not by dint of "pure cognition" but by developing through life experiences the appropriate cognitive-affective habits (Aristotle), and (3) the default presumption that agents are responsible for their actions is empirically necessary to an agent's learning, both emotionally and cognitively, how to evaluate the consequences of certain events and the price of taking risks (R. E. Hobart, Moritz Schlick). Each of the theses has been controversial and remains so now; each has been the target of considerable philosophical criticism. Now, however, as the data come in from neuropsychology, experimental psychology, and basic neuroscience, the empirical probability of each thesis has increased. Consequently, many important social policy questions must be considered afresh, including those concerned with the most efficacious means, consistent with other human values, for achieving civil harmony. Much, much more needs to be learned, for example about the reward circuits in the brain, about pleasure and anxiety and fear. Philosophically, the emphasis with respect to civic, personal, and intellectual virtue has been focused almost exclusively on the purely cognitive domain, with the affective domain largely left out of the equation, as though the Kantian conception of reasoning were in fact correct. In matters of education and social policy, how best to factor in feeling and affect is something requiring a great deal of informed mulling and practical wisdom. In any case, my hope is that understanding more about the empirical facts of decision making, at both the neuronal and behavioral levels, may be useful as we aim for practical wisdom and ponder improvements in our social policy.

Suggested Readings

Aristotle. 1955. *The Nichomachean Ethics*. Trans. by J. A. K. Thompson. Harmondsworth: Penguin Books.

Bechara, A., A. R. Damasio, H. Damasio, and S. W. Anderson. 1994. Insensitivity to future consequences following damage to human prefrontal cortex. *Cognition* 50: 7–15.

Campbell, C. A. 1957. Has the self "free will"? In his *On Selfhood and Godhood*, 158–179. London: Allen and Unwin.

Churchland, P. M. 1995. *The Engine of Reason, the Seat of the Soul*. Cambridge: MIT Press.

Cooper, J. R., F. E. Bloom, and R. H. Roth. 1996. *The Biochemical Basis of Neuropharmacology*. 7th ed. Oxford: Oxford University Press.

Damasio, A. R. 1994. *Descartes' Error*. New York: Grossett/Putnam.

Damasio, A. R. 1999. *The Feeling of What Happens*. New York: Harcourt Brace.

Dennett, D. C. 1984. *Elbow Room: The Varieties of Free Will Worth Wanting*. Cambridge: MIT Press.

Le Doux, J. 1996. *The Emotional Brain*. New York: Simon and Schuster.

Walter, H. 2000. *Neurophilosophy of Free Will: From Libertarian Illusions to a Concept of Natural Autonomy*. Cambridge: MIT Press.

Wegner, D. M. 2002. *The Illusion of Conscious Will*. Cambridge: MIT Press.

Websites

BioMedNet Magazine: http://news.bmn.com/magazine

Encyclopedia of Life Sciences: http://www.els.net

The MIT Encyclopedia of the Cognitive Sciences: http://cognet.mit.edu/MITECS

II   Epistemology

6 An Introduction to Epistemology

1 Introduction

Epistemology is the study of the nature of *knowledge*. Its core questions are these: *what* things do we know, and *how* do we know them? Two competing traditions, both originating in Greece in the fifth century B.C., contour the intellectual landscape. Plato (427–347 B.C.) and Aristotle (384–322 B.C.) are the principal sources for these separate traditions, for they adopted largely distinct strategies. To grasp the reality behind how things seem to be, Plato bet on mathematical or a priori reasoning from the armchair, while Aristotle bet on exploration of the natural world.

Plato contended that learning is really recollection; most of what we call learning he thought to be the uncovering of innate knowledge. How that innate knowledge got into our heads in the first place he never satisfactorily addressed. Plato believed that coming to understand reality consists in the intellectual apprehension of abstract objects, objects that exist not in the physical world but in a timeless "realm of the intellect," later dubbed "Plato's Heaven." For Plato, the ideal kind of knowledge was mathematical knowledge. Mathematical knowledge, in contrast to observation-based opinion about the natural world, was certain, immutable, systematic, and universal. Or so it seemed to Plato, and to Platonists ever since.

By contrast, Aristotle, Plato's most celebrated pupil, emphasized the importance of delineating successful *methods*—how best to use evidence and reasoning—in acquiring reasonable beliefs about world and how it works. In wondering how we perceive, reason, remember, and learn, Aristotle took a more naturalistic approach. He believed perception and memory to be natural functions facilitating the acquisition of knowledge, and he assumed that their operations could be best understood by observation and experimental manipulation. On the question of how memories are stored, for example, Aristotle suggested that experiences "impress" themselves on the stuff of the mind, thus leaving a semipermanent physical trace. When investigating our capacity for knowledge, Aristotle focused less on *metaphysical* questions, such as whether the soul survives the body's death, and more on concrete "How does it work?" questions asked about eyes and ears.

To a first approximation, the Plato/Aristotle division in strategy has demarcated epistemology ever since. Note, however, that the distinction between the Platonic and Aristotelian methodologies is mainly a difference in *emphasis*, since Platonists perfectly well realize that if you want to know whether it is raining, you have to look, and Aristotelians perfectly well realize that imagination and reasoning are important in figuring out how the world really works.

Where the methodologies really diverge is on problems that cannot be solved just by looking—problems concerning the nature of the reality hidden behind observable appearances. On such matters, those of the metaphysical predilection see the naturalists as fudging the Big Questions, while those with a naturalistic bent see the metaphysicians as stuck spinning their wheels.

With the rise of modern science in the Renaissance, the Platonic strategy was forced to make concessions regarding our knowledge of the physical world. Empirical techniques for determining causal mechanisms for physical processes like burning and breathing were demonstrably more successful than nonempirical methods, such as reading sacred texts or trying to deduce the nature of reality from metaphysical principles that were often both contentious and obscure.

One major development concerned the nature of fire. As a result of his explorations into combustion, the French chemist Lavoisier laid the groundwork for the division between elements and compounds between 1772 and 1785. He figured out that during combustion, an *invisible gas* was *combined* with burning wood. This gas was later referred to as *oxygen*. The long-standing theory that this conflicted with said that combustion involved the *ejection* of a substance called phlogiston, which allegedly gave off heat and light. In other words, the conventional wisdom had the dynamics exactly backwards. With the new understanding of burning in hand, Lavoisier then went on to develop the equally surprising idea that animal respiration too consisted of the combination of oxygen with carbon. This suggested a provocative and rather heretical continuity between mechanisms in living and nonliving things.

Other experimental explorations were equally surprising. By passing light through a carefully constructed prism, Newton (1642–1727) showed ordinary light to be a mixture of colored light, ranging from violet to red. In biology, the allegedly obvious spontaneous generation of flies was demonstrated to be false by enclosing meat in a tightly lidded container and leaving it for a few days. The germ theory of disease gradually overturned the religiously grounded *punishment theory of disease* after Lister and Semmelweis showed that soap scrubs by surgeons reduced lethal infections and Pasteur showed that heat killed microbes in food and water. And what of the mind/brain? Not until the nineteenth century were empirical techniques systematically brought to bear on the nature of *psychological* capacities, including the capacity to know.

2   The Rise of Empirical Philosophy in the Nineteenth Century

In his 1862 treatise, Wilhelm Wundt lamented that psychology, unlike physics and chemistry, had scarcely advanced since Aristotle's explorations almost two thousand years earlier. He urged empirical psychology to liberate itself, first, from the metaphysical preoccupations of philosophers and, second, from the idea that introspection and logic are jointly sufficient to understand the nature of the mind. Wundt's cautions against uncritical reliance on introspection has a modern ring: "self-observation cannot go beyond the facts of consciousness, . . . [and] the phenomena of consciousness are *composite products* of the unconscious psyche" (Wundt, 1862/1961, 57; my emphasis).

Wundt's idea of composite products was a direct challenge to philosophers using naive introspection to identify sensory simples. By "simple," they meant something that could not be analyzed or decomposed or reduced any further. This was important to epistemologists because they assumed such simples must be the foundation for knowledge. From what he knew about the sensory system, Wundt realized that lots of nonconscious processing had to go on before one was aware of a color or shape or sound. And, of course, Wundt was perfectly correct: certain favorite philosophical "simples," such as the pain from a burn, are now known to be combinations of somatosensory and hedonic components processed in different brain regions. (See pp. 117–118.) These components are dissociable with drugs or by lesion.

Besides encouraging replicable empirical studies of perception and memory, Wundt realized that the empirical study of the mind needed to develop in three areas in particular: cognitive development in childhood, comparisons between the cognition of humans and other animals, and the effects of social interaction on individual cognition. This latter study he called "Volkerpsychologie," translated as "folk psychology." His three-fold proposal, like his caution concerning introspection, was a masterstroke, though mainstream epistemology, especially in the twentieth century, largely ignored all three domains characterized by Wundt.

The early techniques for the empirical investigation of the mind/brain were somewhat crude, at least as judged against today's toolbox. There were no MRI machines, no computers, and no microelectrodes for recording or stimulating single neurons. Indeed, not until the end of the nineteenth century were neurons finally identified as the cellular units of nervous activity, and even then, the nature of the intricate communication between neurons remained a mystery.

Despite these handicaps, the pioneering psychologists—such as Helmholtz, Wheatstone, and Wundt—realized that to get significant results in a science of the mind, they needed well defined, well controlled experiments and the instrumental means for measuring and quantifying the results. And stunning discoveries were indeed made. Thomas Young, actually quite early in the nineteenth century, had already figured out that color vision must depend on merely three types of light-sensitive receptor (red, green, and blue). Wheatstone demonstrated for the first time that depth perception exploits the fact that each eye gets a slightly different image of the world. Helmholtz showed how the sound-induced vibration of the hairs embedded in the wide-to-narrow basilar membrane of the cochlea was the physical basis for the audible tones ranging from low to high pitches. Helmholtz also realized that what we are immediately aware of in perception involves cognitive filtering—what he called "unconscious inferences."

Some philosophers, especially Alexander Bain, William Hamilton, and others in the so-called Scottish school, recognized the potential in a scientific study of the mind, and they pushed hard for its development.[1] Metaphysically inclined philosophers, on the other hand, tended not to regard any of this as progress in *epistemology*. They considered the important philosophical work to lie elsewhere; for example, in figuring out a priori the "necessary conditions for the possibility of knowledge" (the Kantians) or how a normatively justified knowledge structure could be built on a foundation of self-justifying sensory simples (the British Empiricists). For reasons we shall discuss presently, the nonexperimental stream was the one that survived as the officially recognized discipline of philosophy. Alexander Bain and the Scottish school are names unknown to most contemporary philosophers. Like Wundt and Helmholtz, they are now considered unimportant to the central concerns of *genuine* philosophy, however important they might be to psychology or physiology.[2]

3   Empirical Philosophy and Darwin

Darwin's theory of natural selection has profound epistemological implications. If humans and human brains are the product of eons of Darwinian evolution, and if human capacities for perceiving, learning, and knowing are capacities of the brain, then these capacities are products not of divine creation, but of our evolutionary history. In particular, if humans are born with not mere *capacities* but also a priori *knowledge*, then such knowledge would have to have its origin in our evolutionary history, not in divine engineering. So the existence, character, and accuracy of inborn representations, if such there be, has to fit within a comprehensive biological framework that includes what we know about neural development in individuals and comparisons between human and nonhuman brains (figures 6.1 and 6.2). This point was made earlier in the introduction to metaphysics. I make it again and develop it further in this chapter because mainstream epistemology, arguably the backbone of the academic discipline of philosophy, continues to do business as though Darwin never happened. That is, the profound discoveries of evolutionary biology have scarcely touched mainstream epistemology.

Darwin published *The Origin of Species* in 1859. Selective breeding of domestic animals such as dogs, horses, and sheep was a practice well developed by farmers long before the nineteenth century. Beginning with wolves, humans conducted generations of selective breeding to produce dogs as different as cocker spaniels, bassets, greyhounds, and Newfoundland retrievers. There are individual differences in offspring, and animal breeders select among individuals for breeding those whose traits—color, ear length, water-loving—they want to see in later offspring.

Darwin realized that an entirely *natural* process of selection, without a breeder's controlling selection of the breeding pairs, could also result in selective breeding, albeit much more slowly than breeding by farmers. *Natural selection*, Darwin argued, could occur if an animal happened to have traits that enhanced its capacity to thrive in a particular environment and it survived to reproduce and pass on those favorable traits to its offspring. Most important, he realized that variation among individuals in the offspring sometimes includes mutations, with the result that natural selection can eventually yield *completely distinct, noninterbreedable species*. By and large, he knew, mutations are deleterious, but occasionally a mutation may occur that results in a trait that happens to be beneficial to an animal in a particular environment. Over

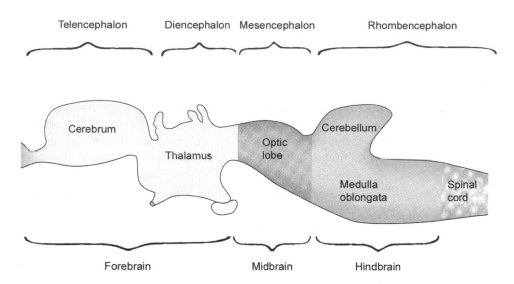

Figure 6.1 Evolution of the vertebrate brain. Ancestral regions of the vertebrate brain—the forebrain, midbrain, and hindbrain—are subdivided in animals that appeared later in evolutionary history. In mammals, the forebrain radically increased in size relative to the olfactory lobe, midbrain, medulla, and thalamus.

long periods of time, highly distinctive species could emerge, while others might disappear, elbowed aside, as it were, by their more successful competitors. And just as natural selection can yield animals with fur or feathers, so it can yield animals with very fancy nervous systems.

Humans, just like other organisms on the planet, must compete for resources to survive and reproduce. Adaptation to the environment through the evolution of brain-based capacities, especially the capacities to perceive, learn, predict, and solve puzzles was undoubtedly significant in the survival of our species. Obviously, some of the capacities demonstrated by modern humans, for example the ability to read or juggle or skate, were not selected for *as such*. Rather, these culturally enabled capacities arise from other more general capacities, such as intricate pattern recognition and motor learning, that presumably did play an important role in the life of primitive hominids.

What is selected is really the *whole animal*, and that means the whole package—weaknesses and strengths, warts and all. So if a trait is to become common in a population, the whole animal that has that trait must reproduce to yield offspring that also have that trait. DNA is the heritable material. Genes are segments of DNA that code for proteins. No gene can code directly

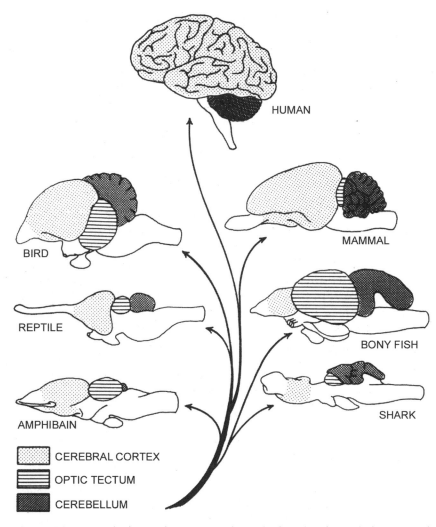

HUMAN

MAMMAL

BIRD

REPTILE

BONY FISH

AMPHIBAIN

SHARK

CEREBRAL CORTEX

OPTIC TECTUM

CEREBELLUM

Figure 6.2 Lateral views of seven vertebrate brains showing relative expansion of major brain divisions. In humans, the olfactory bulb is not visible from the lateral aspect, since it lies on the ventral aspect of the frontal lobes, which are greatly expanded in humans relative to reptiles and rodents. Brains are not drawn to scale. (Based on Northcutt 1977.)

for an organ or a capacity or a trait; *genes can code only for stuff: specific proteins or RNA.*

It is, of course, common to speak loosely of particular functions being selected by Darwinian evolution. Unless we are careful, this shorthand can suggest that natural selection is a bit like a fairy godmother who reaches down into an animal and its DNA, makes base-pair changes in DNA with a magic wand, and lo, a whole new trait appears or an old trait is miraculously optimized. That, of course, is Cinderella-style magic; it does no work in the real biological world. Consequently, it is implausible to suppose that human language or consciousness or decision making are owed to a wholly new *software package* that just happened to get plugged into existing hardware. Certainly, human software *engineers* might design a wholly new software package and install it in a modestly upgraded computer. Biological evolution, however, works very differently from technological evolution (figures 6.3 and 6.4).

Are human brains similar to the brains of other mammals? Indeed they are, and the closer humans are to another species genetically, the closer the similarity in brain anatomy. Humans and chimpanzees share about 98 percent of their DNA; humans and mice share about 90 percent. The human brain and the chimpanzee brain are, so far as is known, very similar anatomically, but human and mouse brain, apart from size, are also similar organizationally (figure 6.5).

There are some differences between human brains and other mammalian brains, notably in overall brain size and in the size of certain general structures relative to others. Rats, for example, have a cortex largely devoted to olfaction, but the macaque-monkey cortex is largely devoted to vision. We all have essentially the same organization in the spinal cord, brain stem, thalamus, and cerebellum. An early hint of these similarities came from François Magendie and Charles Bell, who independently discovered as early as 1807 that the sensory nerves enter the *dorsal* segments of the spinal cord, and the motor nerves exit the *ventral* segments. This pathway specialization holds for all vertebrates, whether rat, lizard, or human (figure 6.6).

Sensory signals in the gustatory, olfactory, somatosensory, and auditory systems follow the much same routes, even in fish and mammals. For example, signals from taste buds on the palate of humans and catfish travel via the seventh cranial nerve into the medulla to the nucleus of the solitary tract and then upwards to the peribrachial nucleus. In the brain, there are differences. In humans and monkeys, but not in catfish, some fibers go directly from the nucleus of the solitary tract to the thalamus.

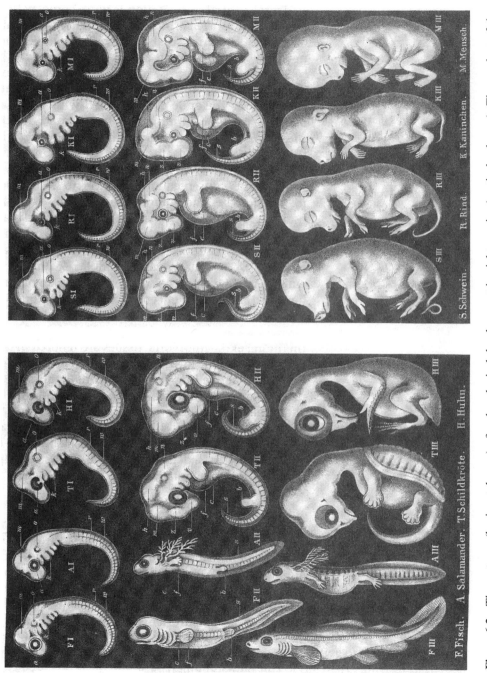

Figure 6.3   Three stages (horizontal rows) of embryological development in eight species (vertical columns). The product of the earliest stages in vertebrate development (the pharyngula, top row) is similar across species, with similar patterns of segmentation and early eye development. In the middle row, limb buds have formed, and although the mammalian embryos (pig, deer, rabbit, and human) are still quite similar to one another, they are now distinct from the fish, salamander, turtle, and chick embryos. In the bottom row, more obvious differences have emerged between mammals and nonmammals, as well as among mammals. (Reproduced from Haeckel 1874.)

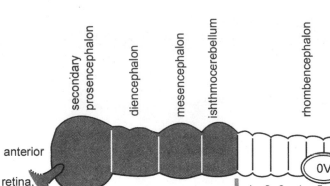

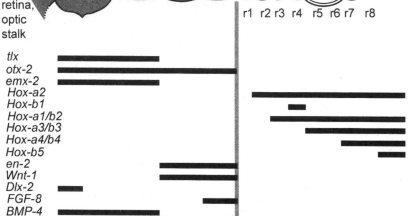

Figure 6.4 The nervous system plan in chordates. Anterior is to the left, dorsal is up. The list to the left identifies specific genes that are expressed (e.g., *Hox* genes) and signal proteins that are secreted (BMP-4, Wnt, and FGF). The gray lines to their right show the regions in which the genes and the signal proteins organize development of specific divisions. (From Gerhardt and Kirschner 1997.)

No unique structures—structures without *any* homologues in other mammals —are in evidence, at least so far as is known. Even frontal regions, long believed to be suggestively larger in humans, relative to other brain structures such as the cerebellum and thalamus, appear in recent anatomical measurements to stand in much the same ratio to other brain structures across all primates and even across all mammals. That is, we do have a larger prefrontal cortex than rats, monkeys, and chimpanzees, but we also have a larger cerebellum, brainstem, sensory cortex, and motor cortex than rats, monkeys, and chimpanzees (see again figure 5.1).[3]

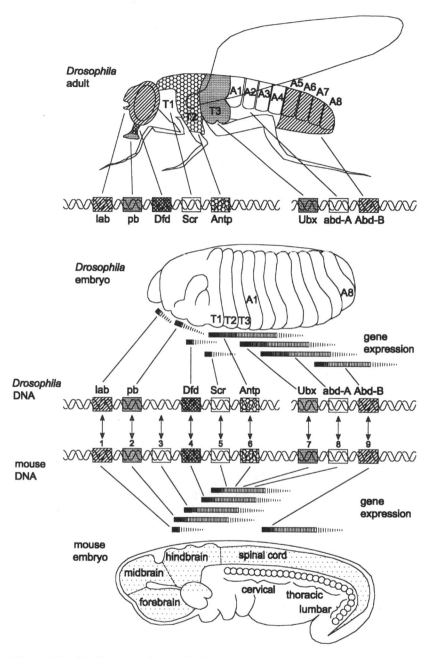

Figure 6.5 Similar spatial organization of compartments by *Hox* gene expression in arthropods and chordates. Top: *Drosophila* adult. Center: *Drosophila* segmented embryo at about 10 hours (phylotypic stage). Bottom: mouse pharyngula embryo at about 12 days (phylotypic stage). Notice that the anterior to posterior compartment order is the same in the phylotypic stages of both *Drosophila* and the mouse, reflecting the 3′–5′ order of genes on the chromosome. (Based on Gerhardt and Kirschner 1997.)

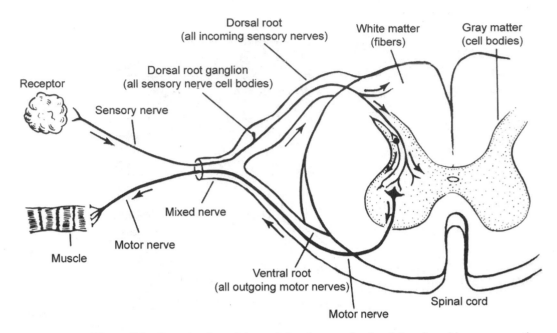

Figure 6.6 Organization of the peripheral nerves in chordates viewed in a cross-section of the spinal cord at right angles to the cord. Sensory signals enter the cord through neurons in the dorsal roots, and motor signals leave the cord via the motor neurons in the ventral roots.

Some behavioral similarities between humans and other mammals indicate similarity of wiring in certain systems. Human babies, monkeys, and even rats "screw up the face" when given something sour to taste. They one and all smack their lips when given something sweet. And they spit out something bitter. We all learn bait shyness in one trial; that is, if a novel food is followed after some hours by nausea, or if a familiar food in a novel place is followed by nausea, we avoid the novel food or the familiar food in the novel place. This is also true of many nonmammals, including birds, as was first shown by John Garcia and colleagues in 1974. As Darwin emphasized, emotions such as fear, disgust, joy, and anger are expressed in very similar ways across species (figure 6.7).

Molecular analyses have revealed that the very same neurochemicals found in the human brain are found in the nervous system of leeches and worms, as well as reptiles, birds, and mammals.[4] Moreover, the physiology of neurons is largely unchanged throughout the animal kingdom; neurons in spiders work

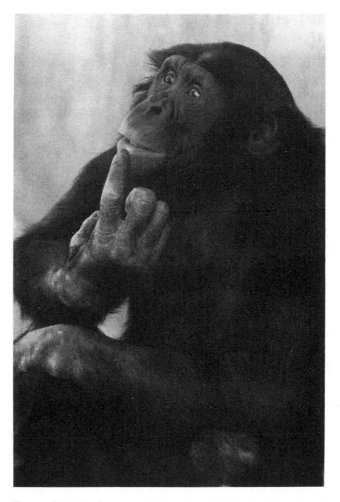

Figure 6.7	Kevin, an adolescent male bonobo from the San Diego Zoo, striking a philosophical pose. (Photo by Frans de Waal.)

essentially the same as neurons in humans. The degree of genetic conservation across species is truly surprising. (See also p. 324.)

Seen naturalistically, the mind is what it is because the brain is what *it* is. The human brain is an evolved device, bearing the stamp of conserved structures and reflecting the natural necessity to eat or be eaten and to mate successfully or not. Some human capacities might have been fancier had a clever engineer designed our brains from scratch. For example, a clever engineer might have given humans a fourth cone type that allowed us to see in the ultraviolet range and also allowed us to discriminate the blues much more finely. A fifth cone type for discerning x-rays and a sixth for microwaves might have been handy as well. It might have been nice to have had built into the material brain the knowledge of mathematics as well as explicit knowledge that the brain, rather than an immaterial soul, is the thing that thinks. Built-in knowledge of what substances make good anesthetics would also have been a great boon to mankind. Personally, I have always wanted to speak Mandarin without having laboriously to learn it. These innate capacities, however, we do not have. Either there was no evolutionary pressure for the development of these capacities, or if there was, no preadaptive structures were in place to be exploited in new ways.

Biological evolution thus raises a very general problem for a priori epistemology. According to the a priori tradition, knowledge about how the mind works is innate. It depends on deduction, introspection, and reflection to be made explicit. The problem is this: Given biological evolution, what could be the Darwinian explanation for the inborn existence of factually correct knowledge about the way the mind/brain works? What could have been the selection pressures? Evidently, there was insufficient selection pressure for innate, factually correct knowledge of the nature of fire, reproduction, disease, the origin of the Earth, and the nature of matter. All these things had to be figured out empirically. Mind/brain function is a natural, biological phenomenon, and here too the likelihood that correct factual knowledge of its mode of operation is *built in* seems far-fetched. Certain perceptual or organizational dispositions might be innate, but a priorists need the stronger claim implied by "innate *knowledge*."

A priori epistemology could command some plausibility when it was thought that the human mind was created by a divine being, who allegedly could plant in the mind whatever he deemed appropriate. At this stage of human understanding, however, divine creation of the mind looks far less probable than its biological evolution. Consequently, such plausibility as a priori epistemology might have enjoyed in the heyday of the theological view of the world evaporates in a scientific view of the world.

4 Why Does Nonempirical Epistemology Still Exist?

Why did traditional (nonempirical) epistemology continue to thrive as a discipline well into the twentieth century? Why do we still have nonempirical epistemology? I discern two main reasons for this, though there are undoubtedly others. The first explanation derives from the fact that the naturalistic project has been very difficult to bring to maturity: brains are complex, fragile, and very difficult to figure out. The second explanation, largely but not wholly independent of the first, concerns the rise of modern logic: its enormous power, its Platonic proclivities, its seductive beauty, and the fact that it is technologically and computationally so very compliant—so very *biddable*, as one might say. Modern logic seemed, for various reasons, to be an ideal tool for a priori epistemology.

4.1 Slow Progress in the Natural Science of the Mind/Brain

What obstacles did the naturalistic program face? These have been touched on in chapter 1, but they can be drawn out a little here. Imagine looking at a slice of cortex under a light microscope. What do you see? Unless the neurons are selectively stained to stand out, not much. The development of stains to render individual neurons visible was crucial to the development of neuroanatomy as a discipline, and it was not achieved until late in the nineteenth century. Suppose that we have applied a Golgi stain to the tissue, so that about 10 percent of the neurons are filled with the stain and hence are visible against the teeming population of other cells (figure 1.4). *Now* what do you see? Unless you are quite lucky, probably not a great deal. Neurons are three-dimensional, and a single slice of neural tissue under a light microscope reveals only a *two-dimensional layer* of the stained neurons. You need slices fore and aft in order to see more of a neuron's axons and dendrites. In a cubic millimeter of cortex, there are about 10^5 neurons and about 10^7 synapses. Synapses are many, and they are small. A synapse (about 1–2 microns) cannot be seen except with an electron microscope, a device not invented until the mid 1950s. An invention of the early 1990s, two-photon laser microscopy allows the experimenter see neurons below the cortical surface, as well as calcium ions moving into a neuron following an action potential.

These are just the merest handful of the challenges facing *anatomists*. What about the *physiology*? There too, highly specialized skills and techniques had to be devised from scratch for extracting meaningful responses from individual *living* neurons and from groups of neurons. Merely preventing the neuron from dying before you got a measure of its activity was a major feat.

A lesion is an area of damaged brain tissue and can occur as a result of stroke, tumor, closed head injury, dementing diseases, and so forth. Studying humans with brain damage was, and still is, an extremely important technique for addressing how the nervous system is organized, what its parts do, and how activity in one part affects activity elsewhere. Nevertheless, in lesion studies, problems constantly arose because the effects of lesions can be markedly different in babies than in adults, because the deficits caused by lesions can change dramatically over time, and because in humans, lesions from stroke, tumors, and so forth, could not be precisely located until autopsy. This meant that interpretation of the behavioral data from lesion studies was persistently problematic. Scanning technology, developed in the last three decades, has largely solved the problem of lesion-localization in living humans (pp. 18–20).

Other obstacles, more subtle perhaps, were due not to technological frustrations but to *conceptual* blocks, that is, to the lack of concepts adequate to thinking about the problem or to articulating the right questions. Concepts are the cognitive lenses we use to see the world and to think about it, and when they are darkened by ignorance and distorted by error, our perception of the world is likewise distorted and confused.

Consider an example. When William Harvey (1578–1657) began research on the heart, his guiding question was this: exactly *where* in the heart are the "vital spirits" concocted? His question reflected the respectable, conventional, too-obvious-to-be-questioned wisdom of his time. According to this conventional wisdom, blood was continuously and copiously made in the liver. The job of the heart was to make vital spirits (by virtue of which life existed) by mixing air from the lungs with blood from the liver. The reason death followed the cessation of heartbeat was that the vital spirits ceased to be concocted.

In one of the great stories of science, Harvey ended up discovering something utterly different from what he sought. He discovered that the heart was actually a meaty pump, blood circulates around the body, and blood is continuously made, but not by the pint per minute and not in the liver at all. Shockingly, Harvey's discoveries implied that almost certainly there were no vital spirits concocted in the heart—or anywhere else either. To come to see this, he had to doff the conceptual lenses of the framework of spirits—vital, animal, and natural—and don a completely different set of lenses. This he did: "Medical schools admit three kinds of spirits: the natural spirits flowing through the veins, the vital spirits through the arteries, and the animal spirits through the nerves, . . . but we have found none of these spirits by dissection, neither in the veins, nerves,

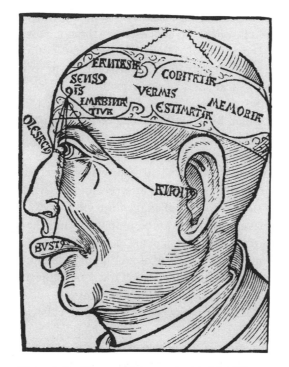

Figure 6.8   The ventricles, as depicted by Hieronymous Brunschwig in the 1525 edition of his book from 1497. (From Finger 1994.)

arteries nor other parts of living animals."[5] Thenceforth the conceptual framework of spirits was in decline.

From Galen (A.D. 130–200) until Vesalius (1514–1564), the conventional wisdom about brains specified that the *ventricles* in the brain—the cavities filled with fluid—were the seat of perception and cognition (figure 6.8). Now, however, we are reasonably sure it is the *neural tissue* that perceives and remembers, with the fluid in the ventricles serving a basically nutritive function. Galen had it just backwards: he thought the *holes* were important for cognition, and the tissue played a supporting role. The ventricular hypothesis was supported by the wider framework of vital spirits—animal and natural. If animal spirits were the wherewithal for cognition, then as *spirits*, they were most likely to be housed in holes, rather than in the meat. Obviously.

Conceptual obstacles included the aforementioned difficulty with specifying mind/brain functions. In probing the mind/brain, nineteenth-century scientists commonly assumed that there were fundamentally three functions: sensory, motor, and the association of ideas. Too simple by orders of magnitude. To others it seemed reasonable to suppose that the complexity in behavior is the outcome of combinations of simple reflexes, such as the eye-blink reflex, the gag reflex, and the knee-jerk reflex. This opinion gave rise to a reflex-based theory of physiological mechanism. Again, this is too simple by orders of magnitude. In this century it has seemed reasonable to suppose that specific functions are handled by dedicated "centers" or modules, which, like different computer applications, operate independently of what is going on elsewhere in the brain. Again, too simple by orders of magnitude.[6] Until the 1980s and 1990s, it also seemed plausible that neurons passively receive signals in the dendrites, integrate the signals, and at a certain threshold of current, the axon sends an active signal. This is called the "integrate-and-fire" model. Alas, dendrites are not passive, signals can be amplified, and the spike sent down the axon can be propagated back up the dendrites. Additionally, more distant dendritic segments have the means of amplifying their signals so that such signals do not decay by the time they reach the soma. Integrate-and-fire is far too simple, even if a reasonable starting point. This has suggested to some neuroscientists that in fact the basic processing unit is not the *neuron* but segments of *dendrite*.[7]

The daunting nature of the problems, conceptual and experimental, has left much scope for creative theorizing, and as noted in chapter 1, that is what philosophy was in its heyday in ancient Greece. Evidently, theorizing, on a small scale and grand scale, is one thing neurophilosophers—along with neuroscientists and empirical psychologists—must *still* do.

From the vantage point of hindsight, a lot of theorizing seems to be an utter waste of time. In a certain sense, it is. Nonetheless, even getting things wrong is not a waste of time, since falsification at least helps narrow the search space. Groping for a torch is what you have to do when you are in the dark, and until some light appears, nothing is obvious. Exploration of conventional wisdom, of the received framework—questioning it, beating on it, and seeing what alternatives look like—is just part of what has to occur until the science is sufficiently established that it does not need such tumult anymore. Perhaps, of course, even *seemingly established* sciences continue to benefit from some tumult, simply because "well established" is never equivalent to "certainly true." The smug claims in the nineteenth century that physics was complete remind us of that particular lesson. Nevertheless, some stages are more tumultuous than others.

Benefiting from a handful of sensible hunches, Democritus in the fifth Century B.C. argued that the reality behind the apparent diversity of objects and substances must be "atoms"—indivisible, invisible units that hook up together in different ways to yield different kinds of stuff, such as gold or hair. A waste of time, perhaps, and yet it was a speculation that nipped at the heels of natural philosophers until, lo and behold, by the time Dalton and Lavoisier started to ponder the nature of elements and change, Democritus's speculation could be seen to be on the right track. Many other speculations, including some that rose to orthodoxy, turned out to be dead wrong, such as that fundamentally there are four elements—earth, air, fire, and water—or that fundamentally, diseases arise from possession by devils or as divine punishment.

Getting the science even more or less right, however, is very, *very* hard, and it is inevitable that most theories will end up on the scrap heap. What we cannot do, however, is get along without theories altogether. We need some concepts with which to see and think about the world; we always need *some* hypotheses to frame the questions that motivate research. *Pure* observation does not really exist, and *idle* observation generally doesn't take you very far. Since there are no algorithms for creating correct hypotheses, there are bound to be many false starts. But without false starts, there are likely no starts at all.

In sum, although it has been difficult to make progress in psychology and neuroscience, the strategy of pursuing epistemology in isolation from scientific data is, I modestly opine, unwise. Managing as best as one can with meager data is very different from turning your back on relevant data while justifying such back-turning on grounds that philosophy is, after all, an a priori discipline. On the positive side, philosophers have thoroughly explored the potential for a priori theorizing about the nature of the mind. Thus its shortcomings, as well as strengths, are clearly visible.

4.2   Logic, Recursion, and Cognition

So far my explanation of why epistemology endures has focused on the technical and scientific obstacles besetting a natural (i.e., scientific) theory of the mind/brain. Although this explains why slow progress might have discouraged some philosophers, it does not explain why a priori epistemology eclipsed empirical epistemology in the twentieth century. There are undoubtedly a number of pertinent sociological factors, such as the personal magnetism of Oxford philosopher G. E. Moore (1873–1958).

Moore set a trend in philosophy that exalted what he called "common sense." In his view, common sense was to be valued not merely over foolish enthusiasms, but even over scientific theories or philosophical theories that were inconsistent with commonsense ideas. By "common sense" Moore did not mean, however, just what the common person means; he had in mind an understanding achievable by paying close, *very* close, attention to precisely what we really mean (or perhaps *should* mean) by particular words. Clarity is, to be sure, a good thing. But Moore's strategy inspired the idea that analysis of the meaning of the word "*x*" led to the *truth* about the *nature* of *x*. Thus philosophers could claim to have a "method" that was not only a priori but even more fundamental than the methods of science. This was sometimes referred to as the linguistic turn in philosophy, though it was also derided by a few as philosophy's turning into a dead end. And now enter modern logic.

The dedicated—even celebrated—isolation of philosophy from the empirical sciences of the mind/brain was also connected, I suspect, to a great achievement: the rise of modern logic. Logic was typically understood within an essentially Platonic framework: it supposedly captured universal logical laws, true independently of any actual human reasoning, laws true in any possible universe.

The rise of modern logic is a story about a beautiful idea that braided together several threads: (1) An algorithm is a "mechanical" procedure that can be applied a finite number of times to crank tremendously complex structures out of very simple elements.[8] (2) If you identify the right set of basic elements and algorithms and pound out the right definitions, arithmetic and mathematics *generally* can be shown to be a system whose truths are *reducible* to the truths of *logic*. The envisioned reduction would be a great achievement, because then mathematical truth would not be so mysterious; it would be just a part of logic. This reductionist program is known as *logicism*. (3) Logic itself, and reasoning *generally*, is just a complex structure resting on a finite set of basic elements and definitions, with a finite set of rules or algorithms for cranking out complex structures out of simpler structures. If this is true, then we can understand the fundamentals of *reasoning*—and perhaps *knowledge* as well—by figuring out the basic elements, rules, and definitions.

Bound together, these three ideas were appealing, for they implied that logic is a well-defined *system*, composable and decomposable by dead-simple mechanical rules. Since Aristotle, logic had been a kind of hodge-podge of useful rules of thumb. Modern logic pulled together a coherent and powerful *system* out of the unconnected bits and pieces of ostensible logical truths. Cranking out logical complexity from logical simplicity by recursion was surprisingly fruitful for another reason: to the imaginative, such as Charles Babbage and later John von Neumann and Alan Turing, it suggested *mechanical computation*, which suggested computers, which suggested mechanical *thinking*.[9]

The logicians realized that even if mathematics were reduced to logic, what made *logical* truths *true* still had to be explained. Here Platonism—the theory that the truths of logic are true because they inhabit Plato's heaven—still appealed to some logicians, most notably Frege. Others, such as Carnap, preferred to find an account with a lighter metaphysical burden. One attractive idea was that logical truths are true by virtue of the *meanings* of their terms. Roughly, this means that the axioms were definitionally true and the theorems were guaranteed true by the rules operating on the axioms. The beauty of this approach was that logical truth, and hence mathematical truth, no longer requires the semimystical objects in Plato's heaven. They require just understanding the *meaning* of terms in the language and using rules. Much mystery about logic and mathematics seemed on the verge of disappearing. Thus *meaning*, in the story as told by Carnap, came to take center stage.

Carnap believed that the systematic power of mathematical logic had unheralded potential, and he pushed to extend the application of the resources and methods of logic from the reduction of mathematics to broader philosophical issues. In particular, Carnap, as well as others with less interest in science, such as G. E. Moore, suggested that *meaning* and *analysis* of the meanings of terms were the keys to making progress not only about logic and reasoning, but also about terms used in reasoning, such as "belief," "desire," "reality," and so forth. This meaning-oriented, language-dominated approach is usually referred to as *logical empiricism*, and in its later incarnations, as *analytic philosophy*. The explanation for the pair of names reflects the epistemology this approach embraced. The crux of the approach can be summarized in three claims:

- Human knowledge is made up of sentences, of which there are two kinds: (1) *analytic* sentences, whose truth depends *solely* on the meanings of the terms they contain, and (2) *synthetic* sentences, whose truth, given the meanings of the terms, depends on how the world is.

- There are two kinds of knowledge: (1) *a priori* knowledge (essentially logic plus knowledge of the meanings of words) and (2) *a posteriori* knowledge (knowledge of how the world is). The foundation of all synthetic knowledge, including therefore scientific knowledge, consists of primitive observation sentences whose truth we know directly, such as "This is round" or "This is yellow." Belief in any nonprimitive empirical sentence ("This is a lemon") is justified by logic and definitions. The two kinds of truth (analytic and synthetic) map onto the two kinds of knowledge (a priori and a posteriori).

■ Many, perhaps most, philosophical problems disappear when the logic of the language and the meanings of terms are properly *analyzed*. The meanings of terms may not always be obvious. Much subtle analysis may be required to reveal the deep meaning below the surface. Analysis consists of reflection, consideration of counterexamples, thought experiments, and reasoning. It requires philosophical training.

This set of convictions launched a program concerning how to do philosophy and how to address classical philosophical issues. For one thing, the approach had an appealing clarity. At the very least, it seemed far less obscure than the theories pushed by neo-Kantians and Hegelians, who were wont to debate issues about the unreality of space and time. Notice, however, that despite including the word "empiricism" in its name, logical empiricism was, in certain crucial respects, more Platonic than empirical in spirit. To begin with, the new logic was really designed to make a hand-in-glove fit with *mathematics*, not with the psychology of perceptual processing or with spatial or temporal problem solving or with the use of images in reasoning. It was the reduction of *mathematics to logic* that motivated the development of the new logical machinery, and the logical machinery was shaped accordingly.

For another, questions about knowledge were walled off from empirical studies about how people and other animals actually know and learn. "Linguistic" epistemology was largely restricted to a priori reflection on the meanings of such words as "knowledge," "justification," "person," "mind," and their deductive environments, as revealed through reflection. Thought experiments, as opposed to results from actual experiments, were considered to have a special role in revealing so-called *conceptual necessities*, such as the "necessary conditions for having a mind," or the "necessary conditions for the possibility of any knowledge." Conceptual necessities, since they were *necessities*, were supposed to tell us something beyond science about how the mind and its conceptual framework had to work. And that meant "work in *reality*." So the search for conceptual necessities was the disguise philosophers used to sneak past the limitations of talking about what words commonly mean, to talking about how things actually are, without worrying about what science says on the matter.

In the period from about 1910 to 1931 the program of the logical empiricists appeared to go moderately well. Before long, however, several disasters struck. The first was this: it turned out that logic plus definitions are *not* sufficient to reduce mathematics. The reduction also required *set theory*. Well, if set theory is axiomatically as secure as logic, is logic plus set theory so bad? Alas, the needed axioms from set theory were hardly as self-evident as the axioms of logic, such as "No sentence *p* is *both* true and false."

For starters, several *nonobvious* set-theoretic propositions had to be introduced as axioms to avoid crippling paradoxes on the one hand and deductive inadequacies on the other. One such assumption was that there exists an infinity of objects. This assumption not only failed to satisfy the ideal of being self-evidently true or true by virtue of meaning alone, it looked quite possibly *false*. Or at least, if it were true, its truth depends on how the empirical world is, not on the meanings of words, nor on any Platonic objects, for that matter. If you avoided that axiom, other axioms even less self-evident had to be invoked. Alas, these befell a similar fate.

Second and perhaps most devastating, the original goal of Frege and Russell proved to be impossible. Not merely difficult to achieve, but impossible. In 1931, the mathematician Kurt Gödel proved that no matter how you axiomatized arithmetic, as long as the axiomatization was consistent, you could *not* crank out all the truths of arithmetic.[10] In other words, if the axiomatization was *consistent*, it was not *complete*. Hence, Gödel's result is known as the Incompleteness Result. Because the tools of modern logic enabled Gödel to prove his result, the proof was both undeniably brilliant and horribly galling. The logicist program, ironically, was unable to succeed precisely where it had seemed most promising.

These disasters might have motivated a quiet shift to *empirical* epistemology, but oddly enough, they did not, by and large. It was as though the hive decided to try to continue even though the queen was dead. In particular, philosophers hoped that logic could be used to reveal the structure of knowledge of the empirical world and how it rested on a foundation of sensation sentences. If the bagel had a hole in it, they hoped that at least the outside was still fairly substantial.

To keep their hopes alive, the logical empiricists needed to prove their claim that sensation sentences are the foundations of belief structures. The idea was that we have direct knowledge of sensations, but not of objects in space and time, let alone of things like genes and gravity. Direct knowledge was supposed to be unmediated by processes such as inference. (See also pp. 117–118.) So physical-object sentences (e.g., "My cow is brown," "The sun is hot") had to be reduced to or justified by sensation sentences (e.g., "Brown here now" and "Cow smell here now"), plus definitions, along with the resources of logic.

A host of problems undermined the "direct knowledge" of sensation-sentences story. As noted earlier (p. 117), Wundt had realized that the "phe-

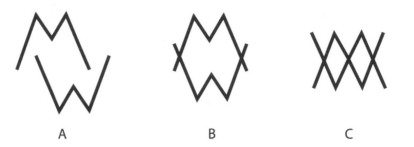

Figure 6.9   The effects of perceptual organization. The letters M and W are obvious in (A), less so in (B), and are fully camouflaged in (C). The stimuli are the same in each case; only the spatial relations change. (From Palmer 1999, with permission.)

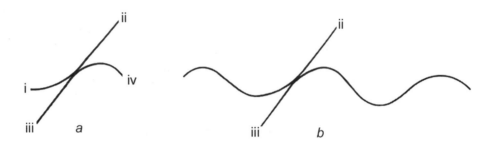

Figure 6.10   A grouping effect studied by Gestalt psychologists. (a) the law of good continuation predicts that subjects visually group (i) and (ii) as forming one object, and (iii) and (iv) as forming a second object. (b) However, when the same pattern is embedded in a larger context, subjects see a line (iii–ii) intersecting a wave. (From Rock 1975.)

nomena of consciousness are composite products of the unconscious psyche." Seemingly direct knowledge is always a product of prodigious nonconscious processing. Because empirical research on perception, learning, and reasoning was assumed to be irrelevant to the business of philosophy, little if any attention was paid to empirical research showing that our "noninferential perceptions," such seeing a set of lines as forming a specific shape (figures 6.9 and 6.10) or smelling an odor as of a rotting carcass, are in fact the results of highly complex processing even though conscious inferences are entirely absent. (For more detail on these problems, see chapter 7.) The "foundations" part of the program was therefore in deep trouble.

So was the project to deduce or otherwise justify truths about objects ("The cow is in the barn") from truths about sensations ("Brown here now").

The envisioned deduction was simply impossible to achieve, even though great ingenuity went into drumming up suitable definitions to fuel the engines for the sought-after deductions. Even softening the criteria for justification still left the object sentences deductively unreachable from the sensation sentences. Not even the more modest attempt of justifying very simple laws of nature (such as "All mammals are warm-blooded") from observations sentences about sensations ("Warm furry thing here") could get to first base. Carnap's heroic but ultimately vain attempt in 1928 to push forward the logicist project in epistemology convinced many philosophers that perhaps the project was fundamentally misconceived. Nevertheless, philosophers by and large still did not see any wisdom in the empirical epistemology of Wundt, Helmholtz, and the Scottish School.

Hopes drifted towards the possibility of dispelling various "philosophical puzzles" by analyzing the meaning of problematic words and laying bare the clean logic of sentences. This was essentially G. E. Moore's strategy, and it got a boost when Wittgenstein abandoned the logicist strategy and turned to the contemplation of meaning and the delivery of obscure aphorisms.[11] Analyses of meaning and thought experiments came to be considered philosophical tools par excellence. Using these contemplative procedures, ill-defined though they were, was advertised as leading to the discovery of so-called "conceptual necessities" or "conceptual truths," which were supposed to reveal a priori truths about knowledge, perception, reasoning, causality, and so forth. They were certainly not truths that one could acquire simply by consulting a dictionary, for the process of meaning analysis required long philosophical training.

Unfortunately, alleged "analyses of meaning" were often thinly disguised propaganda for someone's doctrinal hobbyhorse.[12] Typically, "thought experiments" were unconstrained, poorly defined, and impossible to evaluate. They legitimized a lot of clever but unprofitable wrangling concerning what could and could not be imagined, what the significance of some "thought experiment" was supposed to be, how to weigh counter-thought-experiments, and on and on. Since criteria to evaluate underdescribed thought experiments are a bit like criteria for evaluating the virtues of fairies over gnomes, making recognizable progress was difficult.[13] Probably the most devastating, though largely ignored, criticism was served up by Paul Feyerabend: analysis of the actual meaning of "*x*" only tells you what some people in a certain place and at a certain time believe about *x*s. It does not tell you *anything* about what is true about *x*s.

What decisively weakened the linguistic-analysis program was a set of vexing problems and a counterproject proposed by Harvard philosopher W. V. O.

Quine. Recall that the mainstay of the logical empiricists' approach to meaning was the existence of a principled "analytic/synthetic" distinction. Analytic sentences arc variously specified as *necessarily* true, true by virtue of the meanings of the concepts (which, allegedly, sometimes requires *deep* philosophical analysis). Analytic sentences are said to be *conceptual* truths. The falsity of an analytic sentence is supposed to be *inconceivable, unimaginable,* and so on. Hence the reliance on thought experiments. Synthetic sentences, by contrast, are true by virtue of the facts. If this distinction turned out to be rotten, the program would be in tatters.

In the 1950s Quine realized that the analytic/synthetic distinction was *at best* a continuum, not a genuine two-bin dichotomy. Moreover, he concluded that no distinction between analytic sentences and synthetic sentences *would do the work* that the logical empiricists required. He first observed that the expressions "analytic truth," "necessary truth," "true by virtue of meanings alone," and so forth, were all defined, if at all, *in terms of one another*, holding hands in one suspiciously small circle. This convenient circularity raised the worry that philosophers were deluding themselves into supposing that the claims made for the analytic/synthetic distinction were true and that the a priori epistemology based on those claims was making real progress on the nature of knowledge, representation, learning, and perception.

Having raised this suspicion, Quine then went on to argue that in fact, there was no respectable principle for sorting truths in general into distinct analytic and synthetic bins. The root of the problem, Quine saw, was that what we believe about a phenomenon is not neatly separable from the meanings of the words we use in describing the phenomenon. For example, there seems to be no clean line between the generalizations we believe are factually true of penicillin and what we mean by the word "penicillin." Ditto for "electrons," "DNA," "gravitational fields," "emotions," and "memory." So-called "conceptual necessities" are just firm—sometimes *very* firm—convictions, rather than fundamental truths about the nature of reality as revealed by pure reason. As mere convictions, they were no more instruments of progress than any other conviction.

Cannot one just *stipulate* a boundary between what we believe about a *phenomenon* and what we believe about the *meaning of the word* for the phenomenon? Then the analytic/synthetic story could be salvaged. That strategy is ultimately as useless in propping up the analytic/synthetic distinction as stipulating that the Earth does not move on grounds that what we mean by "Earth" is "thing that does not move." Such a stipulation merely registers someone's decision to hold some sentences—the so-called analytic ones—to be true no matter *what the evidence*. Such stubbornness is indefensible in view of the proclivity of science for discovering very surprising things and overturning very deep convictions. For example, scientists discovered that Earth moves around the Sun, even though obvious observations powerfully suggest otherwise. The issue of whether Earth *does* move around the Sun cannot be settled by the claim, *even if correct*, that part of the very meaning of "Earth" is "thing that does not move." Such facts about meaning notwithstanding, Earth *does* move around the Sun.

Quine's point was that you cannot predict with any certainty how the evidence might eventually go in the future, especially as science discovers surprising new things and develops revolutionary new theories. Declaring some sentences unfalsifiable by *any* evidence either thwarts progress in science or else is futile baying at the moon. Who can predict what evidence science might uncover, or what meaning change might seem most reasonable in the light of revolutionary discoveries.

When people believed—sincerely, fervently, and with complete conviction—that atoms were indivisible, it seemed to them that the sentence "Atoms are indivisible" was unfalsifiable. Part of the original meaning of "atom" is "indivisible basic thing," as reflected by its Greek origins. Once the atom was split, however, physicists said, "Wow! I guess the atom is divisible after all." Here is what physicists did *not* say: "Well, since the sentence 'Atoms are indivisible' is unfalsifiable, we must use a different word for the thing that was split in the cyclotron. Let's call it a 'ratom.' Ratoms *are* divisible, but atoms, obviously, are not." That would have been idiotic, not to say a waste of time. Worse, it would have squandered an opportunity to see the profound ramifications of a brilliant *factual* discovery.

The trouble with the analytic/synthetic distinction, as the logical empiricists hoped to *use* it in epistemology and elsewhere, is that the history of science has many examples of sentences that people were convinced were *necessarily, conceptually* true—true no matter *what* the evidence—but that eventually turned out to be false. For example, "The interior angles of a triangle add up to exactly 180°" and "Parallel lines can never meet" are two sentences considered *necessarily* true by Kant and many philosophers thereafter. Some analytic philosophers insisted that it was part of the very meaning of "parallel" that parallel lines cannot *ever* converge, and hence that all empirical evidence is irrelevant. Period. This intransigence struck Quine as nonscientific and as a sign that so-called *necessary truths* and *conceptual truths* were phony classifications invoked to sustain a phony program.

Kant was convinced that it was *necessarily* true that parallel lines never converge in space. He could not have known that Einstein would come along and propose the general theory of relativity, according to which huge concentrations of mass in space yield a non-Euclidean metric in the space. Near a black hole, for example, parallel lines may well converge. Some philosophers have said, "Well, okay, but then the meaning of 'parallel' has *changed*. According to what Kant meant by 'parallel,' parallel lines in space do *not* converge." This is convoluted, to put it politely. Why not simply say that certain widespread, highly probable *beliefs* about space, large gravitational fields, and straight lines have turned out to be false?

Basically, Quine's challenge is this: if you want to make the analytic/synthetic distinction do a priori work in epistemology, at a minimum you owe us a theory that distinguishes changes in meaning from changes in belief. The distinction will have to draw on a theory of meaning, and that theory will have to have empirical support from psycholinguistics and neuroscience, not just nonempirical invocations of alleged "conceptual truths." Additionally, it will have to work for the tough cases, not just the easy ones, since oodles of dud theories can explain the easy cases.

There are essentially two ways of doing this: (a) declare someone, for example *me*, as Meaning Potentate, with the power to legislate when meaning changes versus when belief changes, or (b) base the theory on actual linguistic practice and scientific development. The first is an example of a dud theory, and no more need be said. As for the second, real examples typically bear out Quine's contention that no sentences are immune to empirically motivated revision, and that meaning is not cleanly separable from unwavering conviction. All of which means that no sentence gets counted as necessarily true, conceptually true, or analytically true.

Responses to Quine flooded the journals. Many of the replies boiled down to variations on the theme that philosophers' belief in and use of the analytic/synthetic distinction can only be explained by its *truth*. Not surprisingly, Quine had foreseen this move. He suggested that a variety of language-based theories could explain why the distinction may *seem* to hold, but really does not. Although Quine's arguments came as close to a rout as anything can in this field, few philosophers took his conclusions seriously enough to change they way they did business. Most tried to find a way to kick up a bit of sand and then carry on as though nothing had happened.[14] This brief account still leaves much to be said on the matter of meaning, but as meaning will be a topic of chapter 8, further issues will be raised there.

4.3   Normative Epistemology and Making Tools

Before ending this chapter, I should note that there is a second, different stream of contemporary epistemology. It survives for completely different reasons. Essentially, this branch survives because it has been successful in making progress and in serving the day-to-day needs of contemporary science. This is the *tool-making* branch of epistemology, and the tools are used for the analysis of data—for suggesting causal theories to explain a large body of observations, for determining what causally significant factors have what degree of importance in the production of a phenomenon, for evaluating the statistical significance of outcomes and strength of evidence supporting an hypothesis, and so on. This is *analysis* in its more customary sense. This subfield of epistemology made productive use of modern logic and modern mathematics, and developed an array of new evaluative techniques.

Many thinkers, including Aristotle (384–322 B.C.), Bacon (1214–1293), and Pascal (1623–1662), addressed some version of the question, What kind of procedures can help us make good progress in understanding the actual nature of the world? What sorts of methods are reliable, in the sense that if we use those methods, we will end up with theories that get us closer to the truth about how things really are? This subfield of epistemology has been remarkably productive, particularly from the middle of the nineteenth century. It includes efforts to establish a sound and sensible mathematics of probability and to characterize what sort of evidence is needed to support causal judgments.

It includes the development of statistical methods for analyzing data and clarifying how we may best interpret the results of an experiment. It includes developments in what are now called "game theory" and "decision theory." It includes trying to understand what *computation* is. The overlap here is with mathematics, mathematical logic, and scientific methodology.[15] Ironically, because powerful technical results have been achieved, results that are broadly used in all sciences, this branch is sometimes considered to have branched off from "proper" philosophy. ("That is not what is *meant* by 'philosophy'" is one way to make a self-sealing claim by invoking the now-abjured analytic/synthetic distinction.)

Whether or not to use the label "philosophy" for this subfield of epistemology is less a substantive matter and more a pointless exercise in linguistic legislation. Do we stop calling a topic "philosophy" as soon as its practitioners get good technical results? Logicians and philosophers of science will say no, while some who favor a "no progress" model of what counts as philosophy will say yes.

5   Toward a Naturalized Epistemology

By the end of the twentieth century, the hope that much could be learned about the nature of knowledge from the logical empiricist or analytical approach had begun to dim. Naturalism—taking relevant empirical data into account when theorizing—has at last acquired respectability within philosophy, though the a priori tradition remains powerful under the rubric of "analytic philosophy."

The convictions of a priori philosophers notwithstanding, progress in empirical psychology and neuroscience continues to narrow the gap between traditional philosophical questions about knowledge and empirical strategies for exploring how brains learn, remember, reason, perceive, and think. The time is right for neuroepistemology. Because cognitive neuroscientists are in fact addressing large-scale (philosophical) as well as small-scale questions, neuroepistemology has its feet well planted, whether or not they be planted in philosophy departments.

As a bridge discipline, neuroepistemology is the study of how brains represent the world, how a brain's representational scheme can learn, and what representations and information in nervous systems amount to anyhow. This characterization must be seen as provisional, however, for it is too early in the game to be very confident that "*representing* reality" is the right way to describe the central function of the mind-brain.

In the next two chapters, we shall look at two main issues in epistemology as they can be considered from within a biological framework. The first concerns whether the notion of representation is needed at all, and if so, how best to understand what representations are and how they relate to whatever it is they represent. The second concerns learning, and in general, the question of adaptation—via evolution as well as via experience-dependent changes in the nervous system. This is the problem of "how meat knows," to put it in its starkest guise. Many of the traditional epistemological foci—skepticism, innateness of knowledge, foundations for knowledge structures—can be usefully reconsidered in the neurobiological context. Other epistemological questions—when are we are justified in believing something; how do we establish that something is true or probably true; how do we falsify a belief—are now more integrated with decision theory and statistics. Will there be overlap between this technical domain of philosophy and cognitive neuroscience on such topics as reasoning, inductive or otherwise? My guess is yes.

One important line in the history of epistemology is the struggle to understand representations and how they relate to reality: the degree to which the one resembles the other, or is caused by the other, or is independent of the other, or yields knowledge of the other. Especially since Kant, an important question is how much the brain itself contributes to the character of what is represented. This question ushers in a problem: if the brain contributes to the character of what is represented, how can *we*, with our brains, separate out what in our representations corresponds to the world and what the brain contributes? If brain organization *dictates* the general form of experience, what do we actually know about the *real* world? I regard these as problems not for pre-Darwinian, a priori epistemology, but for post-Darwinian neuroepistemology.

Suggested Readings

De Waal, Frans. 1996. *Good Natured*. Cambridge: Harvard University Press.

Gibson, Roger. 1982. *The Philosophy of W. V. Quine*. Tampa: University Presses of Florida.

Glymour, Clark. 1997. *Thinking Things Through*. Cambridge: MIT Press.

Glymour, Clark. 2001. *The Mind's Arrows: Bayes Nets and Graphical Causal Models in Psychology*. Cambridge: MIT Press.

Medawar, Peter. 1984. *The Limits of Science*. Oxford: Oxford University Press.

Panksepp, Jaak, and Jules B. Panksepp. 2000. The seven sins of evolutionary psychology. *Evolution and Cognition* 6: 108–131.

Panksepp, Jaak, and Jules B. Panksepp. 2001. A synopsis of "The seven sins of evolutionary psychology." *Evolution and Cognition* 7: 2–5.

Quine, W. V. O. 1960. *Word and Object*. Cambridge: MIT Press.

Quine, W. V. O. 1969. Epistemology naturalized. In his *Ontological Relativity and Other Essays*. New York: Columbia University Press.

Websites

BioMedNet Magazine: http://news.bmn.com/magazine

A Brief Introduction to the Brain: http://ifcsun1.ifisiol.unam.mx/brain/

Encyclopedia of Life Sciences: http://www.els.net

The MIT Encyclopedia of the Cognitive Sciences: http://cognet.mit.edu/MITECS

7   How Do Brains Represent?

We have to remember that what we observe is not nature herself but nature exposed to our method of questioning.
Werner Heisenberg

1   Introduction

However brains work, much of what they do involves *representing*—representing the brain's body, features of the world, and some events in the brain itself. Performing computational operations on those representations serves to extract relevant information, make decisions, remember, and move appropriately. That brains represent and compute are working assumptions in much of cognitive neuroscience. I emphasize that these are indeed *assumptions*, however, not firmly established truths. As science continues to progress, the assumptions may be amplified, revised, or even falsified in favor of better hypotheses, as yet dimly conceived.

The problem of the nature of representations has been attacked from two directions. One is consilient with the neurosciences generally, and is coevolving with them. For convenience, call this the *brain-friendly approach*.[1] It aims to discover how brains map and model the world by looking at all levels of organization from neurons to behavior. The second approach is wedded to the analogy between cognitive operations and software running on a computer (see chapter 1), and hence adheres to the *autonomy* of psychology. Call this the *brain-averse approach*.[2] Because it assumes that cognitive states are a function of their role in the cognitive economy, and hence are independent of any particular hardware "implementation," the brain-averse approach ignores neuroscience as largely irrelevant to the problem of how the mind represents.

Recall that the autonomy-of-psychology thesis assumes that neuroscience can at most reveal something about the implementation of the cognitive software but cannot aspire to revealing anything much about the nature of cognitive processes per se (see pp. 25–28). More extreme versions consider neuroscience an actual impediment to progress. The reason is that neuroscientists routinely ascribe representational functions to neural structures, saying such things as "Neural networks in the superior colliculus represent eye position." Comments like this one are alleged to be worse than confused, since hardware allegedly does not represent anything. As we shall see, brain-averse adherents take a linguistic entity—the *sentence*—as the prototype for all *real* representations. Consequently, those animals that lack the capacity for language are considered to have representations only by courtesy or as a figure of speech, but not literally.

There is also a third approach, which is really a variant of the first. It explores the possibility that in some contexts representation-based explanations for behavior may be replaceable, or at least augmented, by the concepts in the framework of dynamical systems.[3] Like the first, this approach is coevolving with the neurosciences. It is motivated in part by the fact that nervous systems are indeed dynamical systems and in part by the fact that there is no well-developed theory about what exactly *information* and *representation* in biological systems amounts to. Given this dearth of theory, the dynamical-systems approach undertakes to explore how much explanatory ground can be covered without appeal to representations, and how representational accounts, when needed, can best be integrated within a dynamical-systems framework.[4]

As we shall see, there is compelling support for the hypothesis that animals other than humans have representational capacities, and that brains are the platform for those representational capacities. In my opinion, therefore, the brain-friendly approaches are likely to be more productive than brain-averse approaches. As noted in chapter 2, the brain-friendly approaches are also more appealing on sheerly pragmatic grounds, since they consider all data, not just a subclass of ideologically approved data. Additionally, as we shall see, there are certain *fundamental* kinds of representation, such as spatial representation, where cognitive neuroscience is making impressive progress, but where brain-averse approaches are relatively unrewarding.

From an evolutionary perspective, brains are buffers against environmental stress and variability.[5] Early in our history, evolution must have stumbled upon the advantages accruing to nervous systems able to make predictions based on past conditions, while evaluating current circumstances, both internal and external. In short, it helps to have a brain with the capacity to prepare for events that will probably happen, and to organize a behavioral response to something that is not *now* happening but can be expected to happen. If you are a tree, in contrast, there is no advantage to knowing anything about where home is; you have no options about how to hide from a predator or stalk prey, or about which mate to choose. You take what comes. Variations in the weather may affect you, but seeking shelter is not in your repertoire. Animals, however, can move, and hence knowing things and representing things confers a competitive advantage. The hypothesis on offer is that in the service of prediction, neuronal activity maps the various *me-relevant* features of the world—its spatial relations, social relations, food sources, shelters, and so forth. This mapping is usefully considered representational. The next question is how exactly neuronal structures accomplish this.

At the *neuronal level*, a major question driving the field asks precisely *what* features of neuronal activity subserve the coding of information—both encoding and decoding. Neurons exhibit a wide range of activity, and a theory of representing needs to address the problem of how to distinguish genuine *signals* from housekeeping activities and from mere noise.

At the *network level*, the predominant aim has been to find plausible models that will mesh with the facts about neurons and their connectivity patterns, *and* with psychophysical data deriving from behavioral studies. The hope is that network models will be a bridge between what we understand about bodily behavior and what we understand about neurons.

At the *systems level*, a major challenge is to understand how nervous systems integrate information, store information, retrieve task-relevant information and use information to make behavioral decisions. That the nervous system is a complex dynamical system is evident, but figuring out the dynamical principles by which it functions continues to be difficult.[6]

---

2 Do Brains Represent?

What motivates saying that the brain represents *at all*? Why couldn't the story of brain function be told without reference *at all* to representations and computations? (Incidentally, the same discussion would follow whether, instead of the word "representation," we used the word "idea," as Hume preferred, or "thought" [Descartes], or "concepts" [Kant]. "Representation" is just the term currently in fashion.) Although answers can be constructed from different

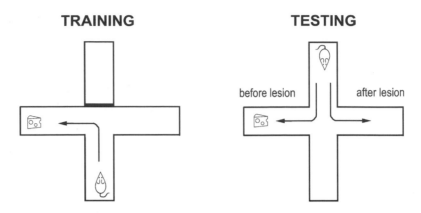

Figure 7.1 Spatial representation in the rat. In the training condition (left), the rat always starts in the same location and learns that food is always in the end of left arm of the maze. In the test condition (right), a block is removed and the rat is placed in the newly opened passage. Rats trained for a normal amount will turn right, correcting for their reversed spatial orientation with respect to the food location. Overtrained rats or rats with hippocampal lesions will turn left. (From Farber, Peterman, and Churchland 2001; based on Packard and Teather 1998b.)

starting points, the most compelling arguments begin with examples of cognitive operations that resist explanation on the stimulus-and-response paradigm. Competence in solving spatial problems will illustrate this explanatory resistance.

Consider a well-controlled and revealing set of experiments by Packard and Teather illustrating that a stimulus-response explanation predicts one result, a representational explanation predicts the opposite, and the latter prediction wins.[7] Put a rat in a T maze for twenty trials, and always bait the left-hand arm. After a few trials, the rat knows where the cheese is (figure 7.1). Next, unblock a barrier at the top, and put the rat in the full maze. If the rat has merely acquired a conditioned response to turn to the left, then when confronted with the full maze, rats should turn left. If the rat has a spatial map for this environment, it will turn right. What do the rats do? They turn *right*, thus turning in the direction opposite to their earlier responses. This behavior implies that the animal is *not* displaying a conditioned response (always turn left), but rather is using a representation of the spatial organization of the maze relative to the room the maze is in. Additionally, to relate the rat's behavior to a specific brain structure, Packard and Teather showed that if the brain's hippocampus is lesioned, either before or after the training trials, the animals *do* show a conditioned response in the test condition: they turn *left*. On the other hand, intact but overtrained rats (*hundreds* of training trials to the left-baited arm) will turn left when put in the full maze almost as though the conditioned response overrides the spatial reasoning when the animal is overtrained (and no longer "thinking"?). Lesions again prove revealing, for when Packard and Teather lesioned the *striatum*, the conditioned response is abolished. Given striatum lesions, even the overtrained rats now turn right, which suggests that when the conditioning circuits are unavailable, the brain again relies on spatial representations.

Additional physiological data about the hippocampus and spatial mapping makes a more compelling case. O'Keefe and Dostrovsky discovered in 1971 that there are *place neurons* in the hippocampus of rats. That is, an individual hippocampal neuron fires when and only when the freely moving rat is in a specific place, such as the upper east corner of the maze (see figure 7.2). Following the pioneer work of O'Keefe and his students, others went on to replicate and extend their results. It was discovered that an individual neuron codes for a place relative to a particular environment—for example, the kitchen versus the living room. That is, a given hippocampal neuron may code for a particular place in the kitchen, and a completely unrelated place in the living room. As expected, rats with hippocampal lesions cannot learn spatial tasks, as indeed humans cannot. Other hippocampal neurons that code for direction of movement in the freely moving rat have also been found.

The above argument for a representational explanation of route-finding behavior in rats has assumed that the only alternative to a conditioned-response explanation is a representational explanation. Although that assumption might be false, the fact is we really do not have any other plausible options at this stage, though theoretical developments could change that.

Many animals, including dogs, horses, bees, and bears, exhibit behavior that shows good spatial representation, such as finding novel routes home. Because many animals can aim for home without benefit of conditioning, and frequently without much in the way of trial-and-error searching, it seems fair to say that they "know where home is," or better, perhaps, they "know *how* to get home" in *some* sense of "know." Nevertheless, describing the matter thus may imply more than is intended, namely, that the animal says to itself "Hey, I know where the cheese is: just over yonder, two left turns from Maggie's nest." Nothing quite so humanlike as self-talk is really implied, however, if only

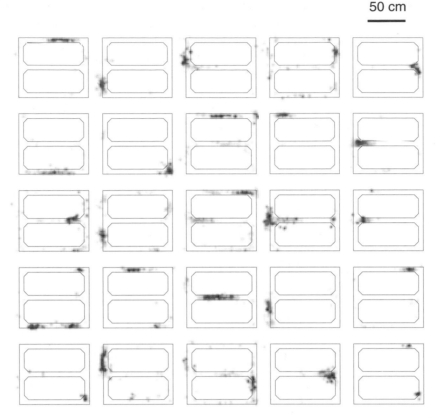

Figure 7.2   Firing-rate maps of 25 hippocampal place cells simultaneously recorded in a rat running on the elevated track of a figure-8 maze. Restricted regions with high firing rates are called place fields. Thus the neuron whose response profile is depicted in the top left box is tuned to respond when the rat is located in the upper rightish region of the maze. Maps were computed from 7 minutes of continuous data. In each plot, scaling is linear, with a 0 firing value corresponding to 0 in the color map and a maximum positive value corresponding to 1. (Courtesy of K. Zhang.)

because these animals do not appear to have a humanlike language in which to talk to themselves. Indeed, it is doubtful that *human* spatial representation is generally languagelike, even though spatial knowledge can sometimes be presented in speech.[8] Consequently, we seek an understanding of representations that does not depend on their being just like words and sentences.

Representing spatial relations is one kind cognitive function, but we commonly consider that the brain represents objects, such as *that barking dog*. When humans plan, imagine, and dream, they represent in the *absence* of the thing they are representing. You can think or dream about skiing down the black-diamond runs at Whistler. Even if you have no skis, or even no legs, you can still produce visual/motor images of skiing down the slopes. Representations are also typically invoked to explain how the brain *perceives*, that is, how the brain makes a perceptual judgment when the relevant object is in full and unobstructed view, in full odor, within earshot, or on the tongue. Why, when the relevant scene *is* present, do neuroscientists say that the brain represents?

Part of the reason is that nervous systems do a lot of processing of signals received at the periphery—at the retina, skin, cochlea, nose, tongue, muscles, tendons, and joints. Information is extracted, augmented, integrated, and generally *worked* so that the perceptual product we are aware of, such as the smell of a wet dog, is really a far cry from the peripheral signals. The brain is not a *passive reflector* of external stimuli; it is in various ways an *active constructor* that builds the animal's perceptual-motor world.[9] Many of the same mechanisms are probably recruited in both visual perception and visual imagery, in both auditory perception and auditory imagery, and in both motor control and motor imagery. A chain of visual examples can illustrate this constructive dimension.

2.1 Contours

In the figure 7.3, devised in 1955 by psychologist Georg Kaniza, we see a white triangle overlying three lines and three black circles. In fact, there are no boundaries demarcating the white triangle; the black areas are actually pacman shaped disk segments. A sensitive photometer run over the figure will detect neither the borders of the triangles nor the increased brightness of the white triangle. Subjective contours, as they are called, are also seen in plate 6.

Plate 6 contains red intersecting lines on the left and, on the right, the very same red intersecting lines with black extensions. Nevertheless, on the right,

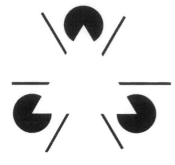

Figure 7.3   Illusory contours. You see an illusory white triangle on a background of partly occluded circles and lines. The interior of the triangle generally appears whiter than the ground, even though it is not. (From Palmer 1999.)

but not on the left, we also see a contour demarcating a light red disk from the background.

Plate 7 is a stereo display consisting of two images, slightly offset, that can be fused to make a single image of a blue semitransparent rectangle hovering over four circles. You can fuse the two images by defocusing your eyes, which is easiest to accomplish by looking at the display as though it were further away than it is. Devised by Ken Nakayama and Shinsuke Shimojo, this illusion is especially striking because the only blue detectable by a photometer consists of little blue arcs on the concentric circles. You will also notice that the filmy blue rectangle curves out slightly toward you.

2.2   Ambiguous Figures

Some stimuli happen to permit two equally good interpretations. The classical case is the Necker cube, investigated by Swiss psychologist Louis Albert Necker in 1832. It can be seen either as having its face oriented up and to the right, or oriented down and to the left (see figure 7.4, B).

2.3   Motion

Your brain will create a perception of motion in the following condition. A light flashes off at one location, and within a very brief time period, a light flashes on at a new but nearby location (figure 7.5). It looks as though a light moved across space from the old to the new location.[10]

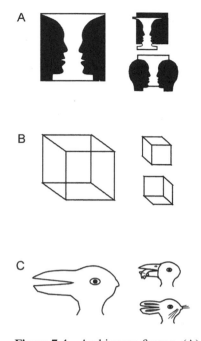

Figure 7.4 Ambiguous figures. (A) can be seen either as a white vase against a black background or as a pair of black faces against a white background (the disambiguated figures can be seen to the right). (B) can be seen as a cube viewed from above or below. (C) can be seen as a duck (facing left) or a rabbit (facing right). (From Palmer 1999.)

Figure 7.5 Subjective motion. A light flashes on first at the position marked O, and then at the position marked X. If the time interval between when the light at O goes off and the light at X comes on is between about 5 and 500 milliseconds, then what is seen is a light continuously moving from position O to position X.

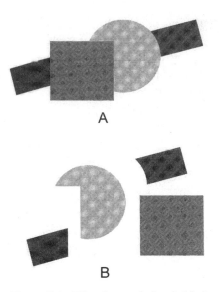

A

B

Figure 7.6   Visual completion behind partly occluding objects. Panel A is perceived as consisting of a square, a circle, and a rectangle, even though the only visible regions are those shown separated in panel B. (From Palmer 1999.)

2.4   Scene Segmentation

In A of figure 7.6 we typically see the bar as behind the circular disk, which is partially occluded by the square. Nevertheless, the only regions that reflect light to the retina are the partial objects shown below in B.

These examples on their own do not provide anything like a *theory* of the nature of representation. Their function is merely to give us a feel for the kinds of job that representations are thought to perform in perception. They show the place in the explanatory scheme of things where representations seem, for now anyhow, to be needed. For this reason, these and other examples provide a modicum of guidance for the investigation. Assuming, therefore, that nervous systems do indeed represent, we now need to ask *how* they represent. Ultimately, we want a theory of representation in nervous systems. As a ground-clearing preliminary, we can first ask what facts from biology, neuroscience, and psychology constrain a theory of nervous-system representation.

3   Some Empirical Constraints on a Theory of Representation

In the early stages of this enterprise, articulating constraints is desirable, since knowing what will *not* work narrows the search space. That the human brain is an evolved organ is, not surprisingly, an overarching constraint on any theory of representation. Proposals that construe representations as literal pictures in the head, to take an unlikely example, are not very promising as a starting place.

3.1   Brains Are Products of Evolution

Because the human brain is the product of evolution, we can expect to find instructive similarities and continuities between representing in infants and adults, and between representing in human and nonhuman animals. A theory that predicts failure of *any* continuity between humans and other animals in, say, spatial or motor or perceptual representation would raise a red flag. A theory that entails a magical origin for complex human representational capacities will raise a red flag. More generally, in science any hypothesis that fills a gap by saying "and then a miracle happened" is not compelling.

3.2   Representations and Language

In humans, language is an important means of communication, and fully verbal humans often use language in thinking. Ultimately, any theory of representations will need also to account for human languages, including the capacity of children to learn language and the range of distinct language deficits seen in humans with brain damage. Even if human language is unique in its complexity and representational power, general considerations from evolutionary biology imply that a theory postulating the absence of any continuity between linguistic representations and *nonlinguistic* representations would need skeptical scrutiny.[11]

A characteristic of humans, one that tends to amplify the differences that do exist between humans and other animals, is cultural evolution. In humans, language, along with cultural institutions, allow later generations to start learning what an earlier generation invented in its maturity. Accordingly, representational skills emerge that are strikingly novel relative to the ancestral versions. Conventions, manners, and ideas newly created by the ancestral generation can seem second nature, logically obvious, and even biologically necessary to the grandchildren who learned them as just part of how the world is.

Unfortunately, we know little about the conceptual resources deployed by hominids 3 million or even 100,000 years ago. Nevertheless, it is sobering to remind ourselves of the many cognitive artifacts that are known to be cultural inventions: reading, writing, mathematics (including the number zero), music, and maps; the use of fire and metals; and the domestication of dogs, sheep, wheat, and rice. We do not know how much of the complexity seen in human language depends on cultural evolution. Structural similarities among human languages are consistent with, but certainly do not entail, that there exists a genetically specified grammar module in the human brain. Such structural commonalities as do exist could be as well explained, so far as is known, as arising from similarities in nonlinguistic representational resources and similarities in fundamental aspects of human experience, such as spatiality, sociability, the need for sequence assembling in forming plans and in behavioral execution, and so forth. As Elizabeth Bates wryly commented, the similarities among humans in getting food to the mouth by using hands rather than feet does not imply the existence of an innate "hands for feeding" module. Rather, the existence of a shared body plan and the ease of hand feeding relative to foot feeding suffice to explain "feeding universals."

3.3 Contrasting Digital Computers and Brains

Although we describe them as computing, brains, in important respects, are profoundly unlike the familiar digital computer. For example, the spatial knowledge of rats is not stored in their "hard drives," because a rat brain does not have a hard drive. Computers have a memory module independent of the structures that process information, but nervous systems do not. More generally, our brains do not have modules in the way our desk-top computers have modules.[12] Brains do, however, exhibit areas of functional specialization, especially at maturity, but the specialization exists with a degree of functional modifiability that is not at all compatible with the idea of "ecapsulated, dedicated modules." A suitably neurobiological sense of module has yet to be characterized in detail, since much about brain organization, function, and development, from conceptus to corpse, is still not understood. Incidentally, inventing a new expression to replace "module" might help us avoid implicitly importing to the neural domain the standard features of modularity in the computer domain.

Other dissimilarities between brains and computers want mentioning:

- Neurons, unlike computer chips, grow and develop, or prune back or die. At least in the hippocampus and perhaps elsewhere, new neurons are generated even into adulthood.

- Neurons are dynamical entities, and they change *structurally* as they learn, making new contacts, abandoning old contacts, strengthening or weakening existing contacts, and so on.

- Changes in neuronal structure often require antecedent changes in gene expression, and certain genes are turned on as a consequence of the level of certain activities in the neuron.[13]

- Neuronal events happen in the millisecond range; events in present-day computers may be four or five orders of magnitude faster.

- Nervous systems have a parallel organization; computers are serial machines.

- Computers have a clock that sets *now* for all components; brains, so far as we can tell, do not have a clock that serves that function.

- Computers were designed by humans to crunch numbers; nervous systems evolved through natural selection to move bodies adaptively. The former is nonsemantic or clean computation; the latter is life-oriented, dirty computation.

- Not all the 10^{12} neurons in the human nervous system are in the representing business. Some, for example, modulate the activity of representing neurons, because they are part of the arousal or attentional systems, or they perform functions we do not yet understand. Others may have a causal role in regulating temperature, heart rate, growth, or appetite, without actually representing any of those things. Since human engineers designed computers, it is relatively straightforward to determine what activities in computers are information-bearing and what not. For brains, however, all of that has to be figured out. You cannot tell by just looking.

4 Coding in Neurons and Networks: A First Pass

Neurons transmit information by virtue of their activity and are believed to store information by changing aspects of their connectivity to other neurons. The prototypical transmission is *point-to-point*; that is, from a site on the

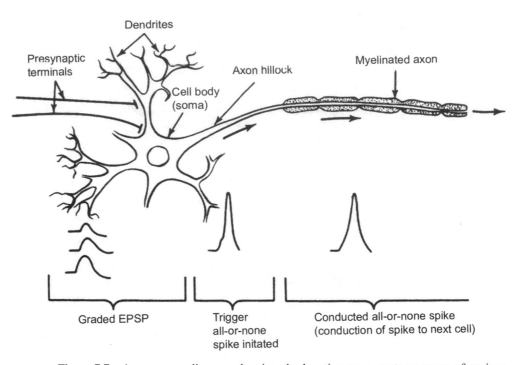

Figure 7.7　A summary diagram showing the location on a motor neuron of various electrical events. In many neurons, dendrites and cell bodies respond with graded excitatory postsynaptic potentials (EPSPs) or inhibitory postsynaptic potentials (IPSPs). The action potential is triggered in the axon hillock and travels undiminished down the axon. (Based on Thompson 1967.)

sending (*presynaptic*) neuron to a site on the receiving (*postsynaptic*) neuron. In the classical paradigm, signals are *received* in the dendrites and cell bodies, and signals are *sent* via the axon to the axonal terminal (figure 7.7). If, as a function of complex interactions in the dendrites and cell body, a sufficiently strong depolarization reaches the axon hillock, then a spike is generated and propagated down the axon to its terminus. With *some degree of probability*, the presynaptic membrane may release neurotransmitter into the synaptic cleft after the arrival of the spike. The probability of transmitter release (also called the synapse's *reliability*) may change as a function of learning.

In classical point-to-point signal transmission, neurotransmitter molecules bind to specialized sites on the postsynaptic cell. These sites are really complex protein molecules than span the neuronal membrane and change their shape when bound by a ligand. This change in shape can allow an influx of positive ions, which will depolarize the postsynaptic membrane, thus exciting the post-synaptic cell. Or, depending on the type of protein channel, it might prevent the efflux of negative ions, which will cause the neuron to hyperpolarize. (See figures 1.5 and 1.6.) Communication between neurons is achieved when the neurotransmitter released from the presynaptic cell affects the postsynaptic cell by either exciting or inhibiting it. Many thousands of postsynaptic sites on a neuron's dendrites may respond with a depolarization or a hyperpolarization within a few hundred milliseconds. Typically, many stimulus inputs are needed to generate a current strong enough to initiate spiking at the axon hillock. Additionally, there are other styles of signaling, some of which occur at non-conventional receptor sites on the receiving (postsynaptic) neuron. Within the last decade, it has emerged that communication in the nervous system spans a continuum of speeds, effect durations, and postsynaptic cascades. These are not just curious exceptions to the old and mainly true story. Rather, they are central elements that profoundly rewrite the classical story.

By recording from individual sensory neurons during the presentation of a stimulus, it has been found that many neurons display a response selectivity when the animal is presented with specific external physical parameters, such as vertical motion of an object (neurons in the visual cortex), or light touch on the thumb (neurons in the somatosensory cortex), or the smell of peppermint (neurons in the olfactory bulb). A neuron's response specificity is often referred to as its *tuning*, and hence a neuron is said to be tuned to visual motion or to peppermint. In a casual manner, we also say that the neuron *prefers* peppermint, or is *driven by* peppermint.

The *receptive field* of a neuron is the area on the receptor sheet (retina, skin, etc.) that, when stimulated, causes the neuron to respond. For example, the receptive field of a neuron in the somatosensory cortex might be a tiny region on the tip of the thumb; the receptive field of a neuron in the visual system might be a particular spot on the fovea of the retina. A neuron may have a small receptive field but be broadly tuned, as is typical of neurons in the primary sensory cortexes. Such a neuron may respond maximally to a bar of light moving vertically, respond slightly less if the light is moving somewhat off the vertical, and respond less and less as the direction of movement of the light converges on the horizontal.

On the other hand, a neuron in a higher[14] visual area, such as the inferior temporal region, may have a *large receptive field* spanning much of the entire visual field and yet be *narrowly tuned* to respond only to faces, or even more narrowly, only to one *individual* face albeit in many orientations. The

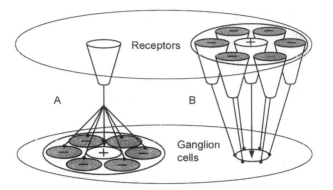

Figure 7.8 Projective and receptive fields. (A) A single receptor projects to many gan-glion cells (via interneurons) in a center/surround organization. The center ganglion cell is excited; the surrounding cells are inhibited. Thus the *projective field* of a receptor is characteized. (B) Each ganglion cell receiving such connections therefore has a center-surround *receptive field*. The illustrated network exhibits an excitatory center and inhib-itory surround, but the opposite organization (inhibitory center and excitatory surround) also exists in the retina. (From Palmer 1999.)

nonclassical receptive field refers to that region around the classical receptive field that can modify the response to stimuli within the classical receptive field. Stimuli *restricted* to the nonclassical region do not, however, drive the cell on their own. The *projective field* refers to the set of neurons to which a given neuron projects (figure 7.8).

Two problems need to be distinguished: (1) What properties in the single neuron carry information? And (2) how is an objective parameter represented by neurons? Traditionally, the dominant hypothesis offered to the first problem has been *rate coding*; that is, the *average firing rate* or spiking frequency of the neuronal axon over a certain interval is what carries information. Although rate coding is one strategy for carrying information, nervous systems probably employ other strategies as well. The list of other possibilities include the *timing of a spike burst* relative to the timing of other neuronal events, the interval *between* spikes in one neuron, the specific *pattern of spikes* in an interval, and the *latency* for the first spike after the stimulus. There may also be other information-bearing neuronal changes that do not involve axonal firing at all. Dendrites, as they receive signals from the presynaptic cell, undergo membrane changes, and these changes must carry information. If they did not, the spike generated from integrated inputs would not carry information either. Dendritic responses are standardly construed as *decoding* the incoming signals, so presumably the states of dendrites are themselves information-bearing. How does *that* work? We are now beyond the well-trodden ground of the conventional wisdom.

For the second problem (how is an objective parameter represented by neurons?) at least two hypotheses command attention. (a) A property, for example, the face of Woody Allen, may be coded by a single neuron, and this neuron normally fires when and only when a Woody Allen face is presented (*local coding*). To avoid losing its entire Woody Allen representation when one neuron dies, the system may have spares; that is, it may have a pool of neurons that *all* respond when and only when the face of Woody Allen is visually presented. Such redundancy is consistent with local coding. One drawback to local coding as a general strategy for the nervous system is that there are too few neurons to account for the huge numbers of things, places, and events we can recognize. Nevertheless, for certain restricted representational purposes, such as coding nonoverlapping values in a small range, local coding could be adequate and efficient.

The second hypothesis, (b), says that some values are coded by a population of neurons whose members are active in different degrees across a range of properties (*vector coding*). As explained below, using vector coding, the brain could represent the face of Woody Allen with a particular *pattern* of responses in the population, and the very same population of neurons, but with a different pattern of responses, may represent the face of Ghandi and the face of Castro.

Although some general points can be made about neuronal coding on the basis of available neurobiological data, many, *many* questions remain unresolved. In particular, neuromodulation, in contrast to classical, fast, point-to-point transmission, is a major feature in all aspects of representational function, from sensory input to motor output. *Neuromodulation* refers to effects on a cell's activity by neurochemicals other than classical neurotransmitters. It can up-regulate or down-regulate sensitivity of the cell, for example. To make matters even more interesting, there appears to be modulation of the modulators. Moreover, neurons appear to have a preferred range of activity, and self-regulating mechanisms kick in once the neuron's activity is shifted out of the preferred range.[15]

Emphasizing this in-progress character of neuroscience is crucial, if a little daunting. At this stage in neuroscience, nothing like a well-established theory of neuronal coding exists. We *will* get there, but we are not there yet. In any case, the range of neurophysiological observations about neuronal responses

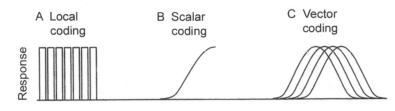

Figure 7.9   Three methods of encoding information. (A) Local coding: a separate unit is dedicated to each feature the system distinguishes. (B) Scalar encoding: features are encoded by the firing rate of a single neuron. (C) Vector coding: features are encoded in the pattern of activity in a population of units that have broad, overlapping tuning curves. (From Churchland and Sejnowski 1992.)

under varying conditions is fuel for future theories. Needless to say, consideration of the neurophysiological data is essential, since unconstrained theories are just guesswork that can be wasteful of time and energy. At the same time, reaching for theoretical perspective is also essential, even when the data are still sparse. Explanatory theories do not automatically waft up from the data; they have to be invented. Moreover, invention of data-inspired theories typically motivates further experiments, with theory-revisions often following in the wake of the experiments. Thus the familiar bootstrapping of science generally.

5   Local Coding and Vector Coding: A Fast Sketch

Conceptually, the basic idea of local coding is relatively simple. A neuron (or pool of response-similar neurons) is dedicated to representing a specific property. If a set of neurons were placed cheek to jowl on a one-dimensional grid, then we could identify a neuron's unique representational job by identifying its unique place in the grid. Taken as a whole, the grid might be a 1 : 1 mapping of locations on a receptor sheet, such as the cochlea of the ear. If the auditory system used this strategy, then middle C, for example, would be represented by the activity of the "middle-C neuron," which would be found at a precise location on the grid. Local coding is also referred to as *place coding*.

Vector coding, by contrast, depends on the idea that features are represented in specific *patterns* of activity in a *population* of units, where each neuron has a tuning curve, perhaps quite broad, and tuning curves overlap, perhaps quite a lot. This is illustrated in figure 7.9. Mathematically, a vector is simply an *ordered set of numbers*, $\langle n_1, n_2, \ldots, n_m \rangle$. The elements in a particular vector are values standing for properties such as the activity levels of each neuron in the relevant population. Let us tentatively make the simplifying assumption that the contribution to the vector made by a single neuron is its average spiking rate over a specified interval, say 100 milliseconds. Each neuron in the relevant population thus contributes some element (= its average firing rate) to the vector. Depending on the stimulus, the neuron may fire a little, a lot, or below baseline firing. Accordingly, a particular vector, say $\langle 16, 4, 22 \rangle$, might represent the hue yellowy orange, while a slightly different vector, say $\langle 16, 6, 14 \rangle$, might represent the hue reddish orange (see pp. 183–187, plate 5). One and the same neuron can participate in the representation of many different items (e.g., hues), and no one neuron represents a property all by itself.[16]

Representation by a population of broadly tuned neurons is economical. For a given number of neurons, vector coding gives you a larger range of values than local coding. Suppose that a system has just five neurons, with four discrete activity levels ranging between 0 and 3. If the system uses *local coding*, the five neurons can represent 20 different values (4×5). If they use *vector coding*, 625 values ($= 5^4$) can be represented. That is, $\langle 3, 1, 0, 1 \rangle$ specifies a particular pattern of activity during a certain time interval and represents one value, $\langle 4, 2, 0, 1 \rangle$ specifies another distinct pattern and a different value, and so on. Greater precision can be achieved with overlapping tuning curves because more fine-grained values of a single external stimulus can be reflected in the joint behavior of the group of cells. Notice that in the limiting case, if a vector has only one element, vector coding and local coding amount to the same thing.

Each placeholder in the vector specifies a distinct dimension of the *parameter space*. When each placeholder is filled with a specific value, the resulting vector delimits a specific point in the parameter space. Thus a three-element vector generates a three-dimensional space; a five-element vector generates a five-dimensional space. The latter is hard to *visualize*, of course, but think of it as just more of the same. If the vector codes for neural activity in a 1,000 neuron network, then the parameter space will have 1,000 dimensions. As with a 5-dimensional space, the mind need not boggle. You can think of this as just a *lot* more of the same (figure 7.10).

What is so tremendously useful about *spatiality* here is that the space (3-D, 10-D or *n*-D) has a metric, meaning that positions in the space can be specified as near each other or far from each other or in-between. And spaces admit of regions, volumes, paths, and mappings. All of this makes it easier to conceptualize representations, relations between representations, and relations between representations and the world.

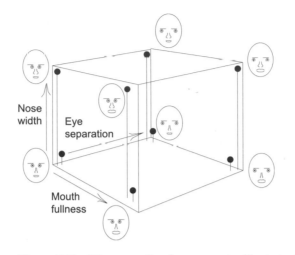

Figure 7.10   Diagram of a face space to illustrate the idea that faces vary along a number of dimensions, represented as axes of the state space, and that a system might code for faces using vectors whose elements represent such features as distance between the eyes, fullness of the mouth, and width of the nose. Obviously, faces have many features that are coded by mammals, and even the three features included here are undoubtedly crude. (Courtesy of P. M. Churchland.)

In the struggle to find useful and coherent ways of *thinking about* how brains represent, the *vector/parameter-space* tool turns out to be conceptually powerful, at least at this early stage. One advantage is that reasonable *explanations* of a range of behavioral capacities displayed by representing animals emerge quite naturally, without ad hoc miracles. In particular, *similarity relations*, the be-all of categories and categorial structures, though difficult to address in other theories, gracefully deliver themselves as neighborhood relations in parameter spaces. To put it crudely, the problem of similarity relations need not be solved with hoked-up mechanisms or structures; they are a relatively simple consequence of parameter-space representation. The color space discussed in chapter 4 (see color plates 3 and 5) illustrated the similarity relations at both the perceptual level and the neuronal level, and showed the fit of perceptual space with neuronal space. A comparable story can be told for tastes (figure 7.11). These and other examples hint that vector coding in some manner or other is really what the basic systems use, and that parameter spaces are in fact one representational strategy brains exploit.

Two jobs are before us: first, we need a closer look at just how the vector-coding and parameter-space story goes, and second, we need to see whether

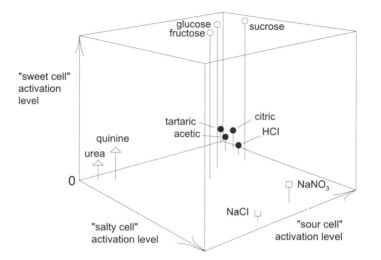

Figure 7.11   Taste space: the position of some familiar tastes. Similar tasting substances are found in similar regions of the parameter space. Thus, sugars form a cluster at the upper middle region, and tart substances are found in the lower rear region. (Based on Bartoshuk and Beauchamp 1994.)

new insights about concepts and *meaning* might be discovered with their help. I shall tackle these tasks in order.

6   Faces: An Artificial Neural Network for Face Recognition

How exactly can neuronal activity *represent* something? The basic ideas of the vector/parameter-space approach to representation can be spelled out in a simplified model, much as one can use a simple model to illustrate basic principles of motion, digestion, or mitochondrial energy production. We shall therefore begin with an artificial neural network (ANN) that can perform recognition tasks on photographs of actual human faces. *Face net*, a three-stage ANN developed by Garrison Cottrell and his colleagues, is schematically portrayed in figure 7.12. Although it is not precisely known how nervous systems do in fact represent faces, the Cottrell network is very useful for demonstrating the basic principles of how a neural network of units *might* represent specific faces.[17] So I will set aside the real details of projection patterns, cell numbers, cell physiology, and so forth as I outline only the *conceptual* resources of ANNs.

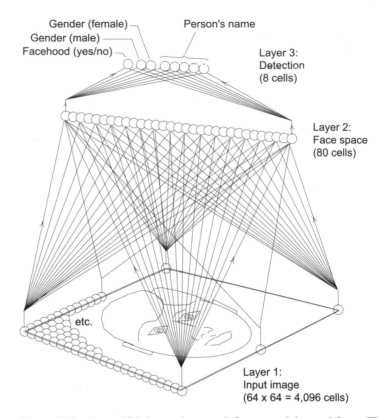

Gender (female)
Gender (male)
Facehood (yes/no)
Person's name
Layer 3:
Detection
(8 cells)
Layer 2:
Face space
(80 cells)
etc.
Layer 1:
Input image
(64 x 64 = 4,096 cells)

Figure 7.12 An artificial neural network for recognizing real faces. The input layer is at the bottom, the output layer at the top. Although this network has 4,184 processing units, it has a very simple organization. Each unit in the input layer connects to every unit in the middle layer, and each unit in the middle layer connects to every unit in the upper layer. (From P. M. Churchland 1995.)

Face net's input layer (for our purposes, a pretend *retina*) is a (64×64)-pixel grid whose elements each admit of 256 different levels of activation or "brightness" according to the light reflected from the region in the photo to which it is sensitive. The network's input consists of gray-scaled photographs (figure 7.13). When initially constructed, of course, the network cannot recognize anything, and its response to any given input is just random noise. It is then trained on 64 different photographs of 11 different faces, along with 13 photos of nonface scenes, after which it can perform specific face-recognition tasks. How is this training achieved?

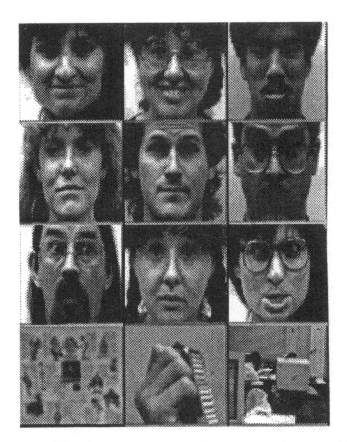

Figure 7.13 Selected input images for training the face-recognition network. (Courtesy of Gary Cottrell.)

Each input unit projects a radiating set of "axonal" end branches to each and every one of the 80 units in the second layer, and this layer maps an abstract space of 80 dimensions (a dimension for each unit) in which the input faces are explicitly coded. (A two- or three-dimensional space is readily understood; now just think of adding axes.) The second layer projects to an output layer of merely eight units. These output units have their connection strengths carefully adjusted so that the units can make a number of discriminations: first, discriminating between faces and nonfaces; second, discriminating between male and female faces; and third, responding with the person's "name" (actually an arbitrarily assigned binary code) when re-presented any face that the network "got to know" during training.

What actually does the work in face net is the overall configuration of "synaptic" connections—positive and negative, weak and strong. It is these, and only these, that progressively transform the initial (64 × 64)-element pattern or vector into a second and finally a third vector that explicitly represents the input's facehood, sex, and name. The fundamental processing format consists of mere vector-to-vector transformations determined by the configuration of connection weights.

A crucial ambiguity must now be resolved. Sometimes "representation" refers to cognitive events happening *now*, such as a visual perception; other times it refers to the *capacity* (*not* now exercised) to have appropriate cognitive events, such as my capacity to recognize an osprey. *Patterns of activity in networks* hook up with the first sense; *configurations of connection weights* (which yield the appropriate patterns of activity when given specific inputs) hook up with the second sense. Think of the first as *displaying* knowledge and the second as the *enduring structure*, or background conceptual framework, that makes the current display possible. (Other terms are "*occurrent* representations" versus "*abeyant* representations.") One caution: because activity can change structure, as in learning, it is wiser to think of activity and structure as different points on a continuum, rather than as utterly distinct things. Some structural features are, in this sense, very slow activities.

As the face net has 328,320 connections, and as its face-recognizing performance depends on how those connections are configured, the question that presses is this: how do the connection weights come to be configured? That question turns out to be much the same question as this: how to you get *information into the structure of a network* so that a fundamentally stupid thing—the network—can display "knowledge"? Needless to say, this is a question about *learning*. Since learning is the topic of the next chapter, the question of *how networks learn* is best addressed later in the more appropriate context of neural learning (chapter 8). The task in this chapter is to understand what conceptual tools are suited to explain how networks that *have learned* do represent. Given that purpose, it may provisionally suffice to know that scientists have discovered a palette of algorithms for adjusting the connection weights in an ANN so that it will end up representing features of the training set and be able to generalize to new stimuli. The existence of such algorithms allows us to comprehend that there are naturalistic solutions to the problem of how neural networks learn. Some algorithms for automated weight adjustment in ANNs are neurobiologically more realistic than others; some scale better than others; some are faster than others. Some involve external feedback; some do not. But applied to a network whose weights are initially set at random, they all yield a network whose structure and dynamics embody information. Regardless of whether any algorithm devised so far truly conforms to one of the brain's methods, we at least understand the sort of procedures that can do the job.

Accordingly, once trained, Cottrell's face net will transform each one of a wide range of possible input vectors (pictures of faces) into an appropriate output vector (see again figure 7.12). The output vector is in effect face net's answer to whether the input is a face at all, whether it is male or female, whether it is Billy or Bob. Cottrell's face net achieved 100 percent accuracy on the 11 images in the training set, identifying facehood, sex, and identity. An interesting question is whether the network can identify the same faces if they appear in different angles, with different expressions, accessories, lighting conditions, etc. On this more demanding test, its accuracy was 98 percent: it missed the sex and identity of one female subject. This is impressive, since it means that the responses are not canned. The network has a kind of flexible competence.

Can face net *generalize* to completely novel (never-before-presented) faces to give correct answers to the questions face/nonface and male/female? Yes. On the novel face/nonface task, it scored 100 percent. On recognizing sex of the novel face, it scored 81 percent, showing a tendency to misclassify some female faces as male. Can it correctly identify a "familiar" face when partially obscured by a bar? Yes, save in one set of cases where the bar was placed so as to obscure each subject's forehead, thus indicating that variations in hair position across the forehead probably played a significant, though not critical, role in identification.

Success on these tests indicates that, indeed, the rudiments of facial representation are embodied in the connection weights. But how does that work, and in particular, how can face net generalize to novel cases? Analysis of the network to determine how each unit responds under various conditions yields the answer. The units whose activity is the focus of analysis are the middle layer of units, sometimes called the *hidden units*. In particular, what we want to know is the "retinal stimulus" to which a given middle unit will give its maximal response. We want to know this because it will tell us something about what stimulus characteristics those units represent and hence how representation is achieved by the population of units in the network.

We might have expected each of these middle-layer cells to become selectively responsive to some localized facial feature such as nose length, mouth width, eye separation, and so forth. Reconstructing the actual "tuning" of the

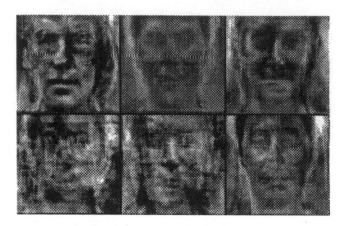

Figure 7.14 Six of many *holons*: the preferred stimuli of some of the cells in layer two of the face-recognition network. Compare these holons to the imput images shown in figure 7.13. Note that each preferred pattern spans the entire input space. (Courtesy of Gary Cottrell.)

80 middle-layer "face cells" reveals that the network settled into a coding strategy very different from this.

Figure 7.14 reconstructs the preferred stimuli for six typical face cells from layer two of Cottrell's network. Notice that each cell comprehends the *entire surface* of the input layer, rather than an isolated facial feature, such as the nose. The result is that each of the units represents an entire facelike structure, which Janet Metcalfe, Cottrell's coworker on this project, calls a "holon." None of these *holon*s corresponds to individual faces in the training set. Rather, they seem to capture somewhat *holistic* characteristics of *facehood*—diffuse, global characteristics for which we do not have applicable vocabulary. A given face presented at the input layer will variously activate each of these 80 cells in the middle layer, as a function of how closely it resembles or *approximates* each of these 80 "preferred stimuli."

Identifications (this is Billy) can be made by the output layer because for each face entered as input, the resulting middle-unit activation pattern (80-element vector) will be unique. Different photographs of the same person will produce highly similar vectors at the middle layer; male/female discrimination reflects the fact that the activation vectors for female stimuli are more similar to one another than they are to activation vectors for male stimuli. Sometimes the network gets it wrong when a female has very short hair, a rather long jaw, etc. Sometimes we get it wrong too.

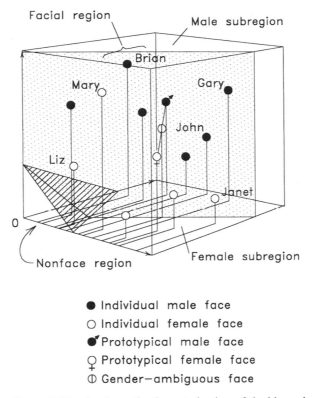

● Individual male face
○ Individual female face
●̷ Prototypical male face
♀ Prototypical female face
⊕ Gender—ambiguous face

Figure 7.15 A schematic characterization of the hierarchy of learned partitions across the neuronal activation space of layer three. (From P. M. Churchland 1995.)

Here, then, is the basic story. The values in the input vector reflect the gray-level values in the photographs, and the configuration of connection weights in the middle-layer vectors embodies what is task-relevant in various aggregations of input values. Input vectors are pushed through the configuration of weights, transformed into abstract representations in a high-dimensional "facial parameter space." These vectors are in turn pushed through the last layer of weights, with the resulting output vector representing answers to "Is it a face or not?" "Is it a male or female?" and "Who is it?"

Figure 7.15 is a three-dimensional diagram of the eighty-dimensional activation space of the of middle-layer units, and each point in it is relevant to representation in the "display of knowledge" sense. By contrast, the overall *partitions* within that space reflect representations in the "capacity for knowledge" sense. They embody the network's background "conceptual framework," within which its fleeting perceptual inputs get integrated. The activation space shows a primary partition into two regions, one for faces, one for nonfaces. The nonface region is small because the middle-layer cells respond minimally to a nonface. Not illustrated is the fact that the boundaries are actually fuzzy. Notice also that there is no cutoff value, in any one dimension, below which the coded subject must fail to be a face. This tells us that a photo may still be coded as a face if it scores zero on one dimension. This is efficient, since allows unusual faces, such as caricatures, to be coded as faces nonetheless.

The face region is further partitioned into male and female subregions, roughly equal in volume. Scattered throughout are the particular faces on which the network was trained. The female subregion's "center of gravity" is the general area of the *prototypical* female face; *mutatis mutandis* for the male subregion. Further subregions might have been found had we asked the network to respond to them—categories such as happy, sad, angry, and frightened. (Metcalfe and Cottrell have trained a network to respond to distinct emotional expressions.[18])

The story so far has been told in terms of *activation spaces* specified by the activation profiles of the hidden units. It is in the configuration of *weights*, however, that the information is stored. Consequently, we can also ask what the *weight space* looks like. In this hyperspace, each "synapse" (weight), and there are roughly 300,000 of them, corresponds to a dimension of the space (300K dimensions) (figure 7.16).

I hasten to add that the network's categories, for example, *male/female*, are scarcely comparable to *my* categories of male and female. Mine are enriched by layers and *more* layers of background knowledge acquired through many years of experience. My brain has vastly more weights than the meager face net, and vastly more categorial understanding. Nevertheless, the *conceptual point* is our focus, and the conceptual point illustrated by face net is that *a network can have categorial representations, which are collectively embodied as positions in weight space and displayed as points in activation space.*

If permitted to speculate, we may imagine that categorial knowledge in real neural networks is likewise embodied in their synaptic-weight configurations and in the resulting set of partitions on their neuronal activation spaces. As weight configurations adjust to conform to the statistics of the input patterns, geometric shapes (the system's categories) are sculpted in the activation spaces. If representation may be so envisioned, then, to a first approximation, my worldly knowledge might be conceived in terms of neural networks, connectivity strengths, and patterns of activation. Undoubtedly, this sketch is too

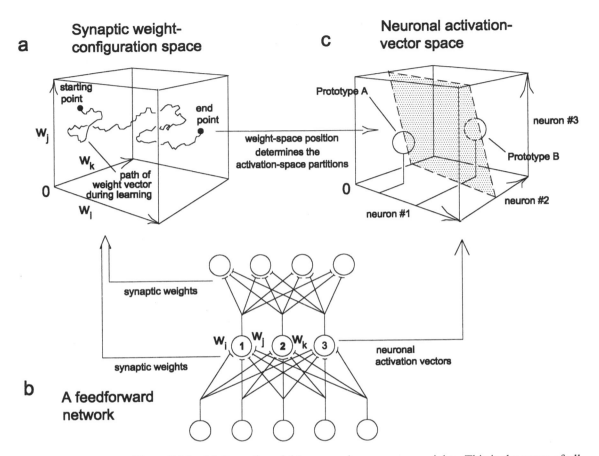

Figure 7.16   (a) Synaptic weight space, whose axes are weights. This is the space of all possible weight combinations from the synapses in the network. (b) A schematic network. (c) Activation-vector space, whose axes are hidden units. This is the space of all possible activation vectors across the population of hidden units. In this ultrasimple case, there is one partition dividing the space, with regions on each side of the partition where the prototypical example is located. (Courtesy of P. M. Churchland.)

crude nine ways from Sunday, but as a beginning, it looks more promising in its consilience with some general properties of nervous systems than various competitors, such as Fodor's representational model, in which representations are sentences written in the mind's encyclopedia.[19] Of the many respects in which it is too crude, one concerns system dynamics. Another concerns the use of time by the nervous system to represent, integrate, and regroup.[20] Although dynamical properties are known to be important, understanding the various ways in which time matters and is managed by nervous systems is difficult, for both technological and conceptual reasons.[21]

7   Neurosemantics

"Semantics" in its most general sense has to do with meaning. In the last sixty years, philosophers have taken *semantics* to cover three problems:

Reference   How can a word, which is one thing, be *about* something, which is *another* thing?

Meaning   What *things* have meaning, what is it for something to *have* meaning, *what* is its meaning, how are *meaning* and *reference* connected, and what is going on when meaning is *conveyed* from one person to another?

Truth   What sorts of *things* are true or false, what *makes* something true or false?

Note that as formulated, the problem considers semantics to pertain *primarily* to language and secondarily to the wider class of representations. This puts the order of problems back-to-front, since *non*linguistic representation is probably the platform for linguistic representation. How did this focus on language as the prototype of representation come to be?

The story involves the development of that powerful tool, modern symbolic logic. The great Polish logician Alfred Tarski (1901–1983) invented *formal semantics* to complement the *formal syntax* of Russell's and Frege's symbolic logic, and he is sometimes credited as the source for the classical approach. Ironically, however, Tarski developed formal semantics precisely because he recognized that in natural languages, syntax, semantics, and background knowledge, along with present context, are inextricably intertwined. Because formal logic was a highly artificial "language," he realized that it needed a complementary artificial semantics stripped of whatever is not formalizable (roughly, not *programmable*). And phenomena like polysemy (multiple meanings), background knowledge, analogy, metaphor, shared assumptions, current conditions, and the like, are not formalizable.

Despite Tarski's caution that formal semantics was no approximation to the real thing, and perhaps because no other approach looked viable, many clever and determined people tried to make it work for natural language anyhow. Perhaps, it was thought, Tarski was wrong.

From the beginning, the fit between natural language and formal logic was problematic at best. Rather like putting an octopus to bed, problems reappeared almost as soon they had been "fixed," and some problems could be tucked away only by pretending that they were not really problems for semantics anyhow, but for some entirely other pursuit, call it "pragmatics."

One tangle of problems derived from the "nonnegotiable" assumption that thought, and representation *generally*, is languagelike. Matters got distinctly worse if the language that all representation was supposed to resemble was the "language" of formal logic. This languagelike assumption created unbridgeable explanatory chasms between human representation and nonhuman representation, between nonverbal children and verbal children, and between sensory perception and imagining on the one hand and linguistic thinking, such as talking to oneself, on the other. One tanker-sized catastrophe occurred over language learning. *Learning* a language obviously requires representations, but all representations were allegedly languagelike, so you cannot learn a language until you have one.

To confront the learning catastrophe, Fodor postulated an innate, and hence unlearned, complete language—a language of thought shared by all humans. According to Fodor, when the infant acquires its cradle tongue, it is learning only a *translation* between its innate Mentalese and its encountered French or English. It is *not* acquiring a language for the first time. This holds even for concepts like gravitational field, neutrino, and virus. For a while, it was hard to tell whether the troubles with the classical approach were just the normal frustrations encountered in getting a theory adequately to explain the phenomena in its domain, or whether they signaled fatal defects that called for a new approach. By the 1980s, however, it looked like the defects were nontrivial.

Withstanding withering scorn, several linguists/psychologists (mainly Ron Langacker, Elizabeth Bates, Gilles Fauconnier, George Lakoff, Jeffrey Ellman and their students) suspected that the flaws were indeed fatal. To test this possibility, they began, each in his or her own way, to challenge the assumptions of the classical approach, including its assumptions about the independence of syntax and semantics, the context-free nature of meaning, the language of thought supposedly used to learn one's natural language. They also challenged the suitability of dumping into so-called "pragmatics" all of the nonformalizable stuff: background knowledge, context, current conditions, analogies, and so forth.[22] The dumping into pragmatics looked entirely too self-serving.

Once detached from the rhetoric and trappings of conventional wisdom, the classical framework tended to look a bit wobbly and unimposing, rather like King George III in his nightshirt. The problems with using formal logic and formal semantics as a model were well understood by the British philosopher Ryle in the 1960s, but with no competing theory of semantics to tempt research in a new direction, Ryle's observations went unheeded.[23]

In simple terms, the new approach, which is often referred to as *cognitive semantics*, suggested that formal logic and formal semantics are *atypical* artifacts of natural language, not its heart and soul. Second, cognitive semantics averred that language is primarily a tool for *communication*, and only secondarily a tool for representation, not the other way around. Third, it said that mental representation has fundamentally to do with categorization, prediction, and action-in-the-real-world; with parameter spaces, and points and paths within parameter spaces. Fourth, cognitive semantics suggests that representing in this manner could be done by something that operated not like a serial computer running a formal logic-like program, but by something with massively parallel networks—something like a brain.

Charting the blow-by-blow history of the debates between cognitive semantics and brain-averse semantics is not germane to our purposes. From my perspective, the important consideration concerns each theory's figures of merit, that is, the comparisons between the power of each approach to explain a wide range of data and mesh with the rest of the cognitive sciences and neurosciences, as well as with evolutionary and developmental biology. Sized up in these ways, the emerging new paradigm appears to have the greater promise as a scientific attack on semantics. For one thing, it loses the absurd complications entailed by the innate-language-of-thought hypothesis (see above). It also fits better with neural-network approaches to representation, though undoubtedly many significant insights made within the classical paradigm can be saved and recycled. For another, it can give unforced and compact explanation-sketches of central semantic phenomena, such as context dependence, counterfactual statements, indexicals, analogy, and polysemy,[24] and these explanation-sketches can be followed with empirical testing.[25]

As with any conflict between paradigms, there has been much posturing, many skirmishes, and many boundary disputes as the brain-averse approach discerned the shape of an impending revolution and cognitive semantics battled entrenched ideology. What will decide the various issues in the long run, however, is neither force of rhetoric nor tonnage of scorn heaped, but evidence and explanatory power. These latter two will be the main focus of my discussion. In the next section, I shall briefly consider an hypothesis to explain how representations can be about things, and how meaning might be rooted in neural network representation.

8 Being about Things

In face net, we saw partitions in the parameter space and specific volumes within the space as fuzzily carving out domains for female faces, males faces, and so on. The configuration of weights, we saw, is the structural matrix that effects the transformation of one activity pattern (vector) into another. Consider now a distinct network, trained on the same set of faces but in a different order and with its various weights in different initial random settings. Even though this net may achieve comparable performance in recognizing those faces, the details of its weight profile may be utterly different from that of the first net.

The important point is this: notwithstanding the differences in "synaptic" details, *comparable partitions in activation space* would be made. The configuration of the activation subspaces for male/female, and of the subspaces for each individual face, would be mutually congruent; that is, *they would map onto each other* (see again figure 7.15). This means that so far as *representing* is concerned, the critical thing is the overall geometry of the subspaces, wherever they happen to be located in the wider activation space of each network. For example, the subregions for each of the learned categories will map onto each other so as to preserve all of the similarity and distance relations between them.

This is significant, because it implies that the two networks represent, say, female faces in much the same way, differences in the details of their learning notwithstanding. In turn, this suggests that having the *same representation* comes to this: there is a relation-preserving *mapping* between configured parameter spaces. Loosely speaking, the two representations are intertranslatable.

Do the networks have to have the same number of units, connections, and weights to achieve this categorial or conceptual similarity? No. If face net α had two fewer middle layer units than face net β, the categorial configurations within α and β can still be very similar, or even perfectly congruent. And so also if face net α is trained on a somewhat different set of faces than face net β, or on different set of nonfaces. Of course, if face net α never sees *any* female faces, or if all the men it ever sees have beards, or if all the women have topknots, it will have a somewhat differently configured space from the more normally trained face net β. The two representational schemes will be at least roughly "translatable," nevertheless.[26]

Perhaps this general picture holds true, very roughly at least, of humans. As toddlers, our limited experience sometimes gives us false expectations. For example, if the only dogs we see are black Labradors, we might predict that *all* dogs resemble black Labradors (as I did). Additional experience with Pomeranians, St. Bernards, poodles, and so forth, along with contrasts with wolves, foxes, coyotes, and raccoons tuned up my neurons so that the categorial configuration of my dog subspaces became a little more closely aligned with those of wider community.

In general, for networks to have congruent subspaces corresponding to a category, they need to pick up on the real similarities in the shared stimuli. For it is the similarity relations that are reflected in the relative positions of the many subspaces: labs are closer to retrievers than either is to schnauzers, and all of these breeds of dog are closer to each other than any dog is to a carrot. My category *bird* may have more distinguishable points in it than yours, but fewer distinguishable points than that of my sister, a devoted bird watcher. Still, there will be sufficient similarity in their internal geometry that we can usually understand each other.

Is it possible that in adulthood your spider subspace and my cow subspace might happen, through pure coincidence, to have an identical geometry? It is extremely unlikely, especially because ours are not spaces with a mere three or four dimensions, but hyperspaces with thousands of dimensions. Sometimes, especially with children, a misunderstanding will arise because by sheer accident the child picked up on the wrong similarities. A toddler's concept of newspaper may apply to anything used to start the fire, the child realizing only later that newspapers are read.

If people are given roughly similar experiences, then superordinate categories, such as animal, vegetable, or furniture, will also be roughly similar in shape and have roughly the same subspaces. Psychological data suggest that barring highly unusual conditions, we and our neighbors share much the same prototypes (carrots and potatoes are prototypical vegetables, chairs and tables are prototypical furniture, and so forth).[27] Such psychological data on category structure could, therefore, be understood as evidence for approximate congruence in hyperspace geometry. It is much more difficult to give a unified account for these and related semantic phenomena in the classical framework.

To a first approximation, a representational framework can be about things in the world because it maps onto the similarity structure of things in world. More accurately, a representational framework maps onto those statistics of its environment that the organism, given its way of life, needs to attend to in order to survive and thrive. Distinctions between individual ravens may be tremendously important to other ravens, but are not something my dog cares much about. Given their way of life, ravens will care quite a lot about the differences between ravens and crows (especially for mating and for cooperative jobs such as harassing a wolf off its kill), between ravens and eagles (especially because eagles can kill ravens), ravens and sparrows (sparrows have yummy eggs but can harass a raven). For my dog, it does not really matter whether the birds stealing his kibble are ravens or crows or jays. Thus the mapping between the animal's world knowledge and the world is not independent of what the animal cares about and pays attention to. This mapping, "me"-relevant and behavior-guiding as it is, makes it possible for an animal's representations to be about things in the world. And the similarity in activation-space geometry between two brains is what makes it possible for one brain to share an understanding with another.

Incidentally, although the face net example used to launch this story involved training by examples, the causal origin of the representational geometry is not my main focus here. Presumably, in animals an important intermixing of genetically driven preparation and experientially driven tuning results in an individual's knowledge (see chapter 8). For the purposes at hand, the main focus is on the question of how representations in brains could be *about* things the world.

Seen through the lens of vector coding and parameter spaces, "aboutness" and meaning in representation are rather like the "aboutness" and meaning of maps. As maps can be richer and more detailed, so with world representations. As maps can have errors, distortions, and omissions, so too can world representations. In maps the internal relationships between the points and regions on the map make it a map of London or the Tatshenshini River or Alaska. Maps are for navigation, for going somewhere and doing something, and thus they can be enriched with task-relevant features. A road map of southern Alaska showing road quality and location of filling stations is less interesting to someone who plans to canoe the Tatshenshini River and needs to know the location and nature of the river's rapids, sandbars, and tributary inflows.[28]

9   Me, This, Here, and Now

The classical approach to meaning and representation was hopelessly outfoxed by indexical expressions such as "I" and "here" and demonstratives such as "this" and "that." These *context-dependent* expressions, so natural and easily usable in natural language, presented a ferocious riddle for the classical approach, with its insistence on contextual *independence*. So the classical story had to cobble together special mechanisms for generating "the view from here," so to speak, from context-free semantics. And a vexing business it was. How much of now is *now*, and how much of here is *here*? How can I crank the equivalent of the term "me" out of a set of descriptions, even a rather long set of descriptions?

Neural-network researchers, however, came to the problem from a different direction. They realized that because the animal's body and its brain are the locus of sensory input, attention, and motor decisions, "my point of view" is the *basic* representational stance. Context-free representation, on the other hand, is a far fancier contraption and a more difficult achievement. A brain can probably take for granted its current context, with its spatial configuration of things and events in relation to "me" and what "I" am interested in and paying attention to. The "me-here-now" trio, therefore, does not need to be specially generated by contrived and devious logical mechanisms out of context-free sentences. So let's have a closer look at how the brain might be organized to handle these matters.

As we saw earlier (chapter 3), *spatiality* is deeply connected to body representation, in both sensory and motor domains, and body representation is fundamental. Understanding where things are in three-dimensional space does not just arise supernaturally, that is for sure, nor is it just *given*, whatever that might mean. Spatial understanding depends crucially on the structural organization of various receptor sheets and on how sensory signals are integrated and represented. And this organization will have been configured to serve the needs of motor skills, and motor control generally.

A range of results from basic neurobiological research, behavioral research, and neural modeling come together in a rather compelling idea developed by Alexander Pouget and Terry Sejnowski. Their hypothesis grounds a strategy for explaining how the primate brain integrates diverse sensory signals and generates an objective representation; that is, a representation of where things are in the space relative to one's independently movable parts—legs, arms, fingers, eyes, and so forth. I devote the next section to sketching their idea, and what is attractive about it.

10   Spatial Representation in Primates

The three brain areas of particular interest here are the hippocampus, prefrontal cortex, and posterior parietal cortex. These three are also highly interconnected, which hints that a consilient, interlocking theory may emerge in the long run.[29] To narrow the discussion, I shall focus on the posterior parietal cortex. This area appears to provide the fundamental "objects-out-there-external-to-my-body" organization critical for primate sensory-motor representation and control. The hippocampus and prefrontal areas likely use these basic parietal representations for additional purposes (e.g., remembering the when and where of goodies, planning movements, generating images of movements, etc.).

The crux of the idea developed by Pouget and Sejnowski (introduced on pp. 77–79) is that certain neural networks in posterior parietal cortex generate a sort of map-on-demand, i.e., a device that takes sensory information from the various modalities and transforms it into information that guides the motor structures. For convenience, I think of this network as an *archmapper*. What does the archmapper do?

Suppose that you have a mosquito on your right elbow that you wish to swat. Something is felt, and your somatosensory cortex registers the sensation in your body-surface-space. Something else, namely your left arm, needs to move from its position at your side to smack your right elbow precisely where the mosquito is feeding. This means that your brain needs to know how to move this object with shoulder, elbow, wrist, and finger joints so that contact is made. That the signal is in the "elbow" position on the somatosensory map does not, in itself, contain that information. Very roughly, your brain's problem, in parameter-space terms, is this: what path in *joint-space* has an endpoint that maps onto the location of the stimulus in *skin-space*? What your brain needs is a *mapping* between joint-space and skin-space. It need, in other words, a transformation from a path specified in joint-angle coordinates to a position specified in skin coordinates.[30]

Or suppose that the familiar whine of the mosquito is detected, and you catch a glimpse in your peripheral vision of a flitting something. In the early stages of the visual system (e.g., V1, V2), the location of the visual signal is specified in retinal coordinates; that is where the signal is on the retina. To move the eyes and head to look at a heard or felt object, or to reach with an arm or tongue or foot for a seen object, the brain needs to know where to go in the appropriate coordinate system. On their own, retinal coordinates will not suffice; cochlear coordinates will not suffice. The brain needs to know, inter alia, where the eyeball is with respect to the head, where the head is with respect to the shoulder and trunk. Coordinate transformations are needed to specify where the eyeball should go to foveate (position the eyeball so that the signal from the stimulus falls on the foveal region of the retina). Normally, we reach our hands and move our eyes to a target effortlessly, and the computational resources needed to pull this off are not part of what the brain has conscious access to. The effortlessness makes the task seem easy, but computationally it is anything but simple. The central point is that sensory coordinates have to be transformed into motor coordinates in order to connect with a sensorily specified target (figure 7.17; see also figure 3.7).

Enter the archmapper. This network has the representational resources to take information from various sensory systems and yield "go to" locations in the corresponding motor frameworks—eyeball, neck-and-shoulder, hand, arm, etc. It can specify what path, given in joint-angle coordinates, will get your arm to the right position in skin space. It can specify what configuration the eye muscles should have so that you can foveate the mosquito. It is not dedicated to any one specific mapping, but integrates fairly abstract sensory signals, and delivers fairly abstract go-to signals to the motor structures. And it seems plausible that a network of this kind provides the wherewithal for the representation of space.

The archmapper can be deployed by different motor structures for distinct motor chores, such as moving the eyes, hands, pinnae (ear flaps), legs, or head. In doing so, it relies on sensory information from retinas, cochleas, joints, muscles, tendon receptors, and so forth. The archmapper is not exactly or merely perceptual, nor exactly motor, nor exactly egocentric (self-centered) or allocentric (object-centered). It combines information from multiple sources in

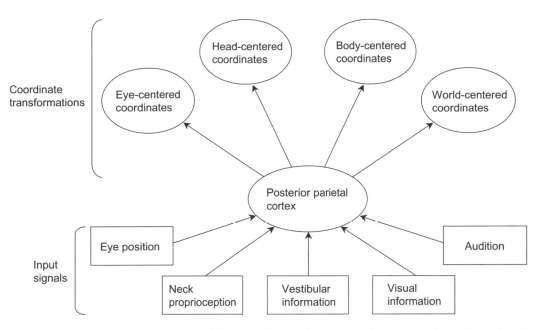

Figure 7.17   The role of the posterior parietal cortex in the transformation of retinotopic visual information into higher-order reference frames. Eye position, head position (determined from neck proprioception and vestibular sources), and gaze position (determined from visual sources) are used to modify retinotopic signals. The posterior parietal cortex is thus positioned to provide an intermediate stage in the conversion of visual and auditory information into eye-, head-, body-, and world-centered coordinate frames. (Based on Andersen 1999.)

a way suited to multiple applications, but cannot neatly be described in everyday terms. This is one of those examples where the function of a neuronal pool does not correspond to any familiar, everyday function. Evidently, however, it is essentially spatial.

Integration of somatosensory "body knowledge," including proprioceptive and vestibular knowledge such as "where-this-body-part-is-in-relation-to-other-body-parts," with visual-auditory "where-things-are-in-relation-to-my-body" knowledge allows for general representations of "me-in-external-space." And structures in the parietal cortex seem to be part of this "me-in-external-space" representation. As noted earlier, the spatial aspects of body representation can be only part of the self-representation story, however, because other aspects, involving various dimensions of feeling and homeostasis, will figure in what it is to have a "me" representation.[31]

The mathematical details of exactly how the Pouget-Sejnowski hypothesis runs take us beyond the scope of this chapter.[32] But some neurobiological evidence is essential as background. Neurobiological studies of area 7a and 7b in the parietal cortex have provided important clues as to how coordinate transformations are accomplished by networks of neurons. Monkeys with bilateral lesions in area 7 show poor reaching to a target (ataxia), misshaping of hands to fit the shape of the target, and slowness of movement. They also show defective eye movements, principally in foveating, and they have other impaired spatial abilities. They are poor at finding the home cage when released, poor at route-finding to a food source, and poor in judging spatial relationships among objects (e.g., "the food source is the box located nearer to the can").

Another region of the parietal cortex, area 5, contains some cells that fire maximally to a signal when the arm is reaching and others that fire selectively to the expectation of a stimulus (figures 7.18 and 7.19). Because a great deal of research has probed the visual properties of this area, one tends to think of these regions as essentially visual. Recent data reveal, however, that they are much more than that. The response patterns of neurons in these areas can be modified by many factors, including auditory, somatosensory, and vestibular signals, as well as attention, intention, expectation, preparation, and execution. This clearly indicates that these neurons are more than just sensory.[33]

Area 7 is multimodal and contains cells individually responsive to either visual, auditory, somatosensory, chemical, vestibular, or proprioceptive signals. Interestingly, auditory cells in this region appear to be mapped in *retinotopic* coordinates. A few cells are multimodal: a given cell may respond to visual and auditory signals, or to somatosensory and visual signals, or to chemical and somatosensory signals.

It is often claimed that our conception of space is unified, and sometimes even that it is *necessarily* unified. Yet it is unclear what introspection, innocent of philosophical indoctrination, actually delivers on this point. Nevertheless, if introspection does present the "oneness" of spatial perception, then that perception is undoubtedly illusory to some degree. Various versions of "where-perceived-objects-are-in-my-body-space" can dissociate (largely without introspective notice) as a function of precisely which perceptual modalities are involved.

The effect has been demonstrated in a variety of experiments. For example, in ventriloquism, speech is perceived as coming from a puppet whose mouth merely moves in synchrony with the speech sounds. In this instance, spatial location via auditory signals is trumped by visual-motion signals associated with

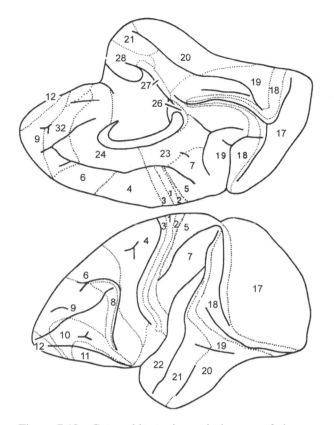

Figure 7.18 Cytoarchitectonic cortical maps of the macaque monkey by Brodman (1909). Note the location of areas 5 and 7. (From Fuster 1995.)

speech. Other examples include changes in visual perception brought about by vibrating the neck muscles (thus stimulating the vestibulum); and Stevens's production of illusory visual motion by paralyzing the eye muscles (see also pp. 85–86).[34] Additionally, *within* vision there can also be dissociation in normal subjects between spatial coding as it is visually experienced and as it is used for grasping.[35]

One intriguing pattern of breakdown in spatial reasoning occurs in *hemi-neglect*, a condition sometimes seen in patients with unilateral lesions of the right parietal cortex. These patients display a marked tendency to ignore the contralesional (i.e., left) side of their body-centered world. They tend to look only to the right, though some can move their eyes to the left if directly asked

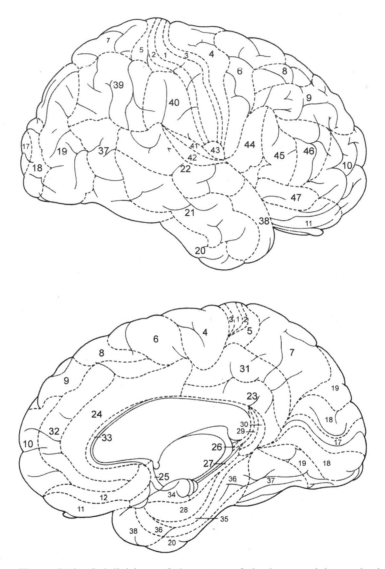

Figure 7.19 Subdivisions of the cortex of the human right cerebral hemisphere into cytoarchitectonic fields according to Brodmann. Note areas 5 and 7. (Based on Nieuwenhuys et al. 1981.)

to do so. Asked to make a drawing or reproduce a figure, they will omit most or all of the left half; asked to "cancel" (cross out) all the lines on a page, they will fail to cancel all the lines left of center; asked to bisect a horizontal line, they will draw the transecting line off-center to the right. (See also discussion of parietal-lobe symptoms in chapter 3.)

In one ingenious experiment (Biziach and Luzzatti 1978), hemineglect patients were asked to imagine that they were standing in a well-known plaza in their city, and to describe what they could see from a given vantage point. Their descriptions omitted objects on the neglected side *relative to the imagined vantage point*: told to imagine they were standing at the north end of the plaza, they would omit the buildings to the east, and when subsequently instructed to repeat the task from the southern vantage point, they would list the eastern buildings and omit from their description all the westerly buildings that they had listed immediately before. This shows that hemineglect is a deficit of spatial reasoning and/or representation at some fairly basic level, and not just a perceptual failure.

There is also a motor component to hemineglect. Neglect patients show little or no spontaneous use of limbs on the left side of the body, though some will reluctantly move the neglected limbs upon direct request. They will also neglect auditory stimuli from the left, sometimes failing to acknowledge others who are speaking to them from that side. This sort of polymodal, perceptuomotor deficit is what one might expect from a lesion of parietal cortex, since it receives and integrates inputs from multiple modalities and is known to be involved in the coordination of perception with action.

Pouget and Sejnowski used hemineglect as a test of the predictive power of their archmapper hypothesis (described above). They created a network model that has the oculomotor input/output structure and response properties that they attribute to area 7a, and then "lesioned" it by removing the units that correspond to the right side of the brain.[36] This left the network with a disproportionately high number of neurons that were most responsive to rightward eye positions and/or right-visual-field stimuli. They then equipped it with a winner-take-all output-selection mechanism and tested it on stimuli similar to those used with neglect patients.

The network output exhibited striking similarities to the human behavioral results. In the line-cancellation task, the network failed to cancel lines on the side opposite the lesion. More important, the line between the cancelled and noncancelled areas was fairly sharp, even though the underlying representation had only a smooth gradient. The network also paralleled human behavior on the bisection task: it was successful before the lesion, but shifted the transection point to the right after the lesion. In other experiments, it was shown to suffer object-centered as well as visual-field-centered neglect. In an experiment where the network received head-position information (instead of eye-position information), the network exhibited the same curious effect found in human patients whereby performance on left-field tasks can be improved by turning the head to the right. Although these phenomena have been problematic for existing theories of hemineglect, Pouget and Sejnowski's model is able to explain how they arise naturally from an organization of response functions that can plausibly be attributed to the human parietal cortex.[37]

To the extent that the experienced "oneness of space" is not illusory, it highly depends on the fact that all of the signals are generated in *one* nervous system, inside *one* body, that has *one* spatially linked source of signals. There is no single objective spatial representation (of the sort standardly presupposed by symbolic models of representation), but a distributed, multimodal representation that fundamentally integrates perception and action, self and world. Where constancies appear across distinct modalities, it becomes possible and even inevitable to understand them as representing an enduring world beyond the body.[38]

Certainly, many questions about the nature of our representation of space remain. In particular, it may be wondered whether the archmapper should be limited to spatial information, or whether the brain would more likely have a *spacetime* archmapper. Probably it should, but fleshing that hypothesis out is a later scientific development. Further research will determine whether the basic Pouget-Sejnowski idea succeeds in pointing us in the right direction.

11 Concluding Remarks

This chapter brings us only to the doorstep of the neurophilosophy of representations. Even then, it provides at most a squinting, keyhole view of the terrain beyond. Neural nets, for example, can be far more powerful and versatile than the simple nets illustrated here. They can have backloops; they can add units and connections, accommodate symbols, develop specialized subregions, and incorporate various activity-dependent and modulatory properties seen in real neurons (figure 7.20).[39] Also undiscussed are surprising discoveries about how smart and computationally deft real neurons are. New results on real

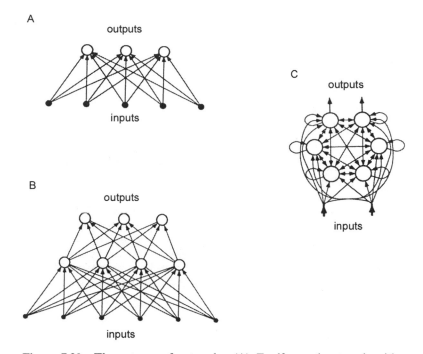

Figure 7.20 Three types of networks. (A) Feedforward network with one layer of weights connecting the input units to the output units. (B) Feedforward network with two layers of weights and one layer of hidden units between the input and output units. (C) Recurrent network with reciprocal connections between units. (From Churchland and Sejnowski 1992.)

neurons and their role in how the brain represents abound; here I list a few: the addition of new neurons to hippocampal and cortical structures, the activation of sequestered synapses as a function of the level of neuronal activity, the modification of receptive-field resolution as a result of attentional influence, the existence of nonspiking computation, self-regulating synaptic receptors, activity-dependent gene expression, and neuromodulation everywhere.

How background knowledge and context figure in ongoing sensory and motor representation is under vigorous study at several levels, as are mechanisms for directing attention. Representation of causality is a monumentally important target of intense research at the cognitive/neuroscience/philosophy interface, though it has not been discussed here. More generally, inference and analogy, though fundamental cognitive operations, have only recently found their place on center stage in cognitive science.[40]

One of the most profound recent developments, sometimes going under the name "situated cognition," has been the realization that brains do not have—and do not need to have—a *complete* representation of the current situation. Instead, brains can selectively represent the world on a *need-to-know* footing and can rely on the fact that the world is mostly stable and continues to be there, available for second looks and closer looks.[41]

Further, the idea of *distributed cognition* depends on the realization that social animals can divide cognitive labor, and that if a brain can represent which person has which competence, this general knowledge is far more economical than representing all of the detailed knowledge in one head. For humans, this strategy gets extended to cultural artifacts, such as tools, stories, books, and knowledge-preserving institutions. Because so much science and know-how is scaffolded onto our environment, I need not learn it all from scratch, or in many cases, I need not learn it at all. I can let the surgeon remove my appendix, the electrician wire my house, and the pilot fly the plane. And the Internet is only the most recent example of artifacts soaked in knowledge.

In canoeing terms, this chapter gets us only to the put-in; the real excitement begins once the canoe is in the river. The recommended readings will help with navigation and will also suggest yet other streams to follow.

Suggested Readings

Abbott, L., and T. J. Sejnowski, eds. 1999. *Neural Codes and Distributed Representations.* Cambridge: MIT Press.

Bechtel, W., P. Mandik, J. Mundale, and R. S. Stufflebeam, eds. 2001. *Philosophy and the Neurosciences: A Reader.* Oxford: Oxford University Press.

Bechtel, W., and A. Abrahamsen 1991. *Connectionism and the Mind.* Oxford: Blackwells. See especially chapter 2.

Churchland, Paul M. 1995. *The Engine of Reason, the Seat of the Soul.* Cambridge: MIT Press.

Clark, Andy. 1993. *Being There.* Cambridge: MIT Press.

Fauconnier, Gilles. 1997. *Mappings in Thought and Language.* Cambridge: Cambridge University Press.

Gärdenfors, P. 2000. *Conceptual Spaces: The Geometry of Thought.* Cambridge: MIT Press.

Geutner, D., K. J. Holyoak, and B. N. Kokinov. 2001. *The Analogical Mind.* Cambridge: MIT Press.

Hutchins, E. 1995. *Cognition in the Wild.* Cambridge: MIT Press.

Katz, Paul, ed. 1999. *Beyond Neurotransmission.* Oxford: Oxford University Press.

Lakoff, George. 1987. *Women, Fire, and Dangerous Things.* Chicago: University of Chicago Press.

Pouget, A., and T. J. Sejnowski. 1997. Spatial transformations in the parietal cortex using basis functions. *Journal of Cognitive Neuroscience* 9 (2): 222–237.

Websites
BioMedNet Magazine: http://news.bmn.com/magazine

A Brief Introduction to the Brain: http://ifcsun1.ifisiol.unam.mx/brain/

Computational Neuroscience Lab: http://www.cnl.salk.edu

Encyclopedia of Life Sciences: http://www.els.net

Living Links: http://www.emory.edu/living_links

The MIT Encyclopedia of the Cognitive Sciences: http//cognet.mit.edu/MITECS

Science: http://www.scienceonline.org.

The Whole Brain Atlas: http://www.med.harvard.edu/AANLIB/home.html

8   How Do Brains Learn?

1   What Is the Problem?

At the heart of traditional epistemology lie two questions: (1) what is the nature of knowledge, and (2) where does knowledge come from? In chapter 7 we considered a neurophilosophical approach to the first problem. The whence and wherefore of knowledge are the targets of this chapter: how does the brain come to represent aspects of the world and, eventually, aspects of itself? More generally, how do we come to know anything?

The range of things in the "knows" category seems as diverse as the range of stuff at a yard sale. Some is knowledge *how*, some is knowledge *that*, some is a bit of both, and some is not exactly either. There are things we can articulate, such as the instructions for changing a tire, and other things we cannot, such as how we retrieve facts from memory or how we distinguish the relevant from the irrelevant in problem solving. To learn some things, such as how to ride a bicycle, we have to *try*. By contrast, avoiding eating oysters if they made you vomit last time *just happens*. Whereas knowing how to install Napster depends on cultural artifacts that are imbued with others' knowledge, knowing how to clap does not.

Even if we have not have considered it before, we know that dolphins do not knit and that Mt. McKinley is not made of yogurt. Presumably, this is because when queried, we *generate* these beliefs from other things we *do* know. Some of what you know are *logical* truths (e.g., it is false that lemons are both yellow *and not* yellow), some are *factual* truths (e.g., bears have not been domesticated), and some a bit of a mix (e.g., you cannot be in two places at the same time). Some knowledge is language-dependent; some is not. Some knowledge evokes strong emotions; some is emotionally pretty much neutral. Some knowledge is conscious; some is not.

Some knowledge (e.g., the nature of electricity) is highly abstract, some (e.g., that nettles sting) is based directly on sensory experience. Some knowledge seems to rely on character traits rather than general intelligence (e.g., how to handle horses, how to make people laugh, how to tell a good tale). Some knowledge is fleeting, but some endures a lifetime.

The dimensions of variation in what we know are legion. Of the miscellany of categories honored in our conventional wisdom, which of them captures a real distinction *from the point of view of the brain* will eventually be revealed through scientific discoveries. That is, new taxonomies will emerge from the coevolutionary interaction of neuroscience and psychology. At this stage of cognitive neuroscience, it is difficult to tell which of our everyday categories have sufficient integrity to endure as they stand and which do not. As I shall suggest below, however, some hypotheses, drawing upon anatomical, behavioral, and physiological results, are beginning to re-fence the landscape of our everyday categorial system for thinking about cognitive matters.

2   Knowledge: Learned and Innate

Historically, much discussion in epistemology concerned how much of what we know is based on "instinct," and how much on "experience." At the extremes, some took the view that essentially all knowledge is innate (the Rationalists). Knowledge displayed at birth is obviously a good candidate for instinctual knowledge. A normal neonate rat scrambles to the warmest place, latches its mouth onto a nipple, and begins to suck. When you touch the cheek of a newborn human, its head turns toward the touch, it nuzzles for a nipple, and sucks efficiently on any warm, nipplelike thing it finds. A kitten thrown into the air rights itself and lands on its feet. Some of these early instinctual behaviors persist through postnatal development; others do not. Other knowledge is obviously learned. That fire is rapid oxidation, that oxygen is an element, how to milk a cow, or how to grow tomatoes are all examples of knowledge acquired by learning, not by instinct.

Such contrasts suggest that everything we know has its origin *either* in the genes *or* in experience, where these categories are entirely separate and exhaustive. Historically as well as currently, debate often revolves around the appropriate criteria for sorting knowledge into the two presumptively separate bins. In the absence of scientific understanding of biological evolution, neuroembryology, and the neurophysiology of experience-dependent modifications to neurons, the debate tends to be rather less productive than intense. The more we know about genes and development and the brain, however, the less we need to rely on speculation and intuitions about what can and cannot be imagined.

Neurodevelopment and neurobiology have essentially laid waste to the very simple *nature or nurture* dichotomy. Biology turns out to be vastly more complicated than the simple dichotomy implies. This two-bins assumption is overturned by a number of considerations, prominent among which is the fact that normal *development*, right from the earliest stages, relies on *both* genes *and* epigenetic conditions. Moreover, paradigmatic examples of long-term *learning* rely on *both* gene expression *and* epigenetic conditions. This does not entail either that there is no such thing as in-born instinct or that there is no such thing as learning. This also does not entail that there are no causally significant differences between, say, the sucking reflex and knowing how to shuck an oyster. Indeed, there are. The important point is that the differences do not neatly line up as *caused by genes versus caused by experience*. Underlying the existence of both capacities are huge numbers of interacting, causally relevant factors, and they do not sort as the simple two-bins assumption demands.

There exist, certainly, causally relevant differences between *prenatal* development and *postnatal* learning, and between *early development* and *later development*, as well as between skill learning, priming, and conditioning. *Genes versus epigenetic conditions* is not a filter for any of those differences. There is, moreover, a compelling explanation why this should be so. The idea, explored for example by Quartz and Sejnowski (1997), is that evolution lucked onto the fact that regularities in the environment mean that the genome does not have to code for everything; rather, it can rely on the existence of certain external conditions to play a consistent role in regulating gene expression. If biological evolution exploits environmental information in building a creature, why not also for a creature's adaptation for environmental change? To put it crudely, why, if you were Mother Nature, would you care about a principled dichotomy between *nature* and *nurture*?

Six important and related developments have chiefly contributed to the appreciation that things are not as simple as the catchy phrase *nature versus nurture* seems to imply.

- What genes do is *code for proteins*. Strictly speaking, there is no gene *for* a sucking reflex, let alone a gene *for* female coyness or Scottish thriftiness or the concept of a hole. A gene is simply a sequence of base pairs whose order contains the information that allows RNA to string together a sequence of amino acids to make a protein. (A gene is said to be *expressed* when it is transcribed into RNA products, some of which are translated into proteins.)

- Natural selection cannot *directly* select particular wiring to support a particular domain of knowledge. Genes are in the cells of animals, and what dies or lives on to reproduce is the *whole animal*, with its own style of perception and motor control. Blind luck aside, what determines whether the animal survives is its *behavior*, and its equipment, neural *and* otherwise, underpins its behavior. If the animal's behavior allows it to outwit or outrun or outmuscle the competition, it has a chance to live on and reproduce. *Representational* prowess can be selected for, albeit *indirectly*, only if the representational package informing behavior was what gave the animal its competitive edge. Hence representational sophistication and its wiring infrastructure can be selected only *via* the motor output it upgrades. Thus the resources, neural and otherwise, for *motor control* exert a powerful constraint on the evolution of representational capacities.

- There is a truly stunning and quite unpredicted degree of *conservation* in structures and developmental organization across *all* vertebrate animals, and a very high degree of conservation in basic cellular functions across phyla, from worms to spiders to humans. (See figures 6.4 and 6.5.) Humans have only about 30,000 genes, and we differ from mice in only about 3,000 genes. Humans and chimpanzees are believed to share about 98.5 percent of their genes. In fact, we share about 110 genes with bacteria. Some proteins, such as histones, actin, and tubulin, are essentially the same in all organisms. Long before the appearance of vertebrates, *all* the major protein superfamilies had formed. Variations and elaborations within superfamilies were seen thereafter, of course, but no completely original protein superfamilies are found in humans that might account for the cognitive differences between us and our closest relatives, chimpanzees, or even between us and simple worms.

- Given the high degree of conservation, whence the remarkable diversity of multicellular organisms? Molecular biologists have discovered that some genes regulate the expression of other genes, and are themselves regulated by yet other genes, in an intricate, interactive, and systematic organization. The systematicity ultimately depends on a clever trick: make some gene expression contingent on the local protein environment. But genes (via RNA) make proteins, so you can regulate the expression of one gene by another gene via sensitivity to protein products. Additionally, proteins, both within cells and in extracellular space, can interact with each other to yield further contingencies that can figure in a regulatory cascade. An example of both the highly conserved nature of developmental organization and of the critical role of regulatory genes is the so-called master gene for the eye in *Drosophila*. This gene regulates some 200 other genes via epigenetic contingencies (conditions that exist at a given time in a given place in the embryo's development). Moreover, this gene is *highly* conserved: the "master gene" for the mouse eye is essentially the same as the "master gene" for eyes in *Drosophila*. Implanted in *Drosphila*, the mouse gene will produce fruit-fly eyes. The emergence of complex, interactive cause-effect profiles for gene expression results in *very* fancy regulatory cascades that can make *very* fancy organisms. Us, for example. Small differences in genes can have large and far-reaching effects, owing to the intricate hierarchy of regulatory linkages.

- Various aspects of development of an organism from fertilized egg to up-and-running critter depend on *where* and *when* cells are born. This includes cell specialization and wiring patterns of the various types of neurons. Neurons originate from a daughter cell of the last mitotic division of precursor cells. Whether such a daughter cell becomes a neuron or a glial cell depends on its epigenetic circumstances. Which type of some *hundred* types of neurons (e.g., excitatory pyramidal, inhibitory stellate, inhibitory basket) the neuron becomes depends on its *epigenetic* circumstances. Notably, the genes, *in and of themselves*, do not specify cell fate. That is, there are no genes for Purkinje cells or for spiny stellate cells, in the sense that a specific gene is necessary and sufficient for the production of specific cell types. Moreover, the manner in which neurons from one area, such as the thalamus, *connect* to cells in the cortex depends very much on epigenetic circumstances, e.g., on the *spontaneous activity*, and later the *experience-driven activity*, of the thalamic and cortical neurons.

- The successful strategy typical in development—an iterated, interactive, organizational cascade—is continuous with regulatory cascades serving the postnatal plasticity we typically call *learning*. Neurotransmitters such as glutamate carry a signal from one neuron to the next, and neuromodulators can regulate the functionality of receptors. Activity cascades, gene-expression cascades, and feedback cascades modulate the modulators and are modulated by other events. Some of the same cascades figure in both learning and development.

For example, the NMDA receptor, a complex transmembrane protein, plays a crucial role in the cascades leading to the synaptic strengthening in certain forms of learning (pp. 345 ff.). But the very same protein, NMDA, also plays a crucial, if quite different, role in brain development. As Corriveau and colleagues have recently demonstrated, in early development, NMDA regulates genes that regulate the transition from proliferation of precursor cells to the differentiation of neurons.[1]

The interaction between genes and extragenetic conditions can be unexpected. In certain species of turtle, for example, the sex of the turtle is determined not at fertilization but by the temperature of the sand in which the eggs incubate. In mice, the sex of siblings adjacent on the placental fetus line in the uterus will affect such things as the male/female ratio of a given mouse's subsequent offspring and even its longevity. Postnatal learning triggers cascades leading to gene expression. For example, as we shall see in section 8.6, this is true of certain cells in the amygdala as the animal is conditioned to expect a foot shock after it hears a tone. We also know that if you are exposed to a new sensorimotor experience during the day, then during your deep-sleep cycle, the gene *zif*-268 is upregulated, and this affects how well you remember what happened to you during the day.

More generally, considerable evidence runs against the idea that brain evolution consists in the selection of anatomically localized functional subsystems (modules) that are *separately heritable* and are gradually optimized over generations. So far as we know, Mother Nature cannot reach into the depths of a contingency cascade to tweak the genes to optimize particular behavioral traits, such as forming the past tense of verbs. Instead, selection is forced to make do with quite general neuroanatomical changes, such as changing the precursor-cell proliferation schedules. These changes are highly constrained. For example, as Steve Quartz (2001) astutely points out, the neocortex does not vary across all dimensions, but retains common organizational themes such as the horizontal 6-layer cortex, the vertical column, the general connectivity pattern of input to layer 4 and output from layers 5 and 6 to other cortical areas and the subcortex, and so on. Strikingly, what *does* change are the numbers of neurons, and hence the numbers and sizes of cortical areas.[2] As a result, functional changes, beneficial or deleterious, may be displayed by large neural regions or even by the brain as a whole. In criticizing alleged examples of domain-specific behavior, such as the human female preference for a mate who is devoted and can provide, Panksepp and Panksepp (2001a) note, "Simple emotional systems with a modicum of some general-purpose cognitive skill may easily yield some of the most striking folk-psychological discoveries of evolutionary psychology."[3]

On the general question of the evolution of the human brain, Quartz sums up his approach thus:

The evidence suggests that the selective forces underlying the evolution of human cognitive architecture were critically connected to highly unstable climes. . . . Based on these considerations, I suggest that an important feature of hominid evolution was a process I have referred to as progressive externalization . . . , whereby the brain's development becomes increasingly regulated by extrinsic factors, likely mediated by variation in the scheduling of various events in neural development. I suggest this process allows for flexible prefrontally mediated cognitive function, particularly in the social domain, and underlies the rapid changes in social structure that was a response to the need for buffering ecological instability. The upshot of this process was symbolic culture, which plays a central role in shaping the structures underlying human cognition. (Quartz 2001)

Bear in mind that many questions in neurodevelopment and brain evolution have not yet been answered, and new discoveries may profoundly change how we think about these matters.[4] What I argue here is that we do know enough to know that the nature versus nurture debate has been substantially misconceived. In sum, postnatal learning and prenatal development share mechanisms; prenatal development relies on epigenetic conditions for gene regulation; and birth allows for a much expanded range of extragenetic conditions to figure in nervous-system self-organization. We are neither blank slates nor bundles of instincts.[5]

One further—mainly *semantic*—point. The description "hardwired" often takes a leading role in discussions about instinct and knowledge. What does this expression mean? As noted earlier, the software/hardware distinction, though applicable to manufactured computers, is hopelessly out of its depth in describing nervous systems. So if "hardwired" means "like my computer's motherboard," then it is meaningless in the context of neuroscience.

If "hardwired" means "a behavior that depends on brain wiring," then we need to ask, "As opposed to *what*?" So far as is known, all behavior depends on brain wiring. If "hardwired" means "caused by genes," we have already seen unqualified versions of this idea wrecked on the shoals of developmental complexity. Sometimes "hardwired" is used to refer to a circuit that is not modifiable postnatally. Typically, this usage too is problematic, since virtually all of a brain's functions are modifiable in one way or another—by expectation, conditioning, drugs, and assorted adjustments of internal or external conditions.[6] This includes perception, motor control, thermoregulation, the vestibulo-ocular reflex, and various "set points" for anxiety, appetite, and aspects of sleep cycles. Even the basic knee-jerk reflex, essentially run on spinal-cord circuitry, though subject to descending influence, is modifiable to a degree. For example, the amplitude of the kick can be affected by something as simple as gritting your teeth, as well as by interruption of descending signals from cortex. Perhaps there exists in some subculture a consistent, useful, and *unambiguous* role for the expression "hardwired," but because it is so heavily encrusted with misconception and misdirection, it is preferable to seek more precise terminology.

Justice cannot be done in this brief section to the large body of research on which these comments rest. But my aim is fairly minimal: to uproot reliance on *outdated* opinions about so-called *innate knowledge* as we move on to questions about learning. To forestall criticism, let me emphasize that I am *not* saying there is *nothing* to the distinction between what is learned and what is innate. Rather, I am saying that the matter is far more complicated than we thought, because of the interdependence of genes and epigenetic factors, prenatally and postnatally.

3   Storing Information in Nervous Systems

The crux of the issue for this chapter is how brains know things. We can begin by addressing the neural basis for *postnatal plasticity*, and more narrowly, for postnatal plasticity that is uncontroversially *experience-dependent*. Hence we shall consider what is more commonly called learning, remembering, forgetting, and adapting.

An appealing idea is that if you learn something, such as how to tie a trucker's knot, then the information will be stored in one particular location, probably along with your other knot-tying knowledge, say between reef knots and half-hitches. That is, after all, the general plan adopted when we store paper files in a particular drawer at a particular location or perhaps when we store electronic files on a computer. It is not, however, the brain's way. This was first demonstrated by American psychologist Karl Lashley in the 1920s.

Lashley reasoned that after a rat learned something, such as a route through a certain maze, *if* the information is stored in a single, punctate location, then by lesioning the rat's brain in the right place, you should be able to take out the rat's knowledge. Where might the right place be? Lashley trained twenty rats on his maze. Next, he removed a different area of the cortex from each animal and allowed the rats time to recover. He then retested each animal in the maze to see which lesion removed the maze-knowledge. Lashley discovered that the rat's knowledge could not be localized to any single region. Instead, it appeared that all the rats were somewhat impaired but all were somewhat competent. To a first approximation, the more tissue removed, the more serious the deficit.

As follow-up discoveries revealed, spatial knowledge was not a particularly good case for Lashley's purposes, since it turns out to involve noncortical structures (the hippocampus) and draws on a range of sensory modalities (smell, vision, touch). Nevertheless, as improved experimental protocols went on to show, Lashley's nonlocalization conclusion was essentially correct. There is no such thing as a dedicated "memory organ" in the brain; information is not stored on the filing-cabinet model at all. Instead, information seems to be distributed over many neurons. Nor is the modular organization of a conventional computer—processing by one component and storage by another—the brain's way. The very same structures that process information are also modified to store information.

If a brain has knowledge, that knowledge depends on wiring, that is, on neurons and how they are connected to other neurons. Additionally, the right neurons must talk to the right neurons. If knowledge is in place prenatally, something has to cause the wiring to be right. If knowledge is acquired in response to experience, then existing wiring has to modify itself in the right way. That is, the informationally relevant changes at the cellular level must be orchestrated so that an overall coherent modification in system output is achieved.[7] Fundamentally, the heart of the problem is to explain *global* changes in a brain's output (behavior) in terms of orderly *local* changes in individual neurons. The local-global problem is part of the more general problem of how to get device-cleverness out of component-stupidity. That is, the device as a whole may respond adaptively and intelligently, but its individual components are not themselves as intelligent as the whole system.

If global learning depends on local changes in cells, how do cells know, without the guiding hand of intelligence, when they should change, by how much, and where? In my discussion of artificial neural networks (ANNs) in chapter 7, we saw how simple units could change so that the network stored information in the pattern of synaptic weights where one set of units meets another set of units (see again figure 7.16). Although neurobiologically unrealistic, these simple ANNs are *conceptually* useful because they successfully demonstrate that the problem *has* a mechanistic solution, and they offer a first-pass explanation of how real neural networks might do it. The basic idea that feedback, such as punishment or reward, can initiate local modifications in connectivity with global import suggests a range of testable hypotheses regarding learning in real neural networks.

There are many possible ways neurons can change. For example, new dendrites might sprout (figures 8.1 and 8.2). There might be some extension of existing branches. Existing receptors could modify their structure (e.g., a change in subunits of the protein that constitutes the receptor). Or new receptor sites might be created. In the curtailing direction, pruning could decrease the dendrites or bits of dendrite, and therewith decrease the number of synaptic connections between neurons. Or the synapses on remaining branches could be shut down altogether. Additionally, there might be modulation of sodium channels to change the spiking profile of an axon as a function of neuron-neuron interactions. These are all *postsynaptic* changes in the dendrites.

There may also be *presynaptic* changes in the axons. For example, there may be changes in the membrane (channels might emerge or be altered), or new axonal branches may be formed or pruned. Repeated high rates of firing will deplete the neurotransmitter vesicles available for release, and that transient depletion constitutes a kind of memory on the order of 2–3 seconds. One important presynaptic change involves increasing or decreasing the probability that a vesicle of neurotransmitter will be released when a spike reaches the axonal terminal of a neuron. The probability of neurotransmitter release when a spike arrives at the terminal is referred to as the *reliability* of the synapse. For example, a synapse may, on average, release transmitter once for every ten spikes reaching the synapse. Reliability can be modified on a time-scale of a few hundred milliseconds. Up-regulating or down-regulating reliability is a fast and flexible way of changing effective synaptic connectivity. The synaptic strength can be increased tenfold in less than a second, without having to build new structures. Other presynaptic changes include changing the number of vesicles released per spike or the number of transmitter molecules contained in each vesicle. Finally, the whole neuron might die, taking with it all the synapses it formerly supported, or in certain special regions, a whole new neuron might be born. Every one of these changes does occur, though precisely how the various changes causally connect to input signals is still under study, and how changes across populations of neurons are *orchestrated* remains baffling.

This broad range of modifiability can be conveniently condensed for this discussion by referring simply to modification of the weights, or *synapses*. The

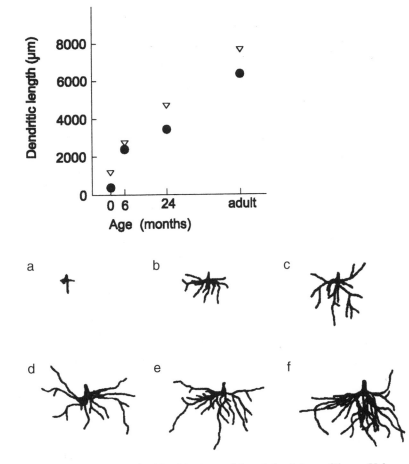

Figure 8.1   Camera lucida drawings of basal dendrites of layer V human pyramidal neurons: (a) newborn, (b) 3 months, (c) 6 months, (d) 15 months, (e) 24 months, (f) adult. (From Schade and van Groenigen 1961.)

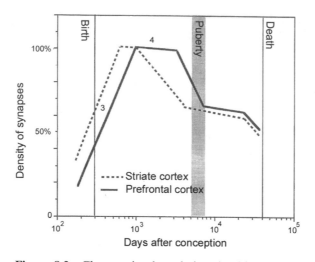

Figure 8.2 Changes in the relative densities of synapses in primary visual cortex (broken line) and prefrontal cortex (continuous line) of the human brain as a function of days after conception (expressed on a log scale on the *y*-axis). Notice that synaptogenesis in the more anterior region continues at a high level after synaptogenesis in the striate cortex has begun to decline. (From Bourgeois 2001; based on data from Huttenlocher and Dabholkar 1997.)

connectivity modifications listed above ultimately involve synaptic change, either directly or indirectly, or can be reasonably so construed.

When and where is the decision to modify synapses made? Basically, the choices are rather limited. Essentially, the decision to change can be made either globally (broadcast widely) or locally (with specific synapses targeted). If it is made *globally*, then the signal for change will be essentially permissive, in effect saying, "You may change yourself now," but not dictating exactly where or by how much or in what direction (stronger or weaker). If global, the decision will likely be mediated by one of the subcortical nuclei that projects very broadly across the cortex and that have a role in regulating arousal, attention, sleep cycles, internal milieu, emotional state, and so on.

On the other hand, if weight change is to be *specific*, we would predict a tight connection in space and time between the cause and the effect. That is, the cause and the effect should be in close spatial and temporal proximity. The next question, therefore, is this: if spatial contiguity is critical, what *temporal* relations might signal a local structural modification with the result that the weights change, and change in the right direction (either stronger or weaker)?

These were the dominant problems raised by psychologist Donald Hebb in his influential book *The Organization of Behavior* (1949). The crux of Hebb's insight, slightly reconstructed, is this: *correlated activity* of pre- and post-synaptic cells should *increase* the strength of the synaptic connection; anti-correlation should *decrease* the strength of the connection. Loosely speaking, the idea is that if activation in the presynaptic cells causes activation in the postsynaptic cell, this should tend to make all of their connections stronger. By changing the strength of the synapse, you increase the probability of the post-synaptic cell firing following the firing of the presynaptic cell. On its own, however, one cell's release of neurotransmitter is unlikely to cause the post-synaptic cell to fire, because the postsynaptic effect of one neuron's transmitter volley is very small. So suppose *two* distinct presynaptic cells—perhaps one from the auditory system and one from the somatosensory system—connect to same postsynaptic cell and fire at the same time. This *joint* input activity creates a larger postsynaptic effect and, if Hebb is right, a strengthening of the con-nection. This general arrangement allows for associated *world* events to be mirrored by associated *neuronal* events.

The actual mechanisms for modifying synaptic weights were not specified in Hebb's proposal, however, since neuroscience had not yet begun to catalogue the assorted structural changes that could yield a strengthening of synaptic connections (e.g., an increase in the number of vesicles released, an increase in the quantity of transmitter per vesicle, an increase in receptor proteins, etc.). A theory of learning mechanisms should itemize and specify the conditions that must be satisfied for information to get stored. For example, it will need to specify whether the *firing* of the postsynaptic cell is necessary or whether mere *depolarization* by some critical amount is sufficient. Only recently have discov-eries at this level of detail been made.

Hebb's principle for synaptic weight change says, "When an axon of a cell *A* is near enough to excite cell *B* or repeatedly or persistently takes part in firing it, some growth or metabolic change takes place in both cells such that *A*'s efficiency, as one of the cells firing *B*, is increased" (1949, 62).

The simplest formal version of the Hebb rule for changing the strength of the weight w_{BA} between neuron *A*, with a firing rate of V_A, projecting onto neuron *B*, with an average firing rate of V_B, is $\Delta w_{BA} = \varepsilon V_B V_A$. This states that the vari-ables relevant to synaptic change are the co-occurring activity levels, and that increases in synaptic strength are proportional to the product of the presynaptic and postsynaptic values. The weight changes, note, are all positive, since the firing rates are all positive.

The simple rule admits of many variations that still qualify as Hebbian. In particular, it can be modified to get a powerful *reinforcement*-learning algorithm, which updates the weights as a function of a Hebbian correlation between a sensory reward (such as nectar) detected *now* and a representation of whether there is an *error* in predicting what that reward *would* be. As we shall see below, this is important because specific neural networks in bees, and probably humans, do learn to expect a specific reward of a certain magnitude at a certain time.

Does *any* kind of weight change count as Hebbian? No. To qualify as Hebbian, the plasticity has to satisfy two criteria: (1) it is specific to the synapse where the pre- and postsynaptic activity occurs, and (2) it depends *conjointly* on both the pre- and postsynaptic cells, but not on the activity of other (connected) cells. Non-Hebbian plasticity will include changes that fail to satisfy either of these two criteria. For example, if the modification occurs to the *whole cell*, rather than to the specific synapse where the activity occurs, then the plasticity is non-Hebbian. If it involves general instructions for cells to up-regulate their synaptic connections, such plasticity is non-Hebbian.

To a first approximation, early development is characterized by mainly *non-Hebbian* plasticity, whereas Hebbian plasticity probably characterizes much of postnatal plasticity, including classical examples of *learning*.[8] In early child development, both kinds of plasticity probably have an important role.

Some inquiries into how postnatal brains build world models are likely to be more fruitful than others. One may be especially fascinated, for example, by how human adults learn to construct proofs in modern symbolic logic. This is unlikely, however, to be the most auspicious place to try to develop neurobiological hypotheses regarding learning. The main problem is that animal models for any but the simplest logical capacities are not available, but animal models are essential to neural-level exploration, and neural-level exploration is essential for discovering learning mechanisms. Starting with simple forms of learning will probably pay off faster and also yield clues to the solution of the more difficult problems. More tractable learning problems than theorem proving are reinforcement learning (operant conditioning), fear conditioning, and spatial learning.

The "simple first" strategy has rarely appealed to philosophers, who tend to feel that simpler forms of learning are irrelevant to "real" epistemology. This is probably short-sighted. From an evolutionary perspective and from what is known about conservation of mechanisms across species, we can infer that fancier kinds of learning procedures are probably modifications, upgrades, and hitch-hikers on the simpler ones. Learning culturally dependent skills, such as reading and theorem proving, undoubtedly engage culturally independent learning mechanisms that are fundamental to honing skills in general, such as visual-pattern recognition, spatial navigation, and problem solving.

4 Reinforcement Learning: An Example

To the casual observer, bees seem to visit flowers for nectar on a willy-nilly basis. It turns out, however, that they forage methodically. Not only do they tend to remember which individual flowers they have already visited, but in a field of mixed flowers with varying amounts of nectar, they learn to optimize their foraging strategy, so that they get the most nectar for the least effort. Do they run through calculations to achieve this economy? No. The neuro-biological basis for this cleverness is now partially understood, and these results suggest some general hypotheses concerning reinforcement learning that may be applicable on a broader scale that includes mammals.

In an experiment designed by Leslie Real, a small field was stocked with two sets of plastic flowers, yellow and blue, each with a well in the center in which precise amounts of sucrose could be deposited.[9] The flowers were randomly distributed around the enclosed field, and were baited with volumes of "nectar" according to the following rule: all blue flowers had 2 µl; 1/3 of the yellow flowers had 6 µl; 2/3 had none. This sucrose distribution ensures that the *mean* value of visiting a population of blue flowers was the same as that of the yellow flowers, though the yellow flowers are more *uncertain* than the blues.

After initially randomly sampling the flowers, the bees quickly fell into a pattern of going to the blue flowers 85 percent of the time. You can change their foraging pattern by raising the mean value of the yellow flowers, for example, by increasing the sucrose in the 1/3 baited yellow flowers to 10 µl. The behavior of the bees displays a kind of trade-off between *reliability* of the source type and nectar *volume* at the source type, with the bees showing a mild preference for reliability. But they will forage *equally* between the blues and yellows when the mean of the yellows is sufficiently high. For our purposes here, what is interesting is this: according to the reward profile acquired in a sample of visits, the bees adapt their strategy. How do bees—*mere* bees—do this?

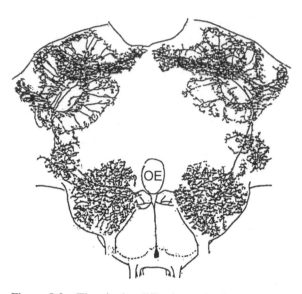

Figure 8.3   The single, diffusely projecting modulatory neuron *VUMmx1* in the bee brain. Neuromodulatory neurons in the bee brain and dopamine projections in the human brain play homologous roles. OE = cell body of *VUMmx1*. Systems like the dopamine system in humans and the octopamine system in bees are called *diffuse neuromodulatory systems*. "Diffuse" because the axons of the neurons are diffusely projecting, making synaptic connections throughout widespread brain regions. "Neuromodulatory" because the neurotransmitters released from these axons are thought to modulate global brain states. Computational models show that neural activity in some of these neurons distributes information about expected rewards based on previous sensory experience. In both species, the diffuse neurons receive precategorized information about rewarding events and combine this with sensory information to construct a scalar signal that represents the error between the expected amount of an reward and the amount actually received. Using this signal to control long-term changes in synaptic weights allows this system to learn and store predictions rather than correlations. (From Hammer 1993.)

The research of neuroscientist Martin Hammer provides an important piece of the puzzle. In the bee brain he found a neuron, though itself neither sensory nor motor, that responds positively to reward. This neuron, called "VUMmx1" ("vum" for short), projects very diffusely in the bee brain, and its activity mediates reinforcement learning (figure 8.3). For example, a particular odor consistently paired with sucrose would change the weights on vum so that eventually vum would fire when that odor occurs alone. But how does the bee's brain allow it to learn the mean value and reliability of source types across a sample?

In an artificial neural network, Montague and colleagues modeled the known and relevant bee anatomy and behavior.[10] They found that the weight-change algorithm operating at vum did not just sum the various synaptic inputs. Instead, the activity of vum represents *prediction error*; that is, the difference between the *goodies expected* and the *goodies received this time*. Here is how it works. Cell vum has input from the bee proboscis, where it sucks up nectar. We can loosely think of this as the reward pathway (figure 8.6). Vum also has inputs from sensory systems, for example visual (for color) and olfactory (for odor). Simplifying a little, the output of vum at a given time t_n is a function of the reward at t_n, which is expressed as $r(t_n)$, plus the combined value of the sensory inputs $(\dot{V}(t_n))$ minus the value those inputs had just previously at t_{n-1}. More formally, the output of vum, $\delta(t)$, is expressed thus: $\delta(t) = [r(t) + \dot{V}(t)] - \dot{V}(t_{n-1})$.

Roughly, a result greater than zero corresponds to "better than expected," and a result less than zero corresponds to "worse than expected." The output of vum is the release of a neuromodulator that targets a variety of cells, including those responsible for action selection. If that neuromodulator acts also on the synapses connecting the sensory neurons to vum, then the synapses will get changed according to whether the vum calculates *worse than expected* (less neuromodulator) or *better than expected* (more neuromodulator) (figure 8.4). Assuming the model of Montague et al. is essentially correct, it turns out that a surprisingly simple circuit, operating according to a fairly simple learning algorithm, underlies the bee's adaptability to foraging conditions. (My account here leaves out various details, but it captures the main ideas. See Montague, Dayan, and Sejnowski 1993.)

Obviously, the bee has more flexibility if it can *learn* the nectar values of flowers than if the nectar values are specified independently of experience. Some years the Honeysuckle might do poorly and have little nectar; new nectar-rich plant species might begin to invade the area; a flood might mean the bee has to find new foraging territory where Indian Paintbrush and Lupin grow instead of Honeysuckle and Campion; and so on. By being modifiable, the bees' neural networks can improve foraging. New pattern recognition (e.g., high nectar in the crimson flowers) enabled by reinforcement learning is a useful thing.

For the bees, the correlations between flower color and nectar reward are essentially *spatial*, but correlations also occur in the temporal domain. A bat, for example, can learn that a certain sequence of tones is a reliable indicator of tasty moths, and a dog quickly learns that one sequence of events predicts

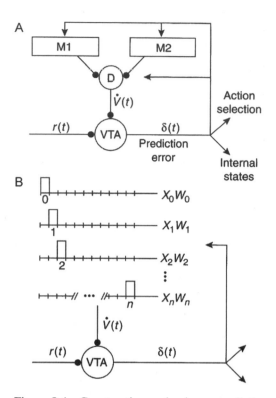

Figure 8.4 Constructing and using a prediction error. (A) Interpretation of the anatomical arrangement of inputs and outputs of the ventral tegmental area (VTA), whose
neurons project very widely and release dopamine. M1 and M2 represent two different
cortical modalities whose output is assumed to arrive at the VTA in the form of a temporal derivative (surprise signal) $\dot{V}(t)$ that reflects the degree to which the current sensory state differs from the previous sensory state. (The overdot indicates the rate of
change.) The high degree of convergence forces $\dot{V}(t)$ to arrive at the VTA as a scalar
signal. Information about reward $r(t)$ also converges on the VTA. The VTA output is a
simple linear sum $\delta(t) = r(t) + \dot{V}(t)$. The widespread output connections of the VTA
make the prediction error $\delta(t)$ simultaneously available to structures constructing the
predictions. (B) Temporal representation of a sensory cue. A cue like a light is represented at multiple delays x_n from its initial time of onset, and each delay is associated
with a separate adjustable weight w_n. The w_n parameters are adjusted according to the
correlations of x_n, activity, and δ, and, through training, come to act as predictions. This
simple system stores predictions rather than correlations. (Reprinted with permission
from Schultz, Dayan, and Montague 1997. Copyright by the American Association for
the Advancement of Science.)

going to the beach, while another predicts hiking on the marsh. Much conditioning depends on temporal associations between events.

The dependency relations between phenomena can be much more complex than such simple correlations as red flowers, high nectar. I may initially note a correlation between dropping eggs and eggs breaking. I think: dropping an egg causes it to break. Then I happen to notice that a dropped egg will not break *if* I drop it on a soft pillow or in newly fallen snow. So the dependency relations are a little fancier than I first thought. With continued exploration, I come to appreciate that even with soft snow to land in, an egg may break if dropped from a sufficiently great height. My simple correlations get upgraded to more complex correlations as I learn about the world. This seems to be true of animals as well. We can learn that one event will *probably* follow the occurrence of another, but not always, and the reason may be completely veiled. Part of what we call intelligence in humans and other animals is the capacity to acquire understanding of increasingly complex dependency relations. This allows us to distinguish *fortuitous* correlations, which are not genuinely predictive in the long run, from *causal* correlations, which are.

Does reinforcement learning in the humble bee have anything to do with *us*? Very likely, since we too have a reward system that mediates learning about how the world works. Wolfram Schultz has found neurons in the monkey brainstem that, like vum, respond to reward, shift their responsiveness to a stimulus that *predicts* reward, and indicate error if the reward is not forthcoming. These neurons release dopamine at their axon terminals (and hence are *dopaminergic*), and the dopamine is believed to *modulate* the excitability of the target neurons to neurotransmitters such as glutamate or glycine.

By recording from single cells, Schultz showed that if an animal gets an unpredicted reward—such as a squirt of juice—the dopaminergic neurons *increase* their firing when the reward is received. With repeated trials where a juice squirt follows the sounding of a tone, the monkey learns that the tone predicts the juice. The response of these neurons tracks the monkey's learning that the tone predicts the juice. That is, the dopaminergic neurons now increase their rate of firing *when the tone is heard*, which thus *predicts* the occurrence of the reward. Should the reward fail to appear when predicted, then activity in these neurons drops markedly below baseline *at the time when the reward should have appeared* (see figure 8.5).

These neurons are believed to be part of the reward system. They arise from areas in the midbrain (the ventral tegmental area or VTA) and the substantia nigra, which receive projections from a wide range of areas. The input probably

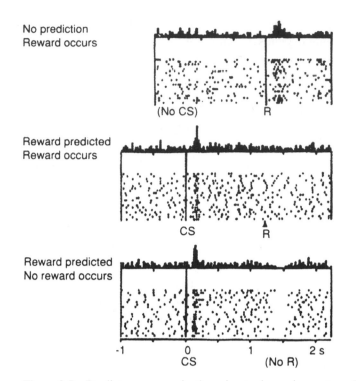

No prediction
Reward occurs

(No CS)   R

Reward predicted
Reward occurs

CS   R

Reward predicted
No reward occurs

-1   0   1   2 s
CS   (No R)

Figure 8.5 Predictor neurons in the primate dopamine system. Each panel shows electrical recordings from individual dopamine neurons from an alert primate during a task where a sensory cue is followed 1 second later by the delivery of a juice reward. Each dot is the occurrence of an action potential, and each horizontal row of dots represents a single presentation of the sensory cue and reward. The histogram on top of each panel is the total number of action potentials in a particular time bin. Top: Presentation of a sensory cue to a naive monkey causes no change in the production of action potentials. Delivery of a juice reward, however, causes a transient increase in the rate. Middle: Presentation of the sensory cue causes a transient increase in spike production, but delivery of the reward causes no change in the firing rate. Bottom: Same as the middle panel except that if the reward is not delivered, the dopamine neurons stop firing when the reward would have been delivered as calculated from previous trials. The interpretation is that the neurons are predicting the time and magnitude of the future reward using information provided by the earliest predictive sensory cue. Abbreviations: CS, conditioned stimulus; R, primary reward. (From Schultz, Dayan, Montague, 1997.)

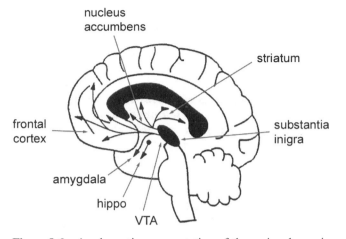

nucleus
accumbens

striatum

frontal
cortex

substantia
inigra

amygdala

hippo

VTA

Figure 8.6 A schematic representation of the major dopaminergic tracts of the human brain. Abbreviations: VTA, ventral tegmental area; hippo, hippocampus.

represents a surprise signal, in the sense that it measures the degree of difference between the current sensory signal and the last sensory signal. The dopaminergic neurons project very diffusely to many regions of the brain involved in goal-directed behavior and motivation, including the striatum, the nucleus acumbens, and the *prefrontal cortex*, which, as we saw in chapter 3, plays a role in emotional valence and in action selection (figure 8.6). The hypothesis is that dopamine delivery regulates the plasticity of those neurons that make action decisions, such as those in prefrontal cortex.

Convergent research indicates that these dopaminergic neurons are indeed involved in reinforcement learning. In the 1950s, James Olds and Peter Milner at Cal Tech devised a set-up whereby a freely moving rat could press a lever to receive a small pulse of current through an electrode implanted in its brain. Depending on the location of the electrode, rats quickly learned to do stimulate themselves by pressing the lever. The only reinforcing reward for the behavior was the pleasure caused by of the stimulation of the neurons. For specific locations, such as the striatum, the nucleus acumbens, and the VTA, the rats found the self-stimulation so pleasurable they would forgo food, sex, and water to continue pressing the lever. Most recently, functional MRI has been used to see whether any particular areas are especially active during reinforcement learning.[11] The results show regionalized increases in activity in the midbrain dopamine system. This suggests that human reinforcement learning may have some features in common with that of other animals.

Additional evidence confirms that the dopaminergic neurons in the VTA and substantia nigra mediate reward and pleasurable feelings, and send prediction error signals to the areas responsible for choice: animals injected with a substance that blocks the activity of dopamine show impaired reinforcement learning; addictive substances such as cocaine and amphetamine increase dopamine levels. It is also important that VTA neurons display the prediction/error profile to *positive* reward, but not to *aversive* stimuli. As we shall see in the next section, a distinct brain region appears to mediate *negative* reinforcement learning.

5   Fear Conditioning and the Amygdala

The amygdala plays a central role in evaluating stimuli as unpleasant. Animals with lesions to the amygdala cannot learn that a certain innocuous stimulus predicts an aversive stimulus, and hence they cannot learn to avoid the aversive event. For example, amygdala-lesioned animals cannot learn that one event, such as a tone, predicts a nasty event, such as a shock to its feet. Unlike normal animals, they do not learn to avoid the nasty event by escaping when the tone sounds (figure 8.7).

The necessity of amygdaloid structures for fear conditioning suggests that some specific change may occur in the amygdala during fear conditioning. Can specific changes in amygdala cells be seen? Yes indeed. The amygdala is not an undifferentiated region, but consists of a number of specialized subregions (figure 8.8). More restricted lesion studies reveal that the subregion relevant to the cellular story of fear conditioning is the lateral amygdala (LA). Within LA is the tiny dorsal subregion, housing two distinct populations of cells with different roles in fear conditioning. In the rat, each population has only about twenty thousand cells.

Cells in one population (A) show a fast and transient change in synaptic strength during the early phase of learning. Cells in the second population (B) change more slowly, and their modification is more permanent. Further manipulations indicate that the learning is Hebbian in both cases, though mediated by distinct mechanisms. Type A cells have several types of receptor channels to which the excitatory neurotransmitter glutamate will bind. One type (the AMPA receptor) opens whenever glutamate binds, thus transmitting a small signal from one cell to the other and causing the receiving cell to depolarize.

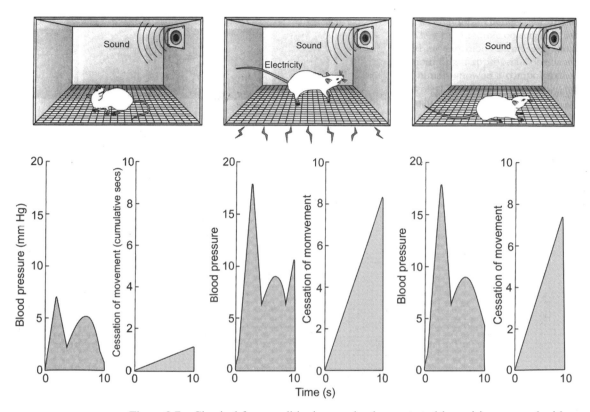

Figure 8.7 Classical fear conditioning can be demonstrated by pairing a sound with a mild electric shock to the foot of a rat. In one set of trials, the rat hears a sound (left panel), which has relatively little effect on the animal's blood pressure or patterns of movement. Next, the same sound is coupled with a foot shock (center). After several pairings the rat's blood pressure rises and the animal freezes; it does not move for an extended period when it hears the sound. The rat has been fear-conditioned. After conditioning, when the sound alone is given, it evokes physiological changes in blood pressure and freezing similar to those evoked by the sound and shock together (right). (From LeDoux 1994.)

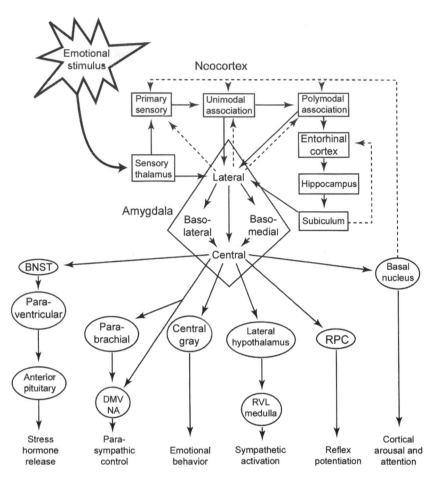

Figure 8.8   A model of the neural circuit involved in conditioned fear. A hierarchy of incoming sensory information converges on the lateral nucleus of the amygdala. Through intra-amygdala circuitry, the output of the lateral nucleus is transmitted to the central nucleus, which serves to activate various effector systems involved in the expression of emotional responses. Feedforward projections are indicated by solid lines, and feedback projections are indicated by dashed lines. Abbreviations: BNST, bed nucleus of the stria terminalis; DMV, dorsal motor nucleus of the vagus; NA, nucleus ambiguus; RPC, nucleus reticularis pontis caudalis; RVL medulla, rostral ventrolateral nuclei of the medulla. (From LeDoux 1994.)

The other protein channel, the *NMDA receptor*, plays the key role in plasticity. (We saw on p. 326 that during early development, NMDA is also involved in regulating precursor-cell schedules.) This receptor is *voltage sensitive*, which means that it will not open unless *two* primary conditions are satisfied: (1) the neurotransmitter glutamate binds to it, *and* (2) the membrane must already be a bit depolarized—typically from a second source. This conjunction of events normally occurs only when a type A cell receives *two distinct inputs*: an innocuous stimulus from one source (the tone), about when it receives a strong stimulus from another source (the shock) (figure 8.12). When these two events happen within a brief time window, the NMDA channel at the "innocuous connection" opens, and stays open for about 100–200 msec. The opening is actually a change in *shape of the protein* that sets free a magnesium ion and permits calcium ions to enter the cell (figure 8.9).

Once calcium enters the cell via the NMDA receptor, a cascade of events is launched that upregulates the response of the cell to the innocuous stimulus. On a subsequent occasion, therefore, when the innocuous event occurs in the absence of the aversive event, the A cells respond roughly as though the aversive stimulus itself had occurred. This causal chain for strengthening the synapse is known as *long-term potentiation*, or LTP. The general characterization of LTP is that the responsivity of the postsynaptic cell is potentiated (increased). The effect can last for many hours. The typical conditions for producing LTP experimentally involve either a conjunction of inputs or a blast from a single input. The NMDA receptor mediates LTP in some, but not all, cells (figure 8.10).

Surprisingly, a crucial component responsible for LTP is *presynaptic*. It consists in increasing the probability that neurotransmitter is released when a spike reaches the axon terminal (i.e., it increases reliability). In some manner, possibly by releasing nitric oxide (NO), the postsynaptic cell signals the presynaptic cell to upregulate its probability of neurotransmitter release (figure 8.11). As noted above, changes in the probability of release is something that can be achieved on the order of a few hundred milliseconds. When the tone is *dissociated* from the shock, LTP does not occur. (If the postsynaptic cell responds even though the presynaptic cell did not send a signal, thereafter postsynaptic responsivity is lowered. This effect is called LTD—*long-term depression*.) In sum, in type A cells of the dorsal region of the LA, we see NMDA-mediated LTP.

What about type B cells, those that exhibit a more permanent change? Instead of the NMDA receptor typical of type A cells, B cells use a voltage-gated

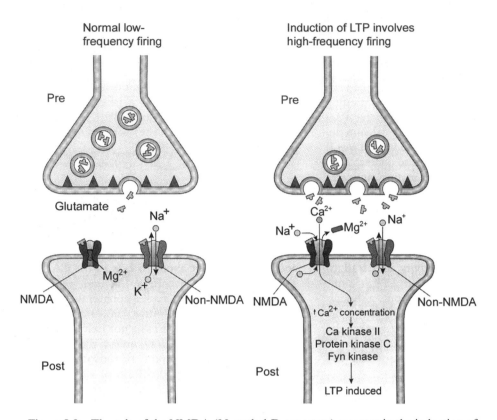

Figure 8.9   The role of the NMDA (N-methyl-D-aspartate) receptor in the induction of a form of neuronal plasticity known as long-term potentiation (LTP). Left: During normal synaptic transmission, when the presynaptic neuron fires at low frequency, the NMDA channels remain blocked by Mg^{2+} ions. Na^+ and K^+ ions can still enter through non-NMDA channels to mediate ordinary synaptic transmission. Right: LTP is induced when the presynaptic neuron fires at a high-frequency (a tetanus) and depolarizes the membrane of the postsynaptic cell sufficiently to unblock the NMDA receptor channel, which allows calcium to enter the cell. (Based on Squire and Kandel 1999.)

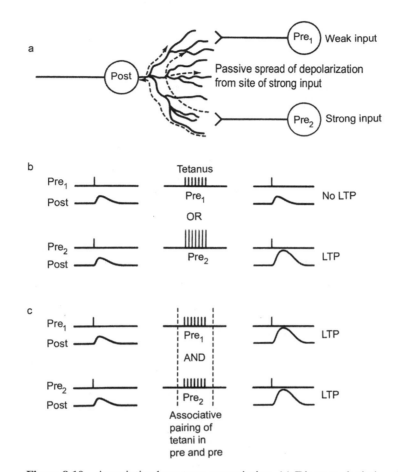

Figure 8.10   Associative long-term potentiation. (a) Diagram depicting the spatial relationships between strong and weak synaptic input. (b) Stimulation of the strong input produces LTP, but stimulation of the weak input alone does not. (c) When the strong and weak inputs are paired, the depolarization produced by the strong input spreads to the site of the weak input, which then contributes to the induction of LTP. (From Levitan and Kaczmarek 1991.)

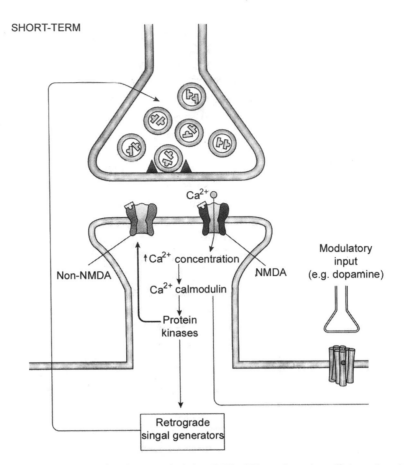

SHORT-TERM

Ca²⁺

↑Ca²⁺ concentration

Non-NMDA

Ca²⁺ calmodulin

NMDA

Modulatory
input
(e.g. dopamine)

Protein
kinases

Retrograde
singal generators

Figure 8.11   Mechanisms underlying LTP. When there is sufficient depolarization to open the NMDA channels in the postsynaptic cell, Ca^{2+} flows into the postsynaptic cell, and protein kinases are activated. Ca^{2+} influx changes the postsynaptic cell by acting on non-NMDA receptors, and it also sends retrograde messages back to the presynaptic cell, telling it to release more transmitter. One of the retrograde messengers is believed to be nitric oxide (NO). (Based on Squire and Kandel 1999.)

calcium channel to trigger strengthening of the synapse. Like NMDA receptors, these receptors are in the plasticity business. Like the type A cells, they require a conjunction of inputs to open, but when they do open and further depolarize the cell, a distinct cascade ensues, ultimately triggering gene expression and therewith the synthesis of proteins. Thus their effect is more permanent and the underlying change is presumably more structural than just regulating the probability of release.

We need to pause and savor how these discoveries add up. Step by artful step, they track the plasticity in fear conditioning from *behavioral changes in the animal's ability to predict shock*, to a particular brain *structure* (the amygdala), then to highly confined *subregions* of the amygdala (the LA) specific to fear conditioning, then to two distinctive *populations* of cells (in the dorsal LA) whose synaptic weights are modifiable on different schedules, then to two specific *voltage sensitive receptor proteins* distinguishing those two cell populations. Opening one type (NMDA) mediates shorter-term memory; opening the other type (the voltage-gated calcium channel) appears to trigger gene expression as part of the process of consolidating memory for the long haul. Thus the story wends its way from behavior down through to specific proteins and changes at the molecular level.

The fear-conditioning studies have been done mainly in rats. As noted in chapter 5, however, in humans, the rare disease Urbach-Vitae causes bilateral atrophy of the amygdala, which thus permits research on the effect of amygdala destruction on humans. Neuroscientist Joseph Le Doux has studied a woman with this disease. Like the amygdala-lesioned rats, she fails to acquire a new fear-conditioned response. In normal subjects, if a mild shock on the hand occurs a few seconds after the appearance of an innocuous blue square on the television screen, in a few trials subjects exhibit a fear response when the blue square appears. Le Doux's subject does not, though she tests normally in other respects. She does respond normally to the mild shock itself, but she shows none of the conditioned responses to the innocuous stimuli that are typical of normal humans exposed to blue/shock pairs: no increase in heart rate, no sweating, and no feeling of apprehension at the appearance of the innocuous stimulus. In response to queries, she says that she does not feel that anything unpleasant is going to happen following the appearance of the blue square. Interestingly, however, after continued trials she does acquire a certain level of understanding, independently of any feeling of fear, based apparently on an intellectual inference that there is a predictive connection between the innocuous event and the unpleasant event.

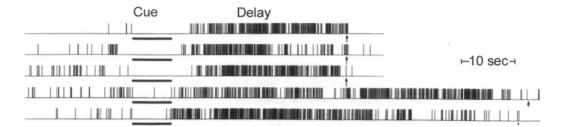

Figure 8.12   Discharge of a cell in the prefrontal cortex of a monkey during five trials in the classical delayed-response task. Arrow marks the monkey's response at the end of the memorization period (delay). Note that the cell is inhibited during presentation of the cue but persistently activated throughout memorization (30 seconds in the upper three trials, 60 seconds in the lower two). (From Fuster 1973.)

The questions driving this chapter are these: Where does knowledge come from? How do we come to represent the world? Learning to avoid damaging stimuli by learning to recognize an event that predicts their occurrence is an important part of learning about the world. As we have seen, neuroscience is beginning to reveal, in research that tracks learning changes through the various levels of brain organization, where knowledge comes from and how we come to represent the world.

Are there other learning capacities whose mechanisms neuroscience is probing? Indeed there are. Working memory—holding information in the ready until the time to act is right—is another capacity where progress has been made at the neuronal level (figures 8.12 and 8.13). This is especially intriguing because of the possible connection between awareness and working memory.[12]

Recollection of events in one's life is another domain where cognitive neuroscience has succeeded in pushing our understanding ahead. As we shall see below, the capacity for recalling life's episodes depends on a set of neural structures distinct from those subserving working memory or fear conditioning.

6   Declarative Memory and the Hippocampal Structures

We can acquire skills, such as how to ride a bicycle or tie a trucker's knot. Memory for skills is referred to as *procedural memory*. Knowledge that a mild shock will follow the appearance of a blue square is distinct kind of knowledge—fear conditioning. Both of these contrast with remembering specific

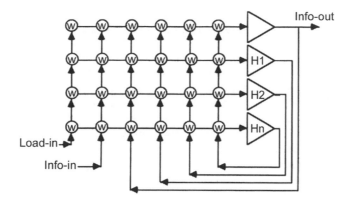

Figure 8.13 The structure of a model of short-term active memory. The soma of each idealized unit is represented by a triangle at the right, and its input dendrite is shown at the left with a row of synaptic contacts of a given strength or weight (*w*). The output unit is the blank triangle at the upper right. The underlying triangles (*H*1, *H*2, *Hn*) represent hidden units, that is, units that mediate transactions within the network and determine its output at any given time in accord with the input it receives and its pre-established (i.e., pretrained) functional architecture. (From Zipser et al. 1993.)

events that happened in the course of one's life, such as that on your sixth birthday you were given a bicycle, or where you parked your car this morning.

Conscious recollection of events and episodes is referred to as *declarative memory*; one can say or "declare" what one remembers about past experiences. It is also called *explicit memory* or *conscious memory*. In ordinary parlance, this capacity is usually what people refer to when they talk about their memory. Recollected events are typically indexed temporally and spatially. That is, we remember, for example, our first kiss with Jerry in the barn after the eighth-grade skating party. Of course, not all details of an episode are bought to mind in conscious recollection, though often the longer we dwell on the event, the more the associated details emerge into awareness.

Recollection of individual events, along with suitable temporal and spatial referencing, requires the *hippocampal structures* in the brain. These include the hippocampus, the entorhinal cortex, the perirhinal cortex, and the para-hippocampal gyrus (figure 8.14). How do we know that these structures are important for declarative memory but not for fear conditioning or positive reinforcement learning?

In the mid-1950s, a groundbreaking discovery was made by two Canadians at the Montreal Neurological Institute, Brenda Milner and William Scoville.

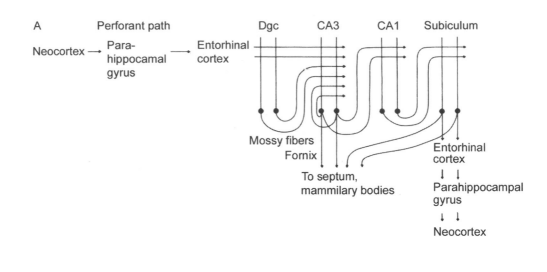

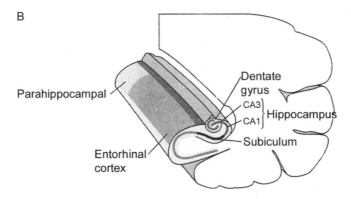

Figure 8.14 (A) A schematic representation of hippocampal circuitry. Note that input from the neocortex reaches the hippocampus via the parahippocampal gyrus and the entorhinal cortex, and output from the hippocampus reaches the neocortex via the entorhinal and the parahippocampal gyrus. Note also a second input path that projects from the dentate gyrus (perforant path). Its axons make synaptic contact with the CA3 neurons below the level at which the entorhinal axons make contact. This arrangement suggests a computational matrix. (From Rolls 1989.) (B) An anatomical diagram showing the location of the hippocampus in the temporal lobe of the brain, as viewed from a coronal section (top is rostral, bottom is caudal), where the hippocampal structures are pulled out from the other tissue to be viewed in depth (facing section is anterior). (Based on Kandel, Schwartz, and Jessel 2000.)

They observed that a 27-year-old surgical patient, H.M., had completely lost declarative memory for all postsurgical events. Nonetheless, his IQ was normal, he retained a normal immediate memory, and had normal memory for events that occurred in his early life. H.M. had undergone a *bilateral* surgery of the medial aspect of the temporal lobe as a treatment for medically intractable epilepsy. A patient with similar lesions, R.B., was discovered by the Damasios in the 1980s and has been intensively studies by their lab over the decades. (In chapter 3, while considering the importance of autobiographical memory to self-representation, R.B.'s symptoms were briefly introduced.[13])

H.M. could not recall an event that happened a minute ago, even when it was a salient and significant event, such as receiving the news that his father had died. This loss of capacity is *anterograde amnesia*. Although he has repeatedly met Milner after his surgery, he cannot remember having met her, even if she left the room only a few minutes earlier. He shows some *retrograde amnesia* for events in the few years preceding surgery, but has good recollection for events in the more distant past. Probing H.M.'s deficits and capacities more deeply, Milner and colleagues discovered that despite his profound anterograde amnesia, H.M. can learn a new sensorimotor *skill*, such as keeping a pencil on a moving target or tracing a star while watching his hand in a mirror. His skill improves gradually, much as it does in normal subjects. Even so, he has no recollection of having encountered the task or having learned the skill. He shrugs off his newly acquired competence with comments such as, "I am good at these sorts of things."

This constellation of data suggested several hypotheses: hippocampal structures are necessary for learning new things, such as how to find the bathroom in a new home, but they are not necessary for retrieval of information that was consolidated when the hippocampal structures were intact, such as how to find the bathroom in your old home or the details of your first kiss. Nor are they necessary for acquiring skills, such as mirror-imaged tracing. This profile of spared and damaged capacities raised fundamental questions: What exactly do the hippocampal structures do? If cells in the hippocampal structures mediate remembering experiences, might they be a test bed for Hebb's hypothesis? How does information come to be *permanently* stored in the cortex, and what is the role of the hippocampal structures in memory?

Targeting all levels of brain organization, from systems and behavior to cells and molecules, labs began to search for answers. Developing animal models was crucial, for otherwise the details of anatomy and physiology remain out of reach. Developing animal models for declarative memory, however, is much

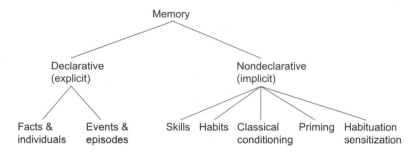

Figure 8.15   A classification of memory. Declarative (explicit) memory refers to conscious recollections of facts and events, and depends on the integrity of the medial temporal lobe cortex. Nondeclarative (implicit) memory refers to a collection of abilities and is independent of the medial temporal lobe. (Based on Squire and Zola-Morgan 1991.)

more difficult than developing them for fear conditioning, since animals cannot be verbally instructed, nor can they verbally declare what they remember. Nonverbal techniques had to be devised, but they had to permit testing of *declarative memory*, not to be confounded with procedural memory or with conditioning. Solving the problems in experimental design required ingenuity in no small degree (figure 8.15).

One widely used test is the Morris water maze, a clever arrangement developed by Richard Morris in Edinburgh. The maze is actually a round tub filled with chalky water containing a small submerged platform. A rat put in the tub swims until he finds a measure of safety on the platform, as rats prefer to avoid deep water. Both normal rats and rats with hippocampal lesions can learn the direct route to the platform, so long as the starting location remains the same. If the *starting location is varied*, normal rats still swim directly to the platform. Rats with hippocampal lesions, however, paddle around the tub searching for the platform as though the task were entirely new (figure 8.16).

If the platform site is then shifted, normal rats learn where to go in one trial, whereas the hippocampal rats require many trials. This one-trail learning of location is a rough analog of declarative memory, and the deficits in hippocampal rats are good, if imperfect, analogs of declarative-memory deficits in hippocampal patients. Incidentally, one advantage of the Morris water maze is that the results are quantifiable, since you can videorecord the search path and directly compare the capacities of the control and experimental rats.

An extremely useful *nonspatial* test was developed by Howard Eichenbaum and colleagues at Harvard.[14] They buried cheerios in cups of sand. Each cup

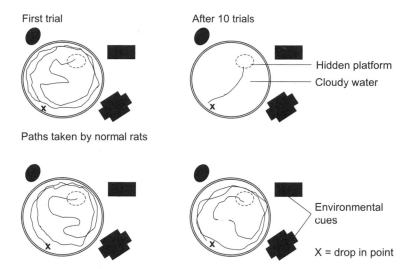

First trial

After 10 trials

— Hidden platform

— Cloudy water

Paths taken by normal rats

Environmental cues

X = drop in point

Paths taken by rats with hippocampal lesions

Figure 8.16   Spatial learning in rats. (A) Rats are placed in a circular arena (about the size and shape of a child's wading pool) filled with cloudy water (the Morris water maze). The arena itself is featureless, but the surrounding environment contains such positional cues as windows, doors, light fixtures, and so on. A small platform is located just below the surface. As rats search for this resting place, the pattern of their swimming (indicated by the traces in the figure) is monitored by a video camera. After a few trials, normal rats swim directly to the platform on each trial. (B) The swimming patterns of rats with impaired spatial memories—induced by hippocampal lesions—indicate a seeming inability to remember where the platform is located. (Based on Purves et al. 2001.)

could be scented with a distinct odor, such as cocoa, coffee, mint, apple, or orange. For rats, odors are a powerful cue. They have excellent odor discrimination and odor memory, which they use to guide behavior. Eichenbaum showed that rats can learn that when, say, coffee-smelling and cocoa-smelling cups are available, the reward is always in the coffee-smelling cup, but when coffee and mint are presented, the reward is always in the mint-smelling cup. And this overlapping-pairing schedule can be extended: in mint/orange pairs, the reward is in orange. Rats display their knowledge by digging only in the cup with the reward (figure 8.17).

This cunning arrangement permits an interesting test: can the rats use stored factual knowledge to handle a new situation? Here is how that can be

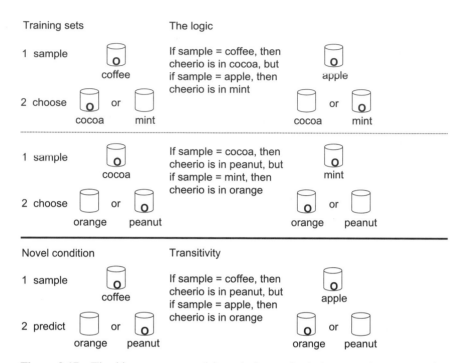

Figure 8.17   The hippocampus and its role in manipulating stored representations to infer what scent predicts the reward. In this experiment, each training phase has two parts: first, the rat is presented with a sample scent (a small cup containing sand, the scent, and a buried cheerio). Second, to get another cheerio, the rat has to choose between two cups with distinct scents and to learn from the sample what smell predicts the reward. The next segment of the training phase requires learning a new prediction, but now the sample scent is the former rewarding scent. Finally, the rat is tested with a novel situation to see whether it can predict which scent contains the reward on the basis of past associative knowledge. There is no *direct* association between a sample scent and the scent predicting the reward in the novel condition. Normal rats can succeed in this task, but rats with hippocampal lesions cannot. This is a matter not of spatial learning but of drawing an inference from earlier experience. (Based on Bunsey and Eichenbaum 1996.)

addressed: if, after learning that in cocoa/coffee pairs, the reward is in coffee, and in coffee/mint pairs, it is in mint, and in mint/orange pairs, it is in orange, present the rat with a *novel combination* of familiar odors: coffee and orange. Can the rat correctly use past knowledge and the logic of transitivity to dig in the mint cup?[15] Normal rats do indeed. Rats with hippocampal lesions perform at chance.

6.1   Anatomy (Very Briefly)

In pondering what neural mechanisms can explain the behavioral data, we need to understand the basic anatomy of the brain in general and the hippocampal structures in particular. In the nervous system, structure is the key to mechanism, and without an understanding of structure, we cannot advance very far in understanding function.

The entorhinal, perirhinal, and parahippocampal cortices are the sites of a convergence of inputs from polysensory regions of the frontal, temporal, and parietal cortices. The hippocampus gets its *input* from these areas, predominantly via the entorhinal cortex (EC), which has reciprocal connections to a range of areas involved in emotions and attention. Hippocampal *output* goes back to EC, via the subiculum. This loopy circuitry, illustrated in figure 8.14A, suggests that information repeatedly circulates through the hippocampus and its associated structures, perhaps involving rehearsal, perhaps involving the selecting and cleaning up of information as it passes through again, perhaps subserving recognition memory by filling in and pattern-completing in response to partial cues.

Neurons in the EC project onto pyramidal neurons in the CA3 field of the hippocampus in a highly regular way: EC projects via the perforant path to the upper dendritic regions, and via the dentate gyrus (DG) to the lower dendritic regions (see again figure 8.14A). The perforant path EC synapses have *NMDA receptors*, the DG synapses do not. Both exhibit LTP. The axons of the CA3 pyramidal neurons go to two places: (1) they project back onto themselves (*recurrent collaterals*) and onto synapses *between* the EC and the DG connections, and (2) they divide into a batch that projects onto the upper regions (apical dendrites) of the CA1 neurons and a batch that projects onto the lower regions (basal dendrites). These synapses have NMDA receptors and exhibit LTP. How does this orderly neuroanatomy serve declarative memory? Now we need the neurophysiology to tell us how cells respond.

6.2   Neurophysiology (Very Briefly)

As discussed in chapter 7, when a rat enters a new environment, specific cells will attach themselves to specific places that the rat visits, and will respond vigorously whenever the rat revisits the preferred location. A cell will respond to its preferred location even when the rat is passively moved in the environment. A cell tuned to respond to a specific location in one environment will respond to an unrelated location in a different environment. As the rat travels among various environments, the cell shows its preference *relative to* the environment it is in. Overall, the spatial layout of the environment is *not* topographically mapped in the hippocampus (see again figure 7.2).

Spatial representation and more

Though place may be a necessary condition for the response, it is not sufficient. Suppose that the rat is trained on a T-maze to get cheese rewards by alternating which arm to choose (if it went left last time, it should go right this time). A hippocampal "place cell" will respond when the rat is in one specific place and plans to go left, but not when it is in that very same place but plans to go right. This implies that the cell is coding for more than just location (Eichenbaum 1998). What precisely do the hippocampal cells code for? That is, what are the dimensions of the parameter space that characterize what hippocampal cells represent? Plan and place? Plan and time and place? Do we even have the *vocabulary* adequate to describe whatever these hippocampal cells are representing?

Learning components: CA1

Using genetic techniques, Tonegawa and colleagues selectively blocked the NMDA receptor in tissue-specific regions of the hippocampus (see Tsien et al. 1996 and McHugh et al. 1996). This means that there is no LTP or LTD in the CA1 cells. Mice that are normal save that they lack functional NMDA receptors only in the *CA1 region* are unable to learn spatial tasks (like the Morris water maze).

Learning components: CA3

Mice that are normal save for lacking functional NMDA receptors on *CA3 pyramidal neurons* have a quite different profile. They *can* learn the spatial task.

If, however, one or more visual cues surrounding the tub are removed, their performance falls off. The fewer the cues, the worse the performance. In addition, after a shift of position of the platform, they cannot learn the new platform location in one trial. Normal rats easily do both. Therefore, the data from Tonegawa's lab suggest that declarative memory can be fractionated into functional components subserved by anatomically distinct regions. From what we know about recurrence in artificial neural nets, we may surmise that the recurrent loops on CA3 pyramidals could subserve pattern completion, and hence are needed if the animal is to retrieve information about platform location with reduced cues. The DG connection on CA3 pyramidals may be crucial for one-trial learning.

Memory consolidation takes time

Inspired by human studies showing that amnesic patients have better recall for *older* memories than for more *recent* events, Larry Squire and Stuart Zola (1996) asked the following question: if you need hippocampal structures to learn new facts, for *how long* after the exposure to the memorable facts must those structures be functional for the facts to be retrievable from memory? This was a fundamental probe into the functional relation between hippocampal structures and cortical structures, and it had a very revealing answer. In monkeys, it turned out that unless the hippocampal structures were intact for about 7–10 weeks following exposure to the to-be-remembered event, the animals' declarative memory was severely impaired. Thereafter, it was normal. Further human data suggested that normal hippocampal structures could be necessary for even longer periods (figures 8.18 and 8.19).

Spatial learning and sleep

Matt Wilson and his colleagues (1994) have shown that during the non-dreaming phases of the sleep cycle, "place cells" in the hippocampus respond as though the rat were actually running through the maze it had explored for reward during the waking period. Although questions remain, this activity looks suggestively like rehearsal. Interference with this activity reduces learning performance. Human data show that deep sleep (stage IV in the sleep cycle) in the early part of the night and dreaming sleep in the later part of the night are necessary for skill acquisition. Moreover, the deep sleep and dreaming sleep must occur within 30 hours of training if learning is to occur, since beyond those limits, catch-up sleep on the second night fails to compensate.[16]

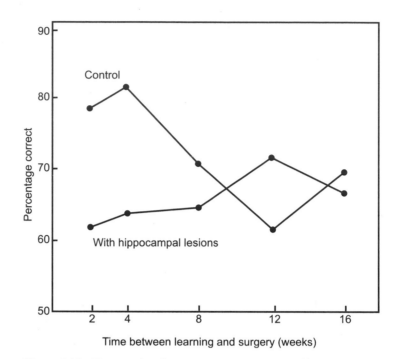

Figure 8.18   Two weeks after surgery to remove the hippocampus, monkeys had difficulty remembering recently learned objects, although their memory for objects learned many weeks ago was as accurate as that of control monkeys not operated on. Chance performance would equal 50 percent correct. (From Squire and Zola-Morgan 1991.)

Learning and neurogenesis

The birth of new neurons (neurogenesis) in adults appears to be restricted to the olfactory bulb and the hippocampus, though this is not known for sure. The level of neurogenesis in the hippocampus increases when the animal explores an interesting environment; it decreases with stress, boring environments, and depression. (New cells can be identified by labeling with an analogue of the DNA base thymidine: *bromodeoxyuridine.* This becomes incorporated into new DNA during cell replication.) What do these new neurons have to do with new memories? Elizabeth Gould and her colleagues (1999) have recently shown that the birth of new neurons in the hippocampus is important for new *trace conditioning,* i.e., learning to associate events that are separated by an *interval of time.* The new neurons appear to be unrelated to learning to associate events that overlap in time (so-called *delay conditioning*). Learning these latter associ-

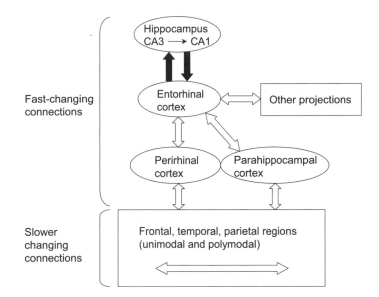

Figure 8.19 Information is transferred from hippocampal structures to neocortical structures, where it gradually becomes consolidated, probably involving such structural changes in connectivity as dendritic growth. The looping pathways between the neocortex and hippocampal structures, together with data on temporally graded amnesia following hippocampal loss, suggests that the hippocampus directs memory consolidation in the neocortex by providing continual input, including, and perhaps most importantly, during sleep. (Based on Squire and Alvarez 1995.)

ations probably depends on the amygdala, not the hippocampus. The Gould lab showed these effects by well-controlled interference with neurogenesis in the hippocampus of rats.[17]

Evidently, the hippocampal story of learning and memory is becoming increasingly detailed, and much more is now known than when Milner began in the mid-1950s to explore what H.M. could and could not learn postsurgically. Nevertheless, there is no shortage of open questions: What *exactly* does the hippocampus do? How is it involved in the consolidation of memory? What mechanisms might be responsible for the consolidation of memory in neural networks external to hippocampal structures? How well connected must new hippocampal neurons be to begin to function in learning? How is the right connectivity established? Why is there a high rate of neuronal turnover in the hippocampus? These are but a handful of questions that should find answers in the coming decades.

7   How Do Networks Learn: A Brief Look

Representations, as we saw in chapter 7, appear to be distributed across many neurons in a network. ANNs, such as Cottrell's face net, have been instrumental in providing a working example of distributed representation, and hence an example of how the brain's representations might be distributed in populations of real neurons. An important question, raised but not answered in chapter 7 (p. 296), asked how the adjustment of individual synaptic weights can be appropriately orchestrated across a population so that the population comes to embody knowledge, such as the knowledge of how to distinguish a male face from a female face or how to identify a face as that of Winston Churchill. In short, we want to know how a neural network learns.

The weights cannot, of course, be hand-set in the brain, and they cannot be hand-set in ANNs either once the number of weights is large enough to service an interesting representation. So we are looking for an automated, brain-plausible weight-adjusting procedure. ANNs are a useful tool for inventing, exploring, and testing various procedures for changing structure to get meaning into processing units in a network. Since we want to know how in fact real populations of neurons adjust their weights, all procedures tested on ANNs must ultimately be tested in the actual nervous system.

A variety of algorithms have been devised for adjusting the connection weights to configure a network to embody knowledge about the properties of the stimulus set. Because these algorithms take a network from a know-nothing state where the weights are randomly configured to a state where the pattern of connection weights embodies information allowing the network to categorize input signals, they are called *learning algorithms*. Learning algorithms for automated weight-adjustment divide into two basic kinds: *supervised* learning algorithms and *unsupervised* learning algorithms. The essential difference concerns feedback. The various supervised learning algorithms use feedback about the network's behavioral performance in determining weight modification, whereas unsupervised learning algorithms use no external feedback.

Supervised learning relies on three things: input signals, the net's internal dynamics, and an evaluation of its weight-setting performance. Unsupervised learning depends only on two things: input signals and the net's internal dynamics. In either case, the point of the learning algorithm is to produce a weight configuration that can be said to represent something in the world, in the sense that when activated by an input vector, the correct answer, or

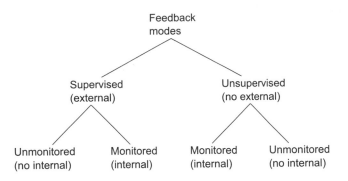

Figure 8.20 Strategies for feedback. (From Churchland and Sejnowski 1992.)

approximately correct answer, is produced by the network. Although unsupervised learning algorithms have no access to external feedback, they can use *internal* error feedback. When the feedback is external to the organism, the learning is called "supervised"; when there is an internal measure of error, the learning is called "monitored" (figure 8.20).

Consider, for example, a net required to learn to predict the next input. Assume that it gets no external feedback, but that it does use its previous inputs to make its prediction. When the next input enters, the net may be able to use the discrepancy between the predicted input and the actual input to get a measure of error, which it can then use to improve its next prediction. This is an instance of a net whose learning is *unsupervised* but *monitored*. More generally, there may be internal measures of consistency or coherence that can also be internally monitored and used in improving the internal representation.

Nets using unsupervised learning can be configured so that the weights embody regularities in the stimulus domain. For example, the weights of a two-layered net can be adjusted according to a Hebb rule, so that gradually, without external feedback and with only input data, the net structures itself to represent the correlation of feature *A* and feature *B*. Beyond the scope of the simple net are higher-order statistical problems, such as "What is the correlation story for $\{A, B, C, D\}$ or for $\{EF, EH, GH\}$?" Going beyond first-order correlations is highly desirable, since mapping causal structure in the world, for example, requires higher-order statistics. To target high-order problems, the simple two-layer architecture must be expanded to include so-called *hidden units* that intervene between external input and behavioral output.

The ability of layers of hidden units to extract higher-order information is especially valuable when the number of input units is large, as it is, for example, in sensory systems. Suppose that an input layer has n units in a two-dimensional array, like the retina, or a one-dimensional array, like the cochlea. If the units are binary, then the total number of possible input patterns is 2^n. In fact, neurons are not binary but many-valued, so the problem is actually worse. Suppose that all patterns (state combinations) are equally likely to occur, and suppose that one hidden unit represents exactly one input pattern (e.g., that H and M are highly correlated). This would make it possible to represent any function in the output layer by suitable connections from the hidden units. The trouble arises when n is very large, e.g., a million, in which case the number of possible states is so large that no physical system could contain all the hidden units. The problem is solvable in part because in this world, not all input patterns are equally likely, and of those that are highly likely, not all are equally interesting to the animal. So only a small subset of all possible input patterns needs to be represented by the hidden units.

Accordingly, the problem for the hidden units is to discover which features systematically occur together or are otherwise "cohorted," *and* among those, which to ignore and which to care about and represent. By means of unsupervised learning, the fundamental correlations can be found, and by means of supervised learning (punishment and reward), the net can learn what correlations it should represent. As the net runs, hidden units may be assigned states according to either a linear or a nonlinear function. If linear, there is an optimal solution called *principal-component analysis*. This procedure is used to find the subset of vectors that are the best linear approximation to the set of input vectors. Although principal-component analysis and its extensions are useful for lower-order statistics, many of the interesting structures in the world can be identified only via high-order statistics. Consequently, we want a learning algorithm that can find high-order features. For example, if luminance is taken as a zeroth-order property, then *boundaries* will be an example of a first-order property, and *characteristics* of boundaries, such as occlusion and three-dimensional shape, will be higher-order properties. Causal relations between three-dimensional objects will be even higher order properties. On the face of it, finding a suitable weight-adjustment rule looks difficult because not only are the units hidden, they are nonlinear, so mere trial and error strategies will not get us there. Fortunately, there are solutions.

Independent-component analysis (ICA) is a technique that uses the statistics of the input signals to identify the independent sources of those signals when the sources of those signals are unknown. ICA has many applications in telecommunications and the analysis of biomedical data such as EEG recordings.

If a system is completely naive about the nature of its signal sources and hence of the parameters of its mixture of input signals, ICA allows it to the find linear, nonorthogonal axes of its parameter space. Thus it can do blind source separation. So if you are a tank commander in midbattle speaking to snipers in the field, for example, ICA can separate the voice out of an extremely noisy background. ICA uses not only first-order statistics, but also higher-order statistics, to find what variables in its "world" are statistically independent; roughly speaking, to find out what in the world is causing its information. It seems rather plausible that nervous systems may, at various stages of development and for various tasks, use ICA learning algorithms to make sense of the booming, buzzing confusion of signals from the sensory periphery. A newborn animal is probably a system that is largely naive about the sources of its sensory signals; it has to find the axes of its parameter spaces. ICA can do precisely that.

Devising a biologically plausible ICA *learning algorithm* for weight adjustment has been both a computational desideratum and a formidable challenge. Fortunately, in 1995 Bell and Sejnowski discovered an elegant and powerful ICA learning algorithm. For example, the Bell and Sejnowski learning algorithm can configure a network to solve face-recognition and lip-reading problems. On neurobiological realism, it also scores well, since it has been tested against a range of real physiological data, including the emergence of organized structures such as ocular-dominance columns in the early visual cortex.

Although research on ICA learning algorithms is still in its infancy, it is a promising attack on the problem of what principles underlie coordinated weight adjustment (learning) in populations of neurons. ICA learning algorithms are powerful, but they are not the whole story, for a variety of reasons. In particular, they assume a stable probability distribution of signals in the world. Because we are constantly moving our eyes, heads, and whole body, the probability distribution is not stable for long periods. So work remains to be done. Nevertheless, even as they stand, ICA learning algorithms take us far beyond what the ANN pessimists predicted.

Supervised-learning algorithms come in various grades as a function of the format of the feedback informing the network on the quality of its performance. The evaluation may (1) merely say "Good answer" or "Bad answer," (2) specify a measure of the size of the error with some degree of precision, or (3) give rich detail, saying, in effect, "You said the answer was $\langle 1, 9, 0, 3 \rangle$, but the answer should be $\langle 4, 9, 3, 3 \rangle$." Given the range available in (2), this allows for a continuum of evaluation formats. As we saw with bee-foraging behavior, diffusely projecting systems such as the dopamine projections from the VTA mediate reinforcement learning. Reinforcement learning—learning via feedback from the environment—is under intense investigation, in both artificial and real nervous systems. As we saw in chapter 3 in the discussion of the Grush emulator, when a brain has an internal model of itself and its environment, it can test tentative plans and, using internal feedback from the model, upgrade it plans. Inner models with inner feedback allow for enormous complexity in learning, and they probably lie at the heart of much reasoning and problem solving.[18]

8   Concluding Remarks

What, the skeptic might ask, has all this to do with epistemology, traditionally conceived? First, note that the philosophical tradition is *multi*tracked. The approach embraced here fits with the tradition that reaches back to Aristotle; it is naturalistic and pragmatic, as opposed to supernaturalistic or a priori. It has links with the philosopher John Locke (1632–1704), who attended lectures and brain dissections by the great British anatomist Thomas Willis (1621–1675). It warms to theories, hypotheses, and models, while at the same time it demands evidence, data, and testing. It looks for coherence and consilience across well-established theories, yet it is open to revision of even the most successful theories.

Together, neuroscience, psychology, ethology, and molecular biology are teaching us about ourselves as *knowers*—about what it is to know, learn, remember, and forget, and about how brains are configured to know, learn, remember, and forget (figure 8.21). These questions are fundamental epistemological questions—really, the *grand questions*—and they are questions that motivated Aristotle, Descartes, Hume, Kant, and Quine. They are also questions that motivated Helmholtz, Darwin, Cajal, E. O. Wilson, and Crick. I see them, one and all, as engaged in *naturalized epistemology*. I don't see that it matters much whether they work in philosophy departments or not.

Not all epistemologists have been so motivated. For some, this is because they believe that what we call external reality is naught but Ideas created in a nonphysical mind, a mind that can be understood only via introspection and reflection on its Ideas. For philosophers who are *idealists* in this technical sense, the new developments in cognitive neuroscience will seem irrelevant. And per-

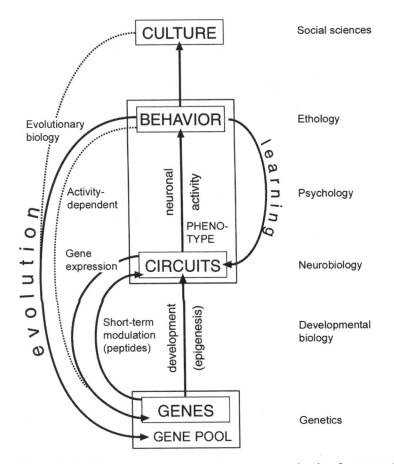

Figure 8.21 The causal interactions between many levels of structural organization involved in cognition, and the particular sciences that address the levels and the connections between them. (After Plotkin and Odling-Smee 1981, Huber 2000.)

haps the idealists are right. Nevertheless, idealism, with its admiration for a priori and introspective strategies, seems to have made little progress on the nature and basis of knowledge. Certainly there is nothing extant in idealism that can hold a candle to the emerging explanatory framework of cognitive neuroscience. This does not mean that idealism is certainly wrong, for it may merely need more time. It does mean, however, that the idealist's introspect-and-contemplate strategy is unappealing for those who wish to make progress in understanding how we know things.

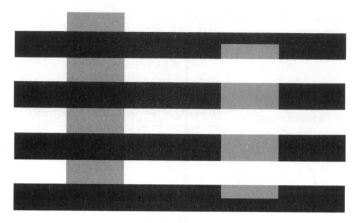
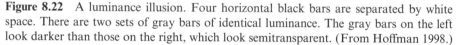

Figure 8.22   A luminance illusion. Four horizontal black bars are separated by white space. There are two sets of gray bars of identical luminance. The gray bars on the left look darker than those on the right, which look semitransparent. (From Hoffman 1998.)

There is one major element of truth in the idealist's approach. As Kant realized, the mind/brain is not just a passive canvas on which reality paints. The brain organizes, structures, extracts, and also creates (figure 8.22). Reality is always grasped through the lens of stacks upon dynamical stacks of neural networks. There is no apprehending the nature of reality except via brains and the theories and artifacts that brains devise and interpret.

From this it does not follow, however, that reality is *only* a mind-created Idea. Rather, it means that we have to keep plugging along, trying to get closer and closer to the nature of reality, and trying to make fewer and fewer predictive errors. Our brains—using whatever equipment is available: conceptual, technological, linguistic, etc.—drum up increasingly adequate models of reality, where the brain, among other things, is part of the reality modeled. We keep questioning, and we build the next generation of theories upon the scaffolding of the last. How do we know the models are increasingly adequate? Only by their relative success in predicting and explaining. We cannot doff *all* lenses—perceptual, conceptual, technological—and make a *direct* comparison between hypothesis and reality.

Does this mean that there is a fatal circularity in neuroscience—the brain uses itself to study itself? Not if you think about it. I use my eyes to study the eye, but nothing very troubling results from this necessity, since I can study the eyes of others and reliably generalize to my own case. The brain I study is seldom my own, but usually that of other animals, and I can reliably generalize to my own case. The enterprise of naturalized epistemology involves many brains—correcting each other, testing each other, and building models that can be rated as better or worse in characterizing the world. If a hypothesis says that no new neurons are made in the adult human brain, that hypothesis can be tested and falsified. If a hypothesis says that memories are one and all stored in the hippocampus, that can be tested and falsified. Figuring out what is *not* true helps us get closer to what *is* true, whether the subject matter is brains or the origin of the Earth.

Is there anything left for the *philosopher* to do? For the neurophilosopher, at least, there is plenty to do. Questions abound: about the integration of distinct memory systems, how nervous systems handle time, how far associationist principles can take us, the nature of representation, the nature of reasoning and rationality, how information is used to make decisions, how information is retrieved, about what information *is* for nervous systems, why sleep and dreaming are necessary for learning, and on and on. These are all Big Questions—big enough for me, anyhow. They are questions where experiment and theoretical insight must jointly conspire, where creativity in *experimental design* and creativity in *theoretical speculation* egg each other on to unimagined discoveries. These are questions with deep historical roots reaching back to the ancient Greeks in 500 B.C. and with ramifying branches extending throughout the history of Western thought. They are, moreover, questions requiring a *synthesis* from psychology, neuroscience, and molecular biology. And *all* this is what makes them *philosophical*. Or so it seems to me.

Suggested Readings

Arthur, W. 1997. *The Origin of Animal Body Plans: A Study in Evolutionary Developmental Biology*. New York: Cambridge University Press.

Clark, A. 1997. *Being There: Putting Brain, Body, and World Together Again*. Cambridge: MIT Press.

Cowan, W. M., T. C. Südhof, and C. F. Stevens. 2000. *Synapses*. Baltimore: Johns Hopkins University Press.

Fuster, J. M. 1995. *Memory in the Cerebral Cortex*. Cambridge: MIT Press.

Gerhadt, J., and M. Kirschner. 1997. *Cells, Embryos, and Evolution*. Oxford: Blackwells.

Grafman, J., and Y. Christen, eds. 1999. *Neuronal Plasticity: Building a Bridge from the Laboratory to the Clinic*. Berlin: Springer.

Heyes, C., and L. Huber, eds. 2000. *The Evolution of Cognition.* Cambridge: MIT Press.

Jeannerod, Marc. 1997. *The Cognitive Neuroscience of Action.* Oxford: Blackwells.

Johnson, M. H. 1997. *Developmental Cognitive Neuroscience: An Introduction.* Malden: Blackwells.

Lawrence, Peter A. 1992. *The Making of a Fly: The Genetics of Animal Design.* Cambridge, Mass.: Blackwells Science.

Le Doux, Joseph. 2002. *Synaptic Self.* New York: Viking.

Nelson, C. A., and M. Luciana, eds. 2001. *Handbood of Development Cognitive Neuroscience.* Cambridge: MIT Press.

Prince, D. J., and D. J. Willshaw 2000. *Mechanisms of Cortical Development.* Oxford: Oxford University Press.

Quartz, S. R. 2001. Toward a developmental evolutionary psychology: genes, development and the evolution of the human cognitive architecture. In F. Rauscher and S. J. Scher, eds., *Evolutionary Psychology: Alternative Approaches.*

Schacter, Daniel L. 1996. *Searching for Memory: The Brain, the Mind, and the Past.* New York: Basic Books.

Squire, Larry R., and Eric R. Kandel. 1999. *Memory: From Mind to Molecules.* New York: Scientific American Library.

Sutton, R. S., and A. G. Barto. 1998. *Reinforcement Learning: An Introduction.* Cambridge: MIT Press.

Websites

BioMedNet Magazine: http://news.bmn.com/magazine

A Brief Introduction to the Brain: http://ifcsun1.ifisiol.unam.mx/brain/

Comparative Mammalian Brain Collections: http://brainmuseum.org

Encyclopedia of Life Sciences: http://www.els.net

The MIT Encyclopedia of the Cognitive Sciences: http://cognet.mit.edu/MITECS

III Religion

9   Religion and the Brain

From a scientific point of view, we can make no distinction between the man who eats little and sees heaven and the man who drinks much and sees snakes. Each is in an abnormal physical condition, and therefore has abnormal perceptions.
Bertrand Russell (1935)

1   Introduction

Progress in science in general, as well as in neuroscience in particular, has had an impact on a range of traditional philosophical issues, including the nature of the mind, the nature of the universe, and the nature of life. One metaphysical matter that looms large for many people concerns supernatural beings, and the existence of God in particular. Is there anything we have learned about the brain that bears upon questions of spirituality?

At the heart of reflections on religion and the brain are three questions: (1) Does God exist? (2) Is there life after death? (3) What happens to morality if God does not exist? One and all, these questions are ancient; one and all, they remain highly current topics of discussion. I raise them here partly because some developments in cognitive neuroscience have an impact on how we formulate possible answers. These questions have both a metaphysical and epistemological dimension, and addressing them pulls together many of the ideas discussed in earlier chapters. Certainly, they are preeminently *philosophical* questions, and the historical tradition is rich with arguments, replies, reformulations, and refutations. In this respect, it resembles the historical tradition of *natural philosophy* generally, as humans struggled to figure out the nature of physical reality and whether their beliefs about fire, life, the Earth, and the mind are likely to be true.

As one's understanding of the world expands, conflicts between beliefs are a regular feature of cognitive life. Some of these beliefs are humdrum (e.g., it looks like the Moon is about as big as a barn; the data show it actually has a diameter of 2,000 miles and is 240,000 miles away). Some are more momentous (e.g., one believes that autism is caused by cold mothering and then discovers that it has a genetic basis). Some have tumultuous personal effects (e.g., you believe that your enduring melancholia is a character flaw and then discover that you have a serotonin deficiency).

Some discoveries bear upon the belief that there is a life after death. More specifically, there is tension between (a) the idea of the *self* as an immaterial *and* immortal soul, created by God, and (b) the idea that the mind is what the brain does, that the human brain is a product of natural selection, and that disintegration of one's brain in disease and death entails disintegration of one's mind. For most of us, it matters how we resolve these tensions, and it matters that we resolve them in a way that is intellectually satisfying rather than flippant or ideological.

For me to live after the death of my brain, I must be independent of my brain. Hence the question of life after death is the springboard question for this chapter. Nevertheless, because the possibility of an afterlife is so closely associated with belief in a Supreme Being, the two matters are, for all intents and purposes, inseparable. In this closing chapter, therefore, we shall take a closer look at all three major questions within the neurophilosophical framework developed for metaphysics and epistemology. My *main purpose* will be to clarify the issues involved, so that the reader can more productively reflect on them and figure out how best to resolve inconsistencies and tensions.

2   Does God Exist?

To reduce ambiguity and confusion, we must, as usual, begin with some preliminary *semantic* geography. Granted that we cannot give a precise definition of God, what *roughly* is meant by "God?" This question does need to be asked, particularly because there are many different religions with many different characterizations of a Supreme Being. Most readers will have some acquaintance with Judaism, Christianity, and Islam. They will consequently have some conception of what, within those religions, is meant by "Supreme Being." Nevertheless, some very large religions, for example, Buddhism, do not really countenance a Supreme Being with metaphysical status in anything like the way in which Christianity, Judaism, and Islam do. In addition, the early Greeks believed in an extended family of humanlike gods. Many North American aboriginal cultures believed in animal-like gods. Some *pantheists* take the view that God is in all of Nature, including lightning, water, plants, and bacteria. Other pantheists consider God to be *equivalent* to Nature as a whole and reject the idea of God as a Supreme Person in any sense. The differences between religious beliefs on the matter of what God *is* are nontrivial.

Significantly, these differences in the belief tend to be culturally dependent. As a matter of sociological fact, if someone has a religious belief, it tends to resemble rather closely the one in which he was raised or to which he was exposed when young. It is less common for someone, having reached adulthood, to canvas the entire range of possible religions and then, on the basis of evidence and moral suitability, to make a choice. Because of this fact and the fact that individuals are prone to the conviction that one's own particular religion is the only true religion, it is all the more important in this discussion to be mindful of the great breadth of religious beliefs.

Despite the diversity of religions and the cultural sensitivity of religious preference, we can continue to make progress on the question by characterizing a deity in terms sufficiently general and minimalist as to be independent of any particular religion, so long as it does espouse, at least and at most, one Deity. It is important to have rough agreement on what we are talking about in order to have common ground for discussion. In keeping with this compromise, suppose that by "God" or "Deity" we mean an entity that has some features of a human being, in the sense that it cares about our welfare, pays attention to prayers, and has high moral standing. In the interests of nonsectarian discussion, let us assume that such a Deity is vastly more capable than a human, perhaps being *omnipotent* (all powerful), *omniscient* (all knowing), and *omnibenevolent* (all good), and that God is responsible for the creation of the universe, its laws, and the things in it. There is some latitude in each of the three descriptions, so the qualifier "more or less" should be taken as implicitly riding along.[1]

Though this characterization is not universally satisfactory, it tries to avoid being empty (as the description "God is everything that is" tends to be), while meeting the religious expectation that God is the supreme creator of the universe, can intervene to change the course of the universe, has a deep understanding of what is going on, cares about our lives and our suffering, and is the source of moral standards.[2] Some such characterization is needed to make sense of the subsidiary belief in the efficacy of prayer, for example. That is, if

God lacked power, there would be little point in praying for help. This characterization does not fit the conception of pantheists (God *is* Nature), but it is consistent with the theist's conviction that praying for intervention is appropriate. The problem with an even more abstract characterization in terms of "the Great All" or "something greater than ourselves," for example, is that for many theists, it undercuts the solace derived from belief in a caring, sympathetic, *personlike* God. It also makes many religious practices, such as worship and seeking redemption, otiose, and it seems too abstract to help out with a belief in an afterlife. So although the three-*omni*s description will be less than satisfactory for some theists, it is minimally satisfactory to many. On that basis, the description is sufficiently adequate to launch a discussion of God's existence.

What are the grounds for believing in a Deity as described? Although there may be almost as many different reasons as there are believers, for simplicity, we can discern three general paths:

Path 1: evidence and analysis   On the assumption that God is a real existing thing, there should be evidence of God's existence, in some form or other. This will yield *empirical* knowledge.

Path 2: revelation   God reveals himself to certain humans, and these persons have *direct* knowledge of God.

Path 3: faith   Belief based on faith is independent of what anyone else observes, believes, or analyzes. Faith may be depicted as "*chosen* knowledge," in the sense that one exercises a choice to believe, perhaps on trust and regardless of evidence and analysis, regardless of revelation or lack thereof.

I turn now to the task of discussing, very briefly, each of the three paths.

2.1   Path 1: Evidence and Analysis

There are two main lines of argument concerning the evidence for the existence of a Deity. The strongest is the *argument from design*, and the second is the *argument from first cause*.

The argument from design

According to the argument from design, the organization of the cosmos, and in particular the existence and organization of the biological world, requires intelligent design. And *that*, the argument continues, requires an Intelligent Designer. Why? Because it is *inconceivable* that material organization, such as the human eye, and biological processes, such as protein manufacture, could have come into existence by mere chance and with no higher purpose.

The main problem with this argument is that as science has progressed, we have come to understand how the organization in matter can come about by entirely natural means. In other words, what *seemed* inconceivable in the middle ages is quite well conceived now. In the biological realm, Darwinian evolution explains how purely natural interactions over many millions of years will result in diverse biological organisms with complex structures.[4] And this has been borne out by comparative physiology, which allows us to see earlier and simpler forms of structures, such as the eye, in organisms that appeared on the planet many millions of years before humans. Variations in a complex structure, such as the ear as it exists in the barn owl, the human, the dolphin, and the bull frog, are best explained in terms of biological adaptations to specific features of an environmental niche through the process of natural selection.

As recently as the later part of the nineteenth century, some eminent scientists, for example Louis Agassiz, thought that the Deity had created all existing life forms at the same time, complete with the structural features that allowed them to function best in their particular environmental niche. The fossil record, the evidence of extinctions, and most recently the discoveries showing physiological homologues and DNA relationships between animals has made this view highly implausible. For example, the oldest (deepest) layers in the fossil record contain no mammalian fossils, and no bony fishes, but only simple organisms, such as trilobites. Dinosaurs, along with many other species, became extinct long before large mammals appeared. In general, the understanding of molecular biology[5] and evolutionary biology[6] has greatly reduced the appeal of the argument from design. This weakness does not yield a proof of the *nonexistence* of God, but it does mean that a traditionally powerful argument *for* the existence of God has lost much of its plausibility.

Nevertheless, adherents of the argument from design might wish to vary the argument by pointing out that there are still explanatory gaps in evolutionary biology. In particular, science has not yet established where the first replicating structures—presumably RNA—came from. We still do not have a satisfactory theory of how proteins fold, or how Monarch butterflies find their ancestral home, or how the human brain, structurally so very similar to the brains of other primates, has the capacity for language. Surely, it may be suggested, these mysteries point towards the intervention of a Supernatural Being. Why? Because it is *inconceivable* that such structural complexity could have come about by sheerly natural means. Our question must be this: *how tenable is the logic*?

As a preliminary point, recall from earlier discussions that what is or is not conceivable varies as a function of what the conceiver already understands and believes. Though it can seem otherwise, conceivability also varies as a function of what conclusion one antecedently finds attractive. The main point is that what is or is not conceivable by me is a *psychological fact* about me, not a *metaphysical fact* about the nature of reality. Consider that vitalists— even twentieth-century vitalists—confidently asserted the inconceivability of explaining what it is to be alive without appeal to the *life force*. Even as late as 1910, many physicians found it inconceivable that diseases could be caused by organisms so tiny that they were invisible to the naked eye. It is not unusual to find people who consider it inconceivable that the continents move. As discussed in chapters 4 and 6, arguments from inconceivability need to be backed up by knowledge, not by ignorance, if they are to make any headway.

Before the development of physical chemistry, molecular biology, and evolutionary biology, the original version of the design argument could lean on inconceivability and resonate with many people. By now, however, the inconceivability argument has lost its luster even as applied to those phenomena that are currently *unexplained*. The problem is that those items still on the list of the unexplained can well be considered as merely *not yet explained*, rather than as items requiring a *supernatural* explanation. For example, since scientists such as Leslie Orgel and Jerry Joyce are hard at work trying to understand the etiology leading up to early forms of RNA, and hence to understand the origin of life, it is all too *conceivable* that they will succeed and answers will be found.[7]

Suppose that scientists such as Orgel and Joyce do not discover an answer. Would that failure constitute evidence for supernatural intervention? No. It would show only that the problem was not solved, not that it is *unsolvable*. Even if the answer were *never* discovered, at most that would show that there is something of which we are ignorant. This is a very banal conclusion, but it is all that the premise supports. From the premise that we *do not know* the originating causes of RNA, can we argue to the conclusion that we *do know* the originating cause was supernatural? Alas, using ignorance as a premise is a fallacy. More precisely, we cannot conclude that we *do know* the cause from a premise asserting that we *do not know* the cause.

There is a further softness in the design argument. As David Hume pointed out, if it is complexity of organisms in the natural world that motivates us to postulate an Intelligent Designer, should we not be *equally unsatisfied* with an unexplained Intelligent Designer?[8] Should we not want to explain where *that* complexity came from? If the existence of *naturally* occurring organizational structure *is* a problem, why is the existence of *divinely* occurring organization structure *not* a problem? If one is *uncomfortable* stopping the chain of causes with scientific explanations of naturally occurring complexity, but *comfortable* stopping with supernaturally occurring complexity, what, Hume inquired, is the rationale? *Why, so far as empirical evidence is concerned, is the existence of natural complexity more in need of explanation than the existence of supernatural complexity?*

The argument from first cause

Hume's objection contains the seeds of a refutation of the first-cause argument. The first-cause argument advances the hypothesis that the chain of causes in the cosmos cannot be infinite. So there must be a first cause and *that*—the *Uncaused Cause*, as it were—must be a Supernatural Being. Hume asked two questions: First, why is an infinitely long chain of causes less plausible than a finite chain whose beginning is supernatural? Perhaps, so far as the empirical data reveal, the chain of causes *is* infinite. Second, if there is a first cause of the events in the cosmos, why is it more plausible that it is supernatural rather than natural, such as the Big Bang? To neither of his arguments is there an empirically grounded, satisfactory response. Notice again that this critical analysis does not constitute a proof of the *nonexistence* of God. It says only that there are logical flaws in the *argument for* the existence of God.

The argument from evil

Hume also challenged the hypothesis that the empirical evidence points to the existence of an omnipotent, omniscient, and omnibenevolent Deity. His principal argument runs as follows: if we are to *infer from available evidence* that God is benevolent, the existence of *natural evil* presents a huge problem. By "naturally occurring evil," he meant such tragedies as infants born with horrible diseases and dying slow and painful deaths. He included the routine struggle for existence that animals endure, as well as the miseries caused by storms, droughts, plagues, insanity, and floods. Listing the miseries of life on the planet, for humans and other animals, is a long, sad business.

Hume concluded that the existence of suffering is prima facie evidence against the Deity *as described*. Either (a) he does not know of the misery in the world, in which case he is not all-knowing, or (b) he does know but cannot prevent it, in which case he was not all-powerful, or (c) he *does* know and *can* prevent it, but *prefers not* to, in which case he is not all-benevolent. The argument does not prove that no such God does exists, but it does show that *if one draws on available evidence*, one would never rationally infer that God is omnipotent, omniscient, *and* omnibenevolent.

A classic set of responses have been made to the argument, essentially all of which Hume anticipated and attempted to refute. First, it might be suggested that if you quantify good and suffering, then on balance there is more happiness than misery. Hume's answer was thorough. First, the estimated ratio of happiness to suffering is, needless to say, only a very rough estimate. Given the evidence of misery on the planet, it is as reasonable to estimate a preponderance of misery over happiness as vice versa. Aside from the difficulties in making the estimate precise, the misery that does exist is, even if counterbalanced by lots and lots of happiness, a terrible lot of misery. Why, Hume asked, is there so much misery? Would not a truly benevolent, powerful God find a way to mitigate much of the pain and suffering of innocents, the misery and horror inflicted on the powerless and virtuous? Therefore, misery blocks any inference to the existence of an omnipotent *and* omniscient *and* omnibenevolent God. Hence the argument from evil cannot be set aside.

A second response suggests that suffering exists because humans have free will and have chosen to do evil things. Misery, therefore, is God's just punishment for sin. Hume's answer was this: even if this response explains the misery that happens to *humans* who have sinned (which he doubted), it does not explain the terrible suffering that befalls innocent human infants or animals.

A third response suggests that evil must exist in the world if humans are to know the difference between good and evil. Hume's answer was this: well, surely a small amount of evil would suffice for that purpose. Additionally, omnipotence is not a trifling capacity, so if the Deity is *omnipotent*, he should be *able* to make that knowledge available without making the innocent suffer. Being omniscient, he should *know how* to achieve this.

A fourth response argues that what we consider evil is not really evil from God's point of view, i.e., that suffering is not really a bad thing from the Divine perspective. Hume suggested that this argument was a shocking refusal to take seriously the theist's own claim that the Deity is genuinely benevolent and cares about our welfare. If, he argued, God does not consider the terminal cancer of an innocent child as a bad thing, then it is hard to see how he can be considered benevolent, in terms of what *we* mean by "benevolent." If such suffering is consistent with supernatural benevolence, then that is a kind of benevolence so alien to us that we recognize it only as evil. If God is not genuinely benevolent, in terms of what we standardly mean by "benevolent," then, Hume suggested, God is not to be embraced as a moral authority.

The argument from evil, as it is called, does not constitute a proof for the nonexistence of a benevolent God. But it does show that if one aims to use reason and evidence to draw an inference about the nature of the Deity, there is a prima facie problem in inferring the existence of a God who is omnipotent, omniscient, and omnibenevolent.

This is a very fast summary of the main positions in the discussion of the existence of a Supernatural Being. One line of evidence not yet considered, however, concerns the possibility that God reveals himself only through a highly select group of humans, who then convey their revelation to others as a basis for religious belief. We turn now to arguments based on revelation.

2.2   Path 2: Revelation

Some individuals claim to have personal contact with a Supreme Being. In the present context, the question is whether the reports are credible, and hence whether one can infer the existence of God on the basis of the individual reports of revelation. Moreover, this question arises whether one has the experience oneself or one knows of the experience only by report. It is well known that many such reports are not credible for any of a variety of reasons. For example, the subjects may be suffering psychiatric disorders, which are identified on completely independent grounds. If so, there are more straightforward explanations of the alleged revelation consilient with the science of the brain. Other subjects may be on drugs, such as LSD, peyote, or other hallucinogens. There are reports of subjects exposed to the elements, such as lost sailors, who, suffering physical exhaustion and the extremes of cold, thirst, and hunger, experience a recurring sense of a nearby rescue boat, looming out of the fog, but invisible. Mountaineers, suffering anoxia (lack of oxygen) also report experiencing the feeling of someone marching along behind, always out of sight, but definitely close by, and occasionally propelling the mountaineer forward. Some subjects have ultimately confessed to fraud or have been shown to have lied for profit. Some subjects have had sexual orgasm in a religious context and mistakenly, if reasonably, have interpreted it as direct contact with God.[9]

Under what conditions should we accept the report of direct knowledge of God as a basis for belief? Since the third path, namely faith, is not yet the topic of discussion, I shall assume that the question concerns when it would be reasonable to think that such a report is highly probably true. Consequently, the standards will be comparable to the standards for reasonable belief generally. That is, what is the evidence for *and* against? Are there other more plausible explanations for the experience or the report of the experience? What other tests could be deployed to see whether the hypothesis survives falsification? And so on. If someone reports an observation of something remarkable, it is always wise to approach the claim in an open-minded but careful fashion.

By the very nature of the case, these claims are hard to test. That is, the experiences are limited to a small number of individuals, the events at issue do not occur with any regularity, and conditions tend not to be replicable. Caution and skepticism are therefore particularly appropriate. It has been claimed, for example, that Mark Anthony was touched by God, though he evidently suffered from epilepsy. Epilepsy has also been suggested as the actual basis for the conversion of St. Paul.

These difficulties notwithstanding, some neurologists have recently suggested that there is a particular class of claims that deserve to be taken seriously as reports of genuine revelations. Because these cases involve subjects with a *neurological* disorder, namely temporal-lobe epilepsy, I am particularly eager to understand and evaluate the arguments for their credibility. First, what are the phenomena?

Epilepsy is a complicated condition in which a large population of excitatory neurons in the cortex fire in abnormal synchrony (figure 9.1). *Focal epilepsy* begins in a restricted area, such as the hippocampus or frontal cortex, and may spread to adjacent areas. During the seizure, the subject may lose consciousness or experience odd feelings. The effect of the seizure depends on the location of the focus. If, for example, the focus is the primary motor cortex, then the subject may display involuntary muscle contractions; if it is the primary somatosensory cortex, there may be tingling or other odd sensory experiences. In a form known as *complex partial seizures*, the regions involved are limbic structures of the temporal lobe, along with the orbitofrontal cortex (figure 9.2). Subjects in whom this form of seizure occurs may briefly display automatized behavior, such as laughter, and even some routinized behavior, such as sweeping the floor. How aware they are during the seizure remains debatable, though they tend to have no memory of events that occurred during the seizure. The

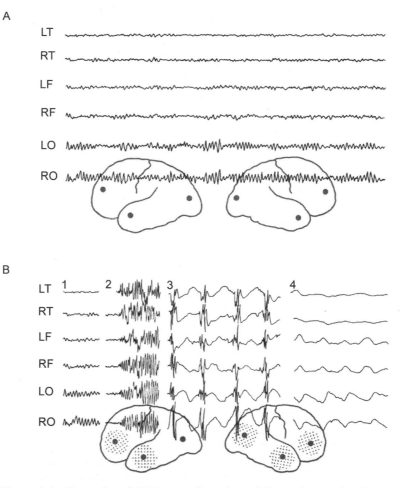

Figure 9.1 Examples of EEG recordings from different forms of epilepsy. Abbreviations: LT, left temporal; RT, right temporal; LF, left frontal; RF, right frontal; LO, left occipital; RO, right occipital. The black dots on the hemispheres indicate the approximate recording sites. (A) Normal adult EEG. (B) Brief excerpts from an EEG taken during a grand mal seizure: (1) Normal recording preceding the attack. (2) A sense of impending seizure, followed by onset of the attack. (3) Clonic phase of the attack during which there may be sudden movements or cries. (4) Period of coma. Shaded areas represent regions picked up by electrodes placed on the scalp. (From Kolb and Whishaw 1990.)

Table 9.1 Manifestations of Complex Partial Seizures

- Affective (fear and anxiety most common)
- Automatisms (perseverative, do novo, gelastic, dacrystic, procursive, and other seemingly purposeful actions)
- Autoscopy
- Cognitive dissonance (e.g., déjà vu, depersonalization, dreamy states)
- Feeling of a presence
- Epigastric and abdominal sensations, indescribable but recognized as outside normal experience
- Hallucinations (any modality)
- Sensory illusions and distortions of ongoing perceptions (e.g., metamorphopsia, separation of color from its boundary, spatial extension of the form constants, paracusia, *umkehrtsehen*, etc.)
- Synesthesia
- Time dilatation and contraction
- Psychosis
- Forced thinking
- Memory intrusions
- Hypersexuality and hyposexuality
- Autonomic dysregulation
- Contraversive movements
- Speech arrest and ictal aphasia

Source: Cytowic 1996.

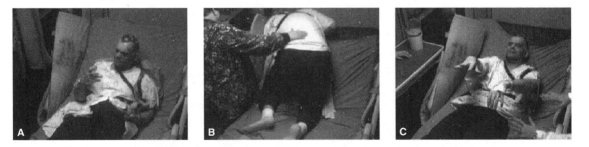

Figure 9.2 A patient with complex partial seizures underwent video-EEG telemetry monitoring, during which several of his usual seizures were recorded. The patient is shown above during different phases of a typical seizure, including his description of the prodromal aura (a foul "sulfurlike" smell and taste) (A), evolving later to confused behavior, left-leg clonic twitching, and an attempt to climb from the bed (B), and postictal (Todd's) paralysis of the left arm immediately following the event (C). (Courtesy of Drs. Erik St. Louis and Mark Granner, Department of Neurology, Roy J. and Lucille A. Carver College of Medicine, University of Iowa).

epileptic focus may be associated with scar tissue, though often the etiology of the focus is unknown.

In *generalized epilepsy*, there is *simultaneous* widespread synchronous activity, and subjects typically lose consciousness. *Grand mal* seizures involve loss of consciousness, and subjects tend to fall down, and their limbs may jerk about. *Petit mal* seizures tend to be briefer, less severe, and do not involve loss of consciousness. Patients seem briefly vacant or "not at home" during petit mal seizures. The root cause of generalized epilepsy is not well understood.

Focal epilepsy can be experimentally produced in animals by applying directly to the cortex drugs that block the activity of inhibitory neurons. For example, high doses of penicillin applied to the surface of the cortex blocks inhibitory neurons and produces seizures. Focal seizures can also be produced by repeated electrical stimulation of the cortex. Generalized seizures are more difficult to produce experimentally. Intravenous doses of penicillin administered over time can result in an animal prone to generalized seizures. In certain baboons, a generalized seizure can be induced by flickering lights. Some breeds of dogs, namely beagles and St. Bernards, are particularly susceptible to epilepsy, and thus constitute an important experimental model. Epilepsy is normally treated with drugs that increase the activity of inhibitory neurons. This treatment is usually effective in controlling the seizures.

Clinicians have long known that a small percentage of subjects with an epileptic focus in the temporal lobe are prone to be hyperreligious. These same subjects may also show hypersexuality and hypergraphia (they tend to write an unusual amount). Dostoyevsky is sometimes cited as one such case, and Ramachandran and Blakeslee (1998) discuss one such subject, Paul. There are also reports from a small percentage of temporal-lobe epileptics that just prior to manifesting an epileptic seizure, they experience unusual feelings. They may say, for example, that they felt a gathering awe and dread or that they felt a huge deluge of emotions. A handful say that their rather indescribable experiences made them feel that they were connected with an overwhelmingly powerful being, that they felt a great presence nearby. Some say that during the seizure, they came in intimate contact with an invisible God. Ramachandran's subject did claim exactly this.

Let us consider now the *possibility* that in this highly restricted class of epileptic patients, God does in fact make himself known to the patient during the seizure, as Paul clearly believed. We need to consider the evidence *for* and *against*. The strongest evidence in favor of the hypothesis is, of course, the sincere reports of honest subjects. How strongly, if at all, does that evidence support the conclusion that subjects who report contacting God during an epileptic seizure *truly do* contact God during the seizure?

One major reservation derives from investigations by neuroscientist Michael Persinger. His strategy was to simulate, albeit weakly, some conditions of a temporal-lobe seizure in normal volunteers by exciting temporal-lobe neurons using an oscillating magnetic field focused on the temporal lobe. His aim was to see whether the experiences described by the special class of temporal-lobe epileptics could be produced in normal subjects.[10]

The results were interesting. Under such activation, subjects did report highly unusual feelings. About 80 percent of Persinger's subjects report feeling as though there was a presence nearby, sometimes just out of view. Others, if they are atheists, may say they feel a "oneness with the universe." At least one person had a visual hallucination involving an angelic appearance—a great deal of light, rushing sounds, sublime feelings. A New York psychiatrist described his feelings in nonreligious terms as a "resolution of binaries."[11]

Persinger's data lend support to the conclusion that these experiences are one and all the result of a particular kind and distribution of neural activity, just as pain, hunger, and fear are neural effects. That seizures in the temporal lobe should produce extraordinary feelings is predictable from the known connectivity of temporal-lobe structures. That is, there are connections to structures known to play a role in experiencing emotions: the amygdala, hypothalamus, brainstem, and orbitofrontal cortex. The amygdala, as discussed in chapter 3, is known to involve feelings of fear. The hypothalamus has subregions involved in sex, hunger, thirst, and other desires and these will be subject to increased activation in a unusual fashion if there is generalized stimulation to the temporal lobe. If the activation spreads, as it does during a seizure, then because of their connectivity, the cingulate and orbitofrontal cortices are likely to suffer abnormal levels of synchronized activity. Random activation of these cortical areas will also have a powerful role in the generation of an odd blend of emotions and feelings. Heightened activity of the hypothalamus, amygdala, brainstem, cingulate cortex, and orbitofrontal cortex may trigger *many strong* feelings all at once, in a composition highly unusual in day-to-day life. For example, there may be feelings of dread, joy, elation, anxiety, hunger, and sexuality all at the same time. This pathological activation of emotion circuitry may be interpreted by the subject in many ways, depending on how his past experiences situate him.

What are we to make of this? Persinger's data raise the possibility that because we can induce the effect in normal subjects by altering neural activity in the temporal lobe, then probably the effect in both normals and epileptics has nothing to do with contact by a Supreme Being. Part of our obligation in evaluating revelation hypotheses is to determine whether other more probable explanations for experiences of God are available. For this reason, Persinger's experiments are very important. They do support a natural (as opposed to *supernatural*), neurally based cause. They do not *prove* it beyond all doubt, of course, but they are supporting evidence. In any case, proof beyond *all* doubt is rare for scientific hypotheses generally.

How might the theist refute these skeptical worries? One strategy is to say that the Persinger data do not *prove* that the experiences of a special class of temporal-lobe epileptics and those of the experimental volunteers have essentially the same cause. Perhaps, it might be suggested, God really does contact the epileptics, but not the volunteers.[12] While this possibility may be worth entertaining, our question is, Which hypothesis is more probable? Given Persinger's results, the burden of proof is now on the theist to show why a natural explanation for both the epileptic and the normal volunteers is not sufficient. Consider a parallel example. Suppose that you believe *your* wounds heal by divine intervention, even if those of everyone else heal by natural processes. Then the burden of proof is on you to show why your case is different, and why one type of explanation cannot serve all relevantly similar examples.

Another strategy for dealing with Persinger's results is to view *all* the experiences—those of epileptics, anoxics, *and* normal volunteers—as confirming contact with God. Although this is a *possible* avenue, it has only a quirky appeal. Both skeptics and believers find it farfetched to suppose that God would choose to manifest himself through one particular pathological condition, namely temporal lobe seizures. And why would he manifest himself via a *simulated* temporal-lobe seizure? Is it reasonable to expect that God's presence can be invoked electromagnetically? Logically, the Persinger results are not, of course, a proof of the *non*existence of God, nor even of the illusory status of the experiences at issue. They are important because they drain *probability* from the hypothesis that the experiences provoking God-reports are truly experiences *of God*. Our question is whether, given the data, that hypothesis is probably true. Given the analysis and the interpretation so far, the hypothesis is not compelling.

Consider now a completely different argument. Suppose we say that the temporal lobe, precisely because its stimulation can, albeit rarely, give rise to experiences described in religious terms, must be specialized *for this purpose*. Just as stimulation of the visual cortex gives rise to visual experiences, so stimulation of the "God module" gives rise to religious experiences. Since purely natural selection cannot account for the emergence of such a cortical specialization in humans, it may be argued, the explanation for its existence must appeal to a Divine Cause. That is, God must have set in place this neurobiological arrangement so that humans could have the capacity to know God directly.

In response, it is important to emphasize again that it is only a tiny *fraction* of subjects with temporal-lobe epilepsy who report their experiences as religious in nature. Second, patients who come to the clinic reporting seizures are normally treated straightaway with seizure-controlling drugs, so the experience they report is typically an *inaugural* event, not a *recurring* event. Consequently, they cannot be observed and tested to see whether rapturous experiences occur on later occasions, or whether there is a correlation between the severity of an episode and its capacity to produce a rapturous experience, or whether the religious denomination of the subject predicts the religious interpretation of the experience. These are human subjects, not experimental animals, and we cannot delay treatment of a potentially dangerous condition to experiment on the nature of rapturous experiences.

A further problem, touched on earlier, is epistemological. In their reports, subjects try to make some sense of the experience. That is, they experience various feelings, and they usually wish to *interpret* those feelings. We know from Persinger's results that the feelings induced by temporal-lobe stimulation are *very* hard to describe. Moreover, as I noted, not everyone interprets the feelings as feelings of God. When they are given strange experiences, people tend to look for explanations that are comparably strange, even though the cause is ultimately neurobiological. We have to remind ourselves that *strange experiences*, such as hallucinations, weird dreams, or out-of-body experiences, may have quite *ordinary explanations* in terms of atypical neural activity. Strange experiences may *seem* to us to be full of meaning and portent, however humble their causal origin, but the strangeness of the experience tells us nothing about whether the *cause* of the experience is equally strange.

Quite likely, cultural factors influence whether one interprets the temporal-lobe-excitation experience as *of* God—*of* an external Supernatural Being—or in some other fashion. That is, you might already have to have religious belief of a certain kind to interpret the experience as *of* God. At least one would want to know whether a pantheist temporal-lobe epileptic interprets the experience in the same way as an epileptic who is a Baptist or Muslim or Buddhist or Satanist or atheist. Consider also that temporal-lobe structures have a role in memory retrieval, and that memory retrieval often involves representation of events or persons not currently present. For example, one can now remember a particularly fearsome first-grade teacher, with all the terror, anxiety, and sense of overwhelming foreboding experienced in early childhood. Is it possible that part of what happens is that the emotion complex generated by Persinger-style temporal-lobe stimulation activates recollections of individual persons who provoked such feelings in the past, such as the fabled first-grade ogre-teacher? This is sheer conjecture, of course, but it is conjecture with an eye toward experiment.

Finally, though the argument depends on the idea that natural selection could not possibly explain the existence of religious feelings, in fact it is very easy to imagine that feelings are part of the more general neurobiological apparatus that serves to bind humans into social groups, where they feel loyalty to a leader and to the group.[13] Consistent with individual variation in biology generally, it may not be surprising if some individuals are more inclined to religious affiliation, just as some humans seem more blessed with mathematical ability or a sense of humor than others. Some individuals may feel strong urges to humble themselves before a great leader or blindly follow his dictates. Others may be strongly independent and find the whole idea of worship and blind loyalty sheerly baffling.

These considerations detract from one's confidence that the reports in question are confirming evidence of Divine Revelation to a select few. They do not absolutely rule out the possibility that the experiences of religious temporal-lobe epileptics are divinely caused, but they do generate skepticism to which there seems to be no convincing counterargument.

2.3   Path 3: Faith

In the previous two sections, I assumed that the issue of whether God exists is best approached by evidence and argument. My assumption itself may be challenged, however, on grounds that the method suitable for religious belief is not evidence and argument, but faith. To a first approximation, this means adopting or rejecting the hypothesis on the basis of private motivation, as opposed to evidence and argument.

To abandon evidence and argument as the basis for religious belief is no small thing, however. For one thing, this means one could as easily have faith that *no* deity exists, or that the deity that does exist is essentially evil, or that there are an infinitely many competing gods, or any number of other variations.

It means that sharing in rational argument to figure out the most reasonable answer thus far is essentially at an end. Against the satanist, who simply has faith in the Devil and his great powers, for example, one then has no argument, since argument is beside the point.

Hume considered this option, and his worry was that it puts an end to the back and forth of exploratory conversation. In its place arise undesirable elements, such as pathology and exploitation. So long as one's religion is personal and private and has no implications beyond the life of the believing individual, this may not matter. But as soon as the believer uses his belief to give him *moral* or *political* authority with respects to others, then, in Hume's view, the trouble begins.

Once you have backed into the faith corner, you have no recourse against terror and repression in the name of religion, no recourse against bigotry, demagoguery, misogyny, or abuse posing as religion. You have no basis for criticism of cruel religions. This is precisely because faith is not a matter of evidence and analysis, not a matter of argument and criticism. It is belief *independent* of those things. If the faith option works for decent folks, it works every bit as well for scoundrels; if faith is acceptable for religion, then deeming it as *unacceptable in other domains* is just special pleading. Faith has been used not only by the charitable and the kind, but also by those who insist on their divine right to unquestioned rule or their divine right to destroy another tribe or enslave women. How can we reason with any of these persons if they claim faith, and faith alone, as the basis of their reasons? As is well known, those who adopt the faith option are often in open conflict on what the right faith is, what range of questions should be decided by faith, and what moral standards ought to be imposed. This is not surprising, since cultures vary and private motivation is as varied as human kind.[14]

Is religious belief, or more specifically, belief in a Deity, *universal*? Is it *innate*? The claim that religious belief is both universal and innate is often raised in a discussion about faith, and in particular, in a discussion of why two individuals have the same faith. Even if such claims are indeed true, it is unclear precisely what conclusion regarding faith is to be drawn. As discussed earlier, innateness of a belief is no guarantee of the truth of the belief. Innateness of a belief is no guarantee even of its utility in survival, since it may be, for example, an innocuous consequence of something else that is adaptive or even a mildly deleterious consequence of something else that is very useful. In any case, there is no compelling reason from child-development studies to think that such a belief is innate. Some children, for example, respond to their first introduction to the idea of a Deity with surprise and incredulity.

Moreover, many entirely normal people lack a belief in a deity. Chinese folk religions and Buddhism joinly have roughly a billion adherents but have no surpraphysical niche for a being like the Christian God. In addition, there are upwards of a billion pantheists, agnostics, atheists, and assorted nonbelievers.[15] This implies that *theism* is not universal. A trap awaiting the unwary is to push the idea that atheists, agnostics, and such are really believers who pretend otherwise. Why? Because belief in a Deity is universal. Unfortunately, the argument has now become circular, since the universality of belief is used to defend the universality of belief.

Even if belief in a Deity is not universal, the personification of nature *is* very common. Personification is a typical response when we do not understand the cause of important events, for example, why the Sun was eclipsed, why a comet appeared, why tornadoes are spawned seemingly from nothing, why bubonic plague kills a quarter of the people in a town, why apple trees are fruitful one year but not another. Bewildered and with no better theory at hand, we fall back on the richest and most powerful explanatory resource we have, namely our framework of mental categories normally used to explain human and animal behavior. That is, we use our *theory of minds*. We ask the storm to subside, entreat the plants to flourish, invoke the good auspices of the Moon to help with fertility, and consider ourselves to be punished by wrathful forces. We make sacrifices in hopes of appeasing anger or currying favor.[16]

My point is not that this is foolish; it is not. It is a worthy attempt to make sense of the universe, using the best explanatory resources at one's disposal. But the progress of science consists in the slow replacement of psychological explanations for natural phenomena by more successful *natural* explanations. Science gives rise to technology and the means for predicting a tsunami or hurricane, for preventing spread of infections, for helping bees to pollinate apple trees in a cold spring, and so on. By and large, these manipulations are more effective than animal sacrifices or prayer. It is useful to remember that most of the dominant religions came into existence in quite ancient, prescientific times, when animal sacrifices to the gods seemed the best way to try to influence fertility, the weather, health, and the course of battle.[17]

I say all this while recognizing that for many people, faith in a deity is a highly positive part of their lives. Their faith may be what sustains them, day after day, in dealing with their own sorrows, anguish, and tragedies. It may be instrumental in defeating alcoholism, coping with depression, and providing courage to do terribly difficult things. I do not doubt that faith, of one kind or another, can be a central element in people's lives. In addition to *religious* faith, the conviction of an athlete that he will win, or of a dancer that he will not stumble, or of a soldier that he will survive, is singularly effective in aiding performance, even if it is no guarantee of success. Engaging the enemy half-heartedly is a recipe for defeat. Nevertheless, in *this* context, in *this* discussion, what is at issue is not so much the psychological role of faith and conviction, but whether what is believed by faith is probably *true* and, more specifically, whether faith that a *deity* exists constitutes *evidence* that a deity exists.

One last, but not minor point. Some have claimed, for example, Paul Davies, that science too has its articles of faith. Davies says that scientists "accept as an act of faith that the universe is not absurd, that there is a rational basis to physical existence manifested as a lawlike order in nature."[18] He thinks that this is essentially the same as faith that a Deity exists.

Davies's suggestion to reduce the intellectual distance between religious faith and science is contrived. *All* scientific hypothesis are evaluated on the basis of evidence and argument, none are considered too sacred to be criticized or investigated or refuted. No instrument is deemed reliable by faith alone, no hypothesis is adopted once and for all on faith alone. If there is order in the universe that we can understand, we do not believe this on faith but because certain laws seem to hold, no matter how stringent the test or how often repeated. On any given occasion, we typically make many assumptions, certainly, but our assumptions are always *defeasible*, that is, we acknowledge that they could be false and may need to be tested on another occasion. Indeed, the history of science is full of examples where it was the seemingly safe assumption that was ultimately overturned. Earth is the center of the universe and does not move—these two assumptions seemed irrefutable, safe, necessarily true, known with absolute certainty, part of the holy plan. And yet Galileo and Copernicus convinced us that they are indeed false. The whole point about faith is that you do *not* criticize or test or marshal evidence and argument. The whole point about science and progress in science is that you *do*.

In the end, one makes up one's own mind about these things. My considered opinion is that no argument for the existence of God is even a little convincing, and to that degree, I find the hypothesis that God exists to be improbable at this time. I do believe this not on faith, but on the basis of evidence and argument. Like Hume, I see the price of the faith option as exorbitant in its moral and political consequences, and hence to be avoided as a moral duty. But we learn new things all the time, and new discoveries can take us by surprise. For all that we can be certain of now, the hypothesis or some variant might someday be rendered probable.

3   Is There Life after Death?

As discussed in earlier chapters, the preponderance of evidence supports the hypothesis that mental states are brain states and mental processes are brain processes. On this hypothesis, what thing exists to survive the death of the brain? What kind of substance would it be, and how could it have the emotions, knowledge, preferences, and memories that the brain had when it was alive? How can it be related to those activities in the brain that make me *me*? Reasonable answers need to be forthcoming if the hypothesis that there is life after death is to win credibility.

So far as I can determine, there are no answers that cohere enough to make some sense of the life-after-death hypothesis. The preponderance of the evidence indicates that when the brain degenerates, mental functions are compromised, and when the brain dies, mental functions cease. The suggestion that the whole body is resurrected after death does address the problem, but so far the evidence for resurrection is not persuasive. Old graves contain old bones, and decaying flesh is devoured by scavengers.

Is there any positive evidence that *something*, we know not what, does in fact live on after the death of the brain? There are, certainly, many reports that purport to provide confirming evidence. Because I cannot consider them all here, I shall restrict myself to the following pertinent observations. So many of the claims that rest on the intervention of a psychic medium have been shown to be fraudulent that a general suspicion of these claims is as prudent as the general suspicion one has toward get-rich-quick investments. Many claims to a previous life are either openly concocted, confabulated, or a matter of unwitting selectivity of evidence. By "selectivity of evidence," I mean that one pays attention to events that, with suitable interpretation, could be construed as confirming one antecedently favored hypothesis, while ignoring or explaining away in ad hoc fashion events that could be disconfirming.

For a made-up illustration of selectivity of evidence concerning an afterlife and a previous life, consider this story. A child draws a picture of a scene with a farmhouse, apple trees in the yard, a dog sleeping under the tree, and so forth. It reminds his mother of Great Grandfather Smith's house. Indeed, little Billy has some of Great Grandfather Smith's physical traits, including his curly red hair and his hot temper. The mother asks the child about his picture, and the source of his ideas. "Do you remember ever seeing a place like this?" she queries. If she *prompts* him, the child will begin to agree, as psychologists have repeatedly shown, that he remembers this place, remembers the dog, and so forth.[19] Later he may quite innocently embellish all these "memories" with details from parental conversation, family albums, and so forth. Billy may even discover, perhaps without conscious knowledge, that he is encouraged to *confabulate* his earlier life, where his confabulations get conceptualized as the *recovery of hidden memories*.

Great Grandfather Smith, in Billy's "recovered memories," killed a grizzly with a mere bowie knife, built a snow house in a blizzard, and talked to quail and coyote. Nobody else remembers these events, but that is not troubling, since Grandfather was somewhat reserved. His mother, we may imagine, does not work hard to test the hypothesis that Billy is the reincarnation of Great Grandfather Smith. When she does ask a question about Great Grandfather Smith's life that Billy *cannot* answer, this is soothingly explained away by saying that Billy has forgotten that particular of his previous life. She ignores countervailing evidence, she tends to notice or remember only confirming evidence. This is not because she is openly mendacious. Quite the contrary. She is inadvertently fooling *herself*. She *wants* to believe. This fable illustrates selectivity in considering evidence, and it is something to which we all are prone. Consequently, we have to work hard to be as tough-minded with respect to hypotheses we *hope* are true as we are with respect to those we *fear* are true.

Whether all accounts of reincarnation share the weaknesses illustrated in the fable is not known, but because so many that have been studied do, and because one does not want to be gullible, we need to exercise careful scrutiny, case by individual case. Why do we not all enthusiastically believe Shirley McLaine's claims of her earlier, colorful lives? Partly, I think, because her accounts seem to suffer from the selectivity-of-evidence problem just outlined, partly because her claims are conveniently untestable, but also because they have the indelible stamp of fantasy. Her "earlier lives" are enviably glamorous; they are not the lives of a poor peasant grubbing about with running sores and bent back. Typically, reports of previous lives are replete with storybook appeal: handsome heroes, beautiful queens, and romantic deeds. Surely, there were many more hungry, stooped peasants than there were pining, gothic princesses, yet these tend not to be the "previous lives" channeling reveals. Or is it perhaps that only glamorous persons are reincarnated and the humble ones stay dead?

Recently, evocative descriptions provided by patients who very nearly died have become a source of interest to our question. Visual experiences involving tunnels with shimmering lights at the far end, feelings of great peacefulness, feelings that one is being led on a journey, and sometimes the experience of seeming to see one's body below on a gurney are typical of experiences called "near-death experiences." These experiences are alleged to be evidence that the patients have experienced the otherworld of the afterlife. As always, we must weigh the evidence for and against, and reflect on whether there might be more down-to-earth explanations.

Several obstacles suggest that caution is in order. First, these experiences seem to be somewhat unusual (about 35 percent) among those patients who are very close to death but who revive. *Selectivity of evidence* makes them seem to confirm an afterlife, despite the existence of other cases where the resuscitated patient reports no such experiences.

Second, the conditions are not those of a controlled experiment, and one wants to know whether any of these patients are *encouraged* to "remember" events that, in their current stressful circumstances, they attribute to experiences "while dead."

Third, the reports are reports from patients whose brains are under great stress; they are anoxic (oxygen deprived) and awash in norepinephrine, precisely *because* they are close to death. Brains under stress may produce many abnormal activities, including involuntary movements, strange speech, unusual eye movements, and unusual experiences. Severe anoxia, for example in drowning, is known to result in feelings of peacefulness, once the panic phase has passed. Some people have used self-strangulation as a means of inducing anoxic ecstasy. Anoxia resulting from breathing nitrous oxide (so-called laughing gas) can produce ecstatic feelings and feelings of having glimpsed profound truths. William James says he experienced "metaphysical illuminations" while intoxicated on nitrous oxide, though what he wrote on these occasions was, by his admission, sheer gibberish. Nitrous oxide stimulates neurons that release endorphins (the brain's endogenous opiates), which is why it can be used as an anesthetic. Endogenous endorphin release, along with some suggestibility perhaps, is the probable cause of ecstatic effects.[20] In this respect, therefore, the problem is similar to the problem with the reports from the cases of temporal-lobe epileptics who experience "religious feelings" during a seizure.

Fourth, as noted in chapter 3, out-of-body experiences, as well as other disorienting and depersonalizing experiences, can be produced artificially, for example with the anesthetic ketamine or with LSD. It is not unlikely that the neuronal explanations for the ketamine experiences and the near-death experiences are very similar. Moreover, as Francis Crick has pointed out in conversation, the out-of-body claims could be tested a little more directly by asking whether the patient saw an object that could be seen only if he was where he said he was, such as floating out the hospital window.[21] So far as I can tell, this sort of test has not been systematically undertaken.

Although the skepticism and caution with respect to claims about past and future lives are justified, we should keep an open mind about the possibility that a genuinely testable case will emerge. If a prima facie case does emerge, it will indeed be of the greatest importance to examine it carefully and systematically, to avoid inadvertent contamination of memory, to do everything possible to rule out fraud, to check the claims against what is known about the facts, to consider other possible explanations, and so forth. The record of examined cases makes one less than optimistic that such a case will survive scrutiny, but one must not rule out the possibility that it will.

But is the prospect of extinction not unsettling? Is it not disappointing and frightening? It may be all these things, but it need not be. One can live a richly purposeful life of love and work—of family, community, wilderness, music, and so forth—cognizant that it makes sense to make the best of *this* life. Arguably, it is less painful to accept that miseries are just a part of life than that they are punishment or trials or that one's prayers are being ignored. Arguably, it is comforting to assume that matters of justice and desert need to be addressed in the here and now, not deferred to an afterlife. Finding peaceful solutions, redressing wrongs, seeking reconciliation and compromise, expressing love, maximizing the significance of each day that one is alive—these things may make more sense than pinning too much hope on an iffy hereafter. When all is said and done, the truth is still the truth, however grim it turns out to be. If there is no life after death—if that *is* the truth—then wishing it were otherwise will not make it otherwise.

4   If God Does Not Exist, What Happens to Morality?

This question is really about the foundations of moral standards. It is a question about why certain behavior is considered wrong or unfair or punishable, and contrariwise, why some behavior is esteemed, praised, or encouraged. It is about what it means to say that an action is wrong. It is a profoundly important question, and one that has been the topic of intense discussion in many cultures since ancient times. In the Western philosophical tradition, we are deeply indebted to the Greek philosophers in the fourth and fifth centuries B.C., for it was they who launched systematic discussion of the problems.

The most insightful and concise examination of the idea of religion as the source of ethical standards is found in Plato's early dialogue *Euthyphro*. Socrates and Euthyphro, a high-born priest-about-Athens, meet on the steps of the law courts. Socrates is awaiting trial for encouraging the young to inquire into everything—orthodoxy, common assumptions, and revered authority. Officially, he is charged with "corrupting the youth of Athens." Euthyphro is at the law courts because he means to prosecute his father for murder. Of the attending circumstances, we learn that his father had punished a servant who, while drunk, had killed a slave. He tied up the servant and left him into a ditch while he went in search of advice concerning what should be done with the miscreant. The servant died before the father returned. In contrast to the ever-perplexed Socrates, Euthyphro is smoothly confident of his moral opinions and certain of his superiority to the common run in moral matters. Euthyphro's legal project intensifies the drama of this dialogue, especially when he reveals himself to be breathtakingly insensitive to the moral ambiguity permeating his action against his own father.

The stage set, Socrates begins his methodical inquiry by asking Euthyphro, "So, in virtue of what is an action right?" Euthyphro has no hesitation: "What is right is what I am doing now; namely, prosecuting the wrongdoer." When Socrates urges him to provide a more general answer, Euthyphro eagerly responds, "What is right is what is dear to the gods." Or, in more contemporary language, what is right is what the gods say is right. Moreover, he candidly confides that he is unusually fortunate in having special knowledge of what is in fact dear to the gods. The theory that religion is the source of morality is now on the table.

In the ensuing conversation, Socrates extracts from the sanctimonious Euthyphro the damaging admission that the gods do not appear to give a single *unequivocal* answer concerning the propriety of Euthyphro's legal action against his father. Described as bringing a murderer to justice, the action may be favored by the gods, at least to judge by some available myths. Described as high-handed action against one's aging and well-meaning father, it is forbidden by the gods, at least to judge by other available myths. Neither myths nor gods converge on a single answer concerning what is right in this case.

In his questioning, Socrates rebuffs the smugly self-righteous, wherever they may be. At the same time, he undermines the pretension to special knowledge of what the gods want, leading us to realize that clerical claims to special knowledge can be crassly self-serving. Additionally, Socrates uses these arguments to show what we all implicitly know and live by, namely that there are recognizably justified, if unlistable, exceptions to any set of rules, whether they are thought to come from the gods or not. We draw upon some deeper understanding of what is right than the rule itself in order to arrive at a reasonable judgment about when we are morally required to deviate from the rule. The rule is only a superficial image of that deeper understanding.

Having shown Euthyphro to be muddled in his conviction that what is right is what the gods say is right, Socrates then lays out the catastrophic problem with Euthyphro's popular answer. He points out that the claim is actually ambiguous, and then asks which one of the two possible interpretations *is* the intended meaning: (1) do the gods *say* something is right because *it is right*, or (2) is something right *because* the gods say so?

On the *second* alternative, morality is sheerly a matter of the decision or decree of the gods. This means that the gods' decree that something is right *makes* it right. For example, if the gods say, "It is right to sacrifice other humans," then it *is* right, regardless of any other feelings or thoughts humans might have on the subject. If, on the other hand, they say it is wrong, then it *is* wrong. On this interpretation, morality depends solely on the choices, whimsical or otherwise, of the gods (or God). This gives morality a decidedly arbitrary character, as though it is only incidentally connected to humans' needs. Moral standards must have more to them than that.

Consider instead the *first*, and more appealing, interpretation, namely, that the gods say something is right because it *is* right. The trouble with this, according to Socrates, is that it implies that the gods are merely spokesmen concerning what is and is not morally appropriate. That is, the rightness of an act derives from something other than the gods. Consequently, on this alternative, what *makes* something right must be *independent* of the gods, in the sense that it would be right whether or not the gods were available to broadcast the news. If so, points out Socrates, then the question concerning the foundation of morality has not even begun to be answered. To put his worry another way, we want to know *why* the gods say of an action that it is right. Whatever the explanation might be, *that* is what we want to understand when inquire into the nature of moral standards. If we cannot make progress on that, then we ourselves do not understand what properties make some actions right and some wrong. So the disappointment with this alternative is that the gods are not the source of moral standards. Socrates also expects us to see the general lesson implicit in his disambiguating the seemingly clear phrase "What is right is what the gods say is right." For it is only by *questioning and reasoned analysis* that he unmasks the flaws infecting each of the two possible interpretations.

This short dialogue is deeply disturbing. Here is Socrates, awaiting trial for less than heinous behavior, namely, his habit of questioning practices and principles that the authorities do not wish to have questioned. We know that he will be found guilty and will be put to death by poison. He is calmly but keenly aware of moral hypocrisy, self-satisfied indecency, and intolerance masquerading as morality. But withal, he is aware of the abiding necessity of morality for civilized community life. He provokes us to see that even though moral decision making is part of everyday life, the everydayness of morality, along with our feelings of moral certainty, should not lull us into thinking we understand the foundations of morality and the origin of moral understanding. More specifically, we should be wary lest we deceive ourselves with self-serving rationalizations about special knowledge derived from special relationships with the gods.

Socrates' argument in *Euthyphro* does not prove that a Supreme Being is *not* the source and basis of morality. It importance is owed to its articulation of the many problems that beset the view that morality is grounded in a Supreme Being. That is, it reminds us that there are (1) evidential problems with the hypothesis that a deity exists, (2) problems with inferring God's benevolence, given natural disasters, suffering, and misery, and (3) problems in knowing precisely what it is that God commands, given the difficulty of access and conflicting accounts. The real power of the argument in *Euthyphro* is that it points us in new directions to understand the nature of morality. It suggests that we entertain a more naturalistic explanation of morality than supernatural command. It also makes us curious to understand what that explanation might be and how it might connect with our evolutionary history.

Socrates' challenge was taken up by Plato and his students, and by many thinkers ever since. In particular, genuine progress was made by Aristotle, who, perhaps better than anyone then or since, grasped the point that the codification of moral rules can at best define the central prototypes, but that the lived moral life requires coming to understand why those rules apply when they do, and when exceptions are justified.[22] Among other things, he grasped that imprecision and inexactness in moral precepts are unavoidable and require us continually to reflect and deepen our moral perspective. Aristotle clearly realized, moreover, that inflexible laws that leave no discretionary room for wise judgment, such as zero-tolerance laws, often do serious harm.[23] He also seems to have understood that impulses of sympathy and caring, and for making a moral community, are just part of our *human nature*, however our natures came to be as they are. Our advantage over Aristotle is that we have some understanding from evolutionary biology of how making a moral community is part of human nature.

The tradition of moral thinkers who have wrestled with Socrates' question is rich indeed. Aristotle, perhaps the greatest of all moral thinkers, I have already mentioned. The tradition also includes Hume, who outlined the fundamental role of emotions; Kant, who tried to understand the authority of reason; John Stuart Mill, who formulated utilitarianism; the pragmatists, John Dewey, and Oliver Wendell Holmes, who were sensitive to evolutionary biology, the provincial nature of a person's moral perspective, and the pragmatic need for democratic institutions; and William Hamilton and Edward Wilson, who gave us insight into the biological basis for altruistic behavior in nonhumans.[24] In the past several decades, some philosophers have tried—by drawing on molecular biology, evolutionary biology, anthropology, and legal history—to achieve a more satisfactory synthesis of the foundations and nature of morality.[25]

An undertaking of great importance, this new synthesis blends the sciences of who we are with pragmatic common sense and the wisdom of lives lived. Will it produce a set of absolute rules, applicable for all times in all places? No. Will it provide an *algorithm* for solving specific moral questions, such as whether stem-cell research is morally acceptable? No. Will it constitute an unquestioned authority of what is right? Not this either.

What it can begin to do is to provide a naturalistic perspective on the foundation of moral judgment, and in so doing, it can help us disentangle ourselves from many myths about morality. In disentangling ourselves from the myths, we may become even more keenly aware of our obligation to think a problem through rather than just react or blindly follow a rule. Ethics, in Aristotle's view, is the most difficult of subjects, not least because the exigencies of life demand that decisions be rendered *now* and actions taken *now*, but also because there is such a thing as moral wisdom, an understanding acquired through long experience and relentless reflection, much of which is scarcely articulable.

In sum, the way things seem to stand is this: (1) There are overwhelming problems with the idea that morality can be grounded in a God. (2) The best modern candidates for understanding the grounding of morality are naturalistic. So (3) morality and moral understanding are unlikely to require the existence of God.

5   Concluding Remarks

There are various kinds of feelings that, for want of a better term, we may describe as *sublime*. Kant used the word "sublime" to characterize those experiences one has when, for example, viewing a wild storm or soaring mountain peaks, though the wilderness is but one source of such feelings.[26] We feel ourselves awed by the immensity or complexity or power of things in various conditions. In its general use, "sublime" means "of outstanding spiritual, intellectual, or moral worth; tending to inspire awe, usually because of elevated quality."[27] In keeping with current usage, sublime feelings might also be described as broadly spiritual, without implying anything about the existence of spirits. They can be associated with different things, including music, art, religion, science, parenting, and intellectual discovery. By temperament, some people may be inclined to enjoy these feelings in the wilderness rather than in church, or in the opera house rather than in the delivery room—or they may enjoy them in *all* these conditions. Whether there is a supernatural *reality* that corresponds to a supernatural *interpretation* of these feelings is, however, a different matter, and in general, the existence of supernatural beings seems rather doubtful.

The point is *not* that these various sublime feelings are unreal. The point is *not* that because the feelings are brain effects, they are unworthy or inconsequential. *Real*, the feelings certainly are. *Worthy*, in and of themselves, they also are—the more so if they inspire kindness and virtue, the less so if they inspire cruelty and terror. Do we *trivialize* a sublime feeling if we appreciate its dependence on the brain? Not in the least. Its significance does not depend on its being a soul state rather than a brain state. Indeed, self-deception is no virtue, and upon reflection, we may find it *un*worthy to give our experiences, wonderful though they may be, an inflated cosmic significance. Isaac Asimov once remarked that astrology narcissistically assumes that the starry universe about us is in fact *about* us.[28] In Azimov's formulation, the astrologer's assumption does seem embarrasingly self-important. Humility bids us to take ourselves as we are; we do not have to be cosmically significant to be genuinely significant. In truth, there is an entirely habitable Aristotelian middle ground between the trivial and the grandiose. There is where humanity lives, and it includes much that is sublime.

Suggested Readings

Albright, C. R., and J. B. Ashbrook. 2001. *Where God Lives in the Human Brain*. Naperville, Ill.: Sourcebook.

Austin, James H. 1998. *Zen and the Brain*. Cambridge: MIT Press.

Black, I. 2000. *The Dying of Enoch Wallace: Life, Death, and the Changing Brain*. New York: McGraw-Hill.

Boyer, Pascal. 2001. *Religion Explained*. New York: Basic Books.

Brugger, P. 2001. The haunted brain. In J. Houran and R. Lange, eds., *Spirited Exchanges: Multidisciplinary Perspectives on Hauntings and Poltergeists*. Jefferson, N.C.: McFarland.

Canup, R. M., and K. Righter, eds. 2000. *Origin of the Earth and the Moon*. Tucson: University of Arizona Press.

Grady, Monica. 2001. *Search for Life*. Washington, D.C.: Natural History Museum/ Smithsonian Institution Press.

Hume, David. 1779. *The Dialogues Concerning Natural Religion*. Edited by N. Kemp Smith. Oxford: Oxford University Press, 1962.

Jacob, François. 1999. *Of Flies, Mice, and Men*. Cambridge: Harvard University Press.

Johnson, M. 1993. *Moral Imagination: Implications of Cognitive Science for Ethics*. Chicago: University of Chicago Press.

Joyce, G. F., and L. E. Orgel. 1993. Prospects for understanding the origin of the RNA world. In R. F. Gersteland, T. Cech, and J. F. Atkins, eds., *The RNA World*. New York: Cold Spring Harbor Laboratory Press.

Loftus, E. 1997. Creating false memories. *Scientific American* 277: 71–75.

McCauley, R. M. 2000. The naturalness of religion and the unnaturalness of science. In F. Keil and R. Wilson, eds., *Explanation and Cognition*. Cambridge: MIT Press.

Menand, Louis. 2001. *The Metaphysical Club*. New York: Farrar, Straus & Giroux.

Orgel, L. E. 1999. The origin of life on Earth. In *Revolutions in Science*, 18–25. New York: Scientific American.

Paine, Thomas. 1794. *The Age of Reason: Being an Investigation of True and Fabulous Theology*. New York: Putnam's Sons, 1896.

Plato. 1997. *Euthyphro*. Trans by G. M. A. Grube. In J. M. Cooper and D. S. Hutchinson, eds., *Plato: Complete Works*, 1–16. Indianapolis: Hackett Publishing Co.

Wilson, E. O. 1998. *Consilience: The Unity of Knowledge*. New York: Knopf.

Websites

BioMedNet Magazine: http://news.bmn.com/magazine

Encyclopedia of Life Sciences: http://www.els.net

The MIT Encyclopedia of the Cognitive Sciences: http://cognet.mit.edu/MITECS

Notes

1   Introduction

1. In his doctoral dissertation, Ilya Farber (2000) focused on the issues involved in what he calls "domain integration," and I shall use his term.

2. Chomsky 1966.

3. Fodor 1974.

4. See, for example, Chalmers 1996.

5. Leibniz, 1989 translation.

6. Güzeldere notes that Searle comes perilously close to epiphenomenalism when he states, "Ontologically speaking, behavior, functional role, and causal relations are irrelevant to the existence of conscious mental phenomena" (Searle 1992).

7. This was first suggested to me in 1982 by Amélie Rorty. Her hypothesis is discussed in A. O. Rorty 1986.

8. Schleiden 1838 and Schwann 1839.

9. See Finger 1994.

10. Kuffler 1953, Mountcastle 1957, Hubel and Wiesel 1959.

11. See Beer 2000, in press; Jeannerod 1997.

12. Functional magnetic-resonance imaging (fMRI) depends on the fact that oxygenated hemoglobin has different magnetic properties from deoxygenated hemoglobin. This give a blood-oxygen-dependent contrast (known as BOLD). On the assumption that blood-oxygen levels vary as a function of neuronal activity (more activity requires more oxygen and more glucose), the BOLD measure indicates varying levels of neuronal activity in different regions in a given time period, such as a second. Recent analyses of fMRI data suggest that the hemodynamics, normally

assumed to be everywhere on much the same time course, may in fact have different time courses. This technique is called "functional" because it maps *activity*, whereas MRI can only map *structure*. Improvements in data analysis, especially independent component analysis (ICA), will help yield more accurate interpretations of the data. (See *The MIT Encyclopedia of Cognitive Sciences*, s.v. "Magnetic Resonance Imaging," for a fuller discussion.)

13. Positron emission tomography maps activity using a positron emitter such as radioactively tagged water (H_2O^{15}). The positron is detected and this data is used to determine the distribution of the emitter in the brain over a specific time period, about 40 seconds. Differences in regional positron counts are correlated with regional changes in blood flow, and hence are indirectly an index of differential neuronal activity. (See *The MIT Encyclopedia of Cognitive Sciences*, s.v. "Positron Emission Tomography," for a fuller discussion.)

14. Logothetis et al. (1999) studied the relation between monkey fMRI signals and single-neuron data in the monkey in an effort to clarify the basis of fMRI signals.

15. For an excellent introduction to imaging, see Posner and Raichle 1994.

16. For a more detailed account, see P. M. Churchland and P. S. Churchland 1991.

17. As an aside, let me say that by "explanation" I mean only that we understand— roughly or in detail—the how's and why's of a phenomenon. Though an imprecise characterization of explanation, this will suffice for present purposes. Attempts to give highly formal, precise definitions of "explanation" have typically traded useful learning-by-example strategies for unusable precision. Scientists have no trouble agreeing on the *prototypical* examples of good explanations and poor explanations, especially in their own subfields. Trying to list a set of necessary and sufficient conditions for something's being an explanation is like trying to list necessary and sufficient conditions for what it is to be polite. In learning a science, one learns to recognize when an explanation on offer is sketchy or weak or bold or not in agreement with data. Seeing hypotheses criticized, amended, rejected, or adopted is part and parcel of learning the science. Similarly, in learning to behave in polite society, one comes to recognize when it is rude to stare or point, when it is polite to decline an invitation, and so on.

18. From the *Oxford Dictionary of Physics* (1996).

19. Rumford 1798. See the discussion by John W. Lyons in his book *Fire* (1985). Lyons notes that Rumford demonstrated his point by making a friction device that was like the cannon borer but did not actually bore. He showed that the device would boil water.

20. See especially Fodor 1974, 1975.

21. The basic idea was first articulated by Hilary Putnam (1967), though he has since recognized its limitations.

22. Dennett often defends this analogy. See Dennett 1978, 1991.

23. For a recent defense of the analogy, but without the claim that neuroscience is relevant, see Pinker 1997.

24. See P. S. Churchland 1986, P. M. Churchland 1988, Churchland and Sejnowski 1992, and P. M. Churchland and P. S. Churchland 2000.

25. See Churchland and Sejnowski 1992 and Bell 1999.

26. See the whole range beautifully discussed in Squire and Kandel 1999.

27. See Hooker 1995 for a discussion of reductionism.

28. For additional discussion, see also P. M. Churchland and P. S. Churchland 1990.

29. See P. M. Churchland 1979, 1993.

30. P. S. Churchland and Sejnowski 1992.

31. Dennett 1991.

32. See, for example, Fodor 1975.

33. See reviews of my *Neurophilosophy* (1986), for example, Corballis 1988, Kitcher 1996.

2   An Introduction to Metaphysics

1. I am grateful to my colleague Georgios Anagnostopoulos for pointing this out.

2. See also Callender 2001.

3. Glymour 1997.

4. Quine 1969.

5. See also Hooker 1995 and G. Johnson 1995.

6. See, for example, Maudlin 1994, Callender and Huggett 2001.

7. Bogen and Vogel 1965, Sperry 1974. For discussion of other disconnection syndromes, see Geschwind 1965.

8. Gazzaniga and LeDoux 1978.

9. See also Bogen 1985.

10. For a brave but unsuccessful attempt, see Puccetti 1981. His basic argument was that since nonphysical souls are not divisible, we all have two souls, one in each hemisphere.

11. Eccles 1994.

12. There are also many examples of nonconscious cognition from human patients with brain lesions. See Weiskrantz 1997.

13. See also Palmer 1999, p. 429.

14. Zajonc 1980, Bornstein 1992.

15. Land and Lee 1994.

16. See, for example, Glymour 2001; Spirtes, Glymour, and Scheines 2000; Pearl 1988; Kelly 1996.

17. For discussion of this episode in science, see Thagard 1998a, 1998b, and especially 1999.

3 Self and Self-Knowledge

1. Portions of this chapter are drawn from P. S. Churchland 2002. Lakoff and Johnson (1999) fully explore the range of metaphors.

2. Flanagan 1992, Metzinger 2000, Llinás 2001, and the essays in Bermúdez, Marcel, and Eilan 1995. See again Lakoff and Johnson 1999.

3. See also Squire and Zola 1996, Squire and Kandel 1999.

4. For an extended discussion of this hypothesis, see C. Frith 1992 and Stephens and Graham 2000. See also Flanagan 1996.

5. See Hobson 2001 and Sharp et al. 2001.

6. Ramachandran and Blakeslee 1998.

7. A person is diagnosed with Body Dysmorphic Disorder if he is preoccupied with an imaginary defect in his appearance to the degree that it impairs his daily functions. The disorder is characterized by the subject's sincere and unalterable conviction that some aspect of his body is extremely ugly, even though others can detect no abnormality at all.

8. See also Jeannerod 1997 and Llinás 2001.

9. MacLean 1949, Damasio 1999.

10. Damasio 1994, Cytowic 1996.

11. Wolpert et al. 1995.

12. Grush 1997.

13. This is a highly simplified account of the problem. For example, arms have mass, and the brain has to take this into account, as well as making postural adjustments

to the whole body, and so on. But I am aiming only to get across the general and basic point that coordinate transformations are needed.

14. See Wolpert et al. 1995.

15. See Jeannerod 1997 and Grush 1997.

16. For a review paper, see Kosslyn, Ganis, and Thompson 2001.

17. See Grush 1997.

18. Although the emulator solution has been the focus of discussion, it should be mentioned that at least for some concrete problems such as grasping the plum, on-line error correction as a solution to the problem is also very possible. See the Ph.D. dissertation of Elizabeth B. Torres (2001).

19. Zigmond et al. 1999, p. 1372.

20. Pouget and Sejnowski 1997.

21. For a discussion on the connection between self-representation and spatial representation, see Grush 2000. For a discussion of spatial representation in the blind, see Millar 1994.

22. See Andersen 1995b, Sakata and Taira 1994.

23. Heinrich 1999 and 2000.

24. Heinrich 2000, p. 300.

25. Blakemore and Decety 2001. An earlier version of this experiment was tried by Larry Weiskrantz (personal communication).

26. For a very different example involving the vestibular system and how predicting self-movement in darkness has a cognitive effect on the feeling of tilt, see Wertheim, Mesland, and Bles 2001.

27. Lotze, Flor, Klose, Birbaumer, and Grodd 1999.

28. Kravitz, Goldenberg, and Neyhus 1978.

29. Meltzoff and Moore 1977, 1983.

30. See Gallese and Goldman 1998.

31. Llinás (2001) emphasizes this point.

32. Damasio (1999) uses the term "protoself" for coherent neural patterns of which we are not aware, and "core self" for nonverbal self-representations. My use of "protoself" does not map perfectly onto his use.

33. See Gopnik, Meltzoff, and Kuhl 1999. See also Meltzoff 1995.

34. Thelen 1995, Butterworth 1995.

35. Sellars 1956. For discussion of Sellars, see P. M. Churchland 1979.

36. Blakemore and Decety 2001.

37. Rizzolatti, Fogassi, and Gallese 2001; Gallese and Goldman 1998.

38. Meltzoff and Gopnik 1993. See the review article by Heyes (2001).

39. Allison, Puce, and McCarthy 2000.

40. Carl Jung, 1959 translation.

41. Willatts 1984, 1989; Leslie and Keeble 1987; Wellman, Hickling, and Schult 1997.

42. See Povinelli 2000, Premack 1988, Tomasello and Call 1997, and the essays in Haug and Whalen 1999.

43. See P. M. Churchland 1979, 1993, 1996b; P. S. Churchland 1986.

44. Bates 1990.

45. See Tomasello 1992, Kagan 1981, and Gopnik, Meltzer, and Kuhl 1999.

46. De Waal 2001.

47. See Tomasello and Call 1997.

48. U. Frith 1999.

49. For a review paper, see Bauman 1999.

50. For a review of the evidence for activation of motor areas during motor imagery, see Jeannerod 2001.

51. Searle 1992.

52. P. M. Churchland 1996b.

53. See especially Damasio 1999.

54. P. M. Churchland 1995, pp. 164 ff.

55. See Tomasello 1999, 2000; Mithen 1996.

4 Consciousness

1. See Allen and Reber 1998.

2. See Flanagan 1992.

3. Portions of this section are drawn from Farber and P. S. Churchland 1994.

4. Dan Dennett also makes this point in *Consciousness Explained* (1991). See also P. S. Churchland 1986.

5. Also see my 1983 paper.

6. Crick 1994; Crick and Koch 1998, 2000. See also P. S. Churchland 1996a, 1997.

7. To experience the bistability in binocular rivalry, go to http://www.psy.vanderbilt. edu/faculty/blake/rivalry/waves.html.

8. Leopold and Logothetis 1999, Blake and Logothetis 2002.

9. For a discussion of this technique, see Purves et al. 2001.

10. Mark Churchland has raised these matters in personal communication.

11. Dennett (1978, 1998) has long believed that having a language is a necessary condition for consciousness, and hence that nonverbal animals are not conscious, or at least are not conscious of a pain in the way that I am conscious of a pain. He argues that to be conscious, the organism has to have a brain organization that it gets after immersion in culture and language. He says, "Other species no doubt achieve *somewhat similar* organizations, but the differences are so great that most of the specualtive translation of imagination from our case to theirs *makes no sense*" (1998, p. 347; his italics).

12. See Sue Savage-Rumbaugh and Roger Lewin's 1994 book on Kanzi, the bonobo chimp studied for many years at the Yerkes Primate Center of Georgia State University.

13. For a fuller discussion, see Glymour 1997.

14. Polonsky et al. 2000.

15. Lumer, Friston, and Rees 1998.

16. Tootell et al. 1995.

17. Ffytche et al. 1998.

18. Dehaene et al. 2001.

19. See also Lumer and Rees 1999, McIntosh et al. 1999. For a brief discussion on interpretive questions regarding fMRI, see Jennings 2001. For a general discussion, see Purves et al. 2001.

20. Lumer, Edelman, and Tononi 1997; Edelman and Tononi 2000.

21. See also P. M. Churchland 1995, O'Brien and Opie 1999.

22. This point was actually appreciated by Immanuel Kant (1797), but also by Wilfrid Sellars (1956) and W. V. O. Quine (1960).

23. P. M. Churchland, in press.

24. Pascual-Leone and Walsh 2001.

25. Crick and Koch, in press, and Crick, in conversation.

26. Meno et al. 1998.

27. For a review of the issues involved in determning the neural correlates of consciousness, see Frith, Perry, and Lumer 1999. It should be added that neuroscientists do typically recognize all these problems. See e.g. Dehaene et al. 2001.

28. For hypotheses concerning the roles of the brainstem and thalamic structures, see Damasio 1994 and 1999; Bogen 1995; Purpura and Schiff 1997; Llinás and Pare 1996; Llinás 2001; Lumer, Edelman, and Tononi 1997.

29. This seems to be favored by Merlin Donald (2001).

30. See McConkie and Rayner 1975, Henderson 1993.

31. Or left if one is reading Hebrew, down if one is reading Cantonese.

32. Dennett (1978) was among the first to see the importance of looking at the problem this way.

33. Dennett 2001b, p. 1.

34. Baars 1989, 2002; Dehaene and Nuccache 2001.

35. Or, to be honest, even very roughly.

36. Dennett 1998.

37. Popper 1959.

38. For example, the hypothesis predicts that the activity in the populations with access to global information will show coherent (synchronous) activity. It is worth noting that evidence of synchrony was first found in the anesthetized (albeit lightly anesthetized) animal, and hence there is some question about the role of synchrony of neuronal activity in perceptual awareness. But see Singer 2000.

39. Thomas Metzinger (2000, 2003) develops a very similar framework. Paul Churchland (1995) and Rosenthal (1997) also argue for a version of this thesis. See also Armstrong 1981 for earlier discussions of this central idea.

40. This line is also developed in Llinás 2001.

41. See also Yates 1985, Flanagan 1992, Metzinger 1995.

42. See also Schore 1994, P. M. Churchland 1995, Lycan 1997, P. S. Churchland 2002.

43. See especially Parvizi and Damasio 2001.

44. Fiset et al. 1999.

45. See also P. M. Churchland, 1987.

46. Portions of this section are drawn from my 1996c paper.

47. McGinn 1994, p. 99.

48. Vendler 1994.

49. Portions of what follows in the section are based on P. S. Churchland 1998.

50. For an amusing but pointed discussion of this and related issues, see also Dennett 2001a.

51. Pages 180–189 are closely based on P. M. Churchland and P. S. Churchland 1997 and also depend heavily on Palmer 1999.

52. For this criticism, see P. M. Churchland 1996a and Perry 2001.

53. On coding and models of color coding, see Lehky and Sejnowski 1999.

54. See pp. 20–25 above.

55. Palmer 1999.

56. See Nagel 1994.

57. For the details behind my reservations, see Grush and Churchland 1995 and the reply by Penrose and Hameroff (1995). See also Putnam 1994; Smullyan 1992; Maddy 1992, 1997. Pat Hayes and Ken Ford (1995) found Penrose's mathematical argument to be so outlandish that they awarded him the Simon Newcombe Award in 1995. They explain that Simon Newcombe (1835–1909) was a celebrated astronomer who insisted in various articles that manned flight was physically impossible.

58. See Feferman 1996; Putnam 1994, 1995.

59. Franks and Lieb 1994; Bowdle, Horita, and Kharasch 1994.

60. Vendler 1994.

5   Free Will

1. Portions of this chapter are drawn from P. S. Churchland 1996b.

2. See Campbell 1957, Kane 1996.

3. In his anonymously published *A Treatise on Human Nature*. Modern edition by Selby-Bigge (1888).

4. Hume 1739, p. 411.

5. P. M. Churchland makes this point in his APA presidential address (in press).

6. See, for example, Kane 1996 and Stapp 1999. For more discussion, see also Walter 2000.

7. See Taylor 1992, Van Inwagen 1975.

8. See more extended explanations in P. M. Churchland 1995.

9. This syndrome is also known as *akinetic mutism*. For a review paper, see Vogt, Finch, and Olson 1992.

10. Damasio and Van Hoesen 1983.

11. Ballantine et al. 1987.

12. For this study, see Beauregard, Lévesque, and Bourgouin 2001.

13. For a fuller discussion, see Hobson 1993.

14. See Bauman and Kemper 1995.

15. For a review paper on the ascending projection systems, see Robbins and Everitt 1995.

16. This was first pointed out to me by Carmen Carillo in a paper for my class and was subsequently discussed in an editorial in *Nature*: Neuroscience, fat, and free will (2000, 3: 1057).

17. See also Walter 2000.

18. See Kagan, *Galen's Prophecy* (1994).

19. Kant actually says, "the rule and direction for knowing how you go about *sharing in happiness*" (my italics), because the matter arises in the context of a teacher-student dialogue about a particular case, namely how to help others and whether to give them what they want. Kant likely intends the point to be general, and hence my more general interpolation.

20. Or as Marge Piercy remarks in *Braided Lives* (1982), "... treats his emotions like mice that infest our basement or rats in the garage, as vermin to be crushed in traps and posioned with bait."

21. See de Sousa 1990, p. 14.

22. Damasio 1994.

23. Saver and Damasio 1991.

24. The GSR measures change in conductivity of the skin as a function of increased sweat on the skin, which is an effect produced by the sympathetic nervous system.

25. Bechara et al. 1994, Damasio 1994.

26. Bechara et al. 1997.

27. Benjamin Libet (1985) came to a similar conclusion using a very different experimental paradigm.

28. Is EVR merely showing frontal perseveration? No, because he does score normally on the Wisconsin card-sorting task, in contrast to perseverative patients. For a much fuller account, see Damasio 1994. See also Raine et al. 1998 and Raine, Buchsbaum, and LaCasse 1997.

29. Anderson, Bechara, H. Damasio, Tranel, and A. R. Damasio 1999.

30. An earlier hypothesis related to this view was suggested by Paul MacLean (1949, 1952). He said, "As a working hypothesis, it can be inferred that the limbic system is for the 'body viscous,' a visceral brain that interprets and gives expression to its incoming information in terms of feeling" (1952). See also Papez 1937; Klüver and Bucy 1937, 1938.

31. Damasio 1999, Brothers 1997.

32. See Schore 1994, Schulkin 2000.

33. P. M. Churchland 1995. See also the Ph.D. thesis of William Casebeer (2001).

34. Recall that Buridan's ass was placed midway between two bales of hay and could not decide which to approach first, and so died of starvation.

35. Damasio 1994, p. 134 ff.; Le Doux 1996, 2002.

36. This view can also be found in the classic essays of Hobart 1934 and Schlick 1939.

6   An Introduction to Epistemology

1. Bain founded the journal *Mind* in 1876. It was launched as an organ of empirical philosophy, though later editors soon transformed it into the very reverse of that.

2. See David J. Murray's book *A History of Western Psychology* (1988) for an illuminating discussion of these developments.

3. For a comparison among primates, see Semendeferi et al. 2002. See also Finlay and Darlington 1995.

4. See the discussion of neurochemicals in Cooper, Bloom, and Roth 1996, and chapter 8 in Zigmond et al. 1999.

5. Quoted in Murray 1988, p. 116.

6. See a discussion of this point by Panksepp and Panksepp, who comment, "From a neuroscience persepctive, 'modularity' is an obselete concept, resembling the 'cen-

ters' concept that was discarded by scientists doing brain research several decades ago" (2001a, p. 3).

7. See chapter 13 by Gordon M. Shepherd in Zigmond et al. 1999.

8. The foundations for algorithms were laid down by the brilliant mathematician Al Khwarizmi, born in Uzbekistan about 800. He published a treatise in 830 called *Al-jabr wa'l muqabala*, from which the name algebra was derived. The term "algorithm" is derived from his name. See Crowther 1969.

9. See the clear and concise lectures by John von Neumann in *The Computer and the Brain*, posthumously published in 1958. (Second edition, 2000.)

10. For a clear and accessible discussion of Gödel's theorem, see Detlefsen 1999.

11. Wittgenstein's *Philosophical Investigations*, published posthumously in 1958, is a rich source of perplexing, but possibly insightful, aphoristic pronouncements that launched a cottage industry devoted to determining what he might have and must have meant. For example, "That what someone else says to himself is hidden from me is part of the *concept* 'saying inwardly.' Only 'hidden' is the wrong word here; for if it is hidden from me, it ought to be apparent to him, *he* would have to *know* it. But he does not 'know' it; only, the doubt which exists for me does not exist for him" (1958, 220e; italics in the original text). On the matter of the conscious experience of pain, Wittgenstein says, "It is not a *something*, but it is not a *nothing* either! The conclusion was only that a nothing would serve just as well as a something about which nothing could be said" (1958, sec. 304, p. 102e.) On philosophy, he says, "Philosophy simply puts everything before us, and neither explains nor deduces anything. Since everything lies open to view there is nothing to explain. For what is hidden, for example, is of no interest to us" (1958, sec. 126, p. 50e).

12. See for example Wittgenstein 1958, Malcolm 1971, and Hacker 1987. Hacker proposes that it is meaningless to say the brain thinks or remembers or sees. Wittgenstein thought that it was meaningless to say, "I know I have a pain," and meaningless to say, "I don't know whether I have a pain." Malcolm argued that it is strictly meaningless to say that people have dream experiences while they are asleep. Dan Dennett shows some sympathy with this approach when he says that the proposition that nonverbal animals are conscious is *senseless* (1996). Such a proposition might, of course, be false, but perhaps it is somewhat excessive to say the proposition has *no meaning*.

13. See Dan Dennett's brilliant attack on thought experiments 1999.

14. This was most evident in work on meaning and language. See especially Fodor 1987, and Fodor and LePore 1992.

15. For a fine sample of this kind of work, see the essays in Glymour and Cooper 1999. See also Glymour 2001 and Kelly 1996.

7   How Do Brains Represent?

1. See, for example, Millikan 1984, Cummins 1996, Elman et al. 1996, Lakoff 1987, Deacon 1997.

2. See especially Fodor 1974, 1994, and Pylyshyn 1984.

3. Beer 2000, Elman 1995.

4. For a general discussion on this topic, see Bechtel 2001.

5. Allman 1999.

6. For developments on this front, see Dayan and Abbott 2001; Beer, in press.

7. Packard and Teather 1998a, 1998b.

8. Farber, Peterman, and Churchland 2001.

9. Llinás and Pare 1996, Llinás 2001.

10. To see subjective motion, go to Don Hoffman's website: http://aris.ss.uci.edu/cogsci/personnel/hoffman/Applets/index.html. For another set of excellent visual demonstrations, see the Stuart Anstis website: http://psy.ucsd.edu/~sanstis.

11. Deacon 1997, Fauconnier 1997.

12. Quartz 1999; Quartz and Sejnowski 1997 and in press.

13. Squire and Kandel 1999.

14. By "higher" I mean that the neurons in the region are a greater number of synapses away from the sensory periphery (the retina) than neurons in V1. A more satisfying account of "higher" will depend on a more adequate theory of brain organization and function.

15. Turrigiano 1999.

16. For a review of population coding in the somatosensory system, see Doetsch 2000.

17. The description that follows is closely based on the description in Paul Churchland's *The Engine of Reason, the Seat of the Soul* (1995, pp. 4–45).

18. It is also noteworthy that other experiments with networks replicated the human "familiarity effect," according to which someone who grew up with Asians finds discriminations among Asian faces easier than discriminations among Caucasian faces, and vice versa for Caucasians.

19. See P. M. Churchland 1979. Dennett long ago in *Brainstorms* (1978) made detailed criticism of Fodor's idea of knowledge as sentences stored in the brain. For an more recent defense of the sentences-in-the-head view, see Fodor 1990.

20. For example, it has been shown that when individuals listen to a complex tone, they may perceive it as a single pitch. Using magnetoencephalography (MEG), Patel and Balaban (2001) show that when different individuals extracted different pitches, the spatial distribution of activity may be quite similar, but the temporal patterns in the activity are different.

21. There are promising breakthroughs. One concerns the use of independent component analysis (ICA) to analyze data from MEG, EEG, and f MRI. See Makeig et al. 1997.

22. A number of neuropsychologists—including Elizabeth Bates, Virginia Voltcrra, Mark Johnson, and their students—had come to similar conclusions, based mainly on infant studies and studies of humans with brain damage. They too had to keep digging out from under the scorn heaped upon them as a new paradigm began to take shape. Among philosophers, the renegades numbered Wilfrid Sellars in the 1960s, followed by Paul Churchland (1979, 2001), Robert Cummins (1996), Jared O'Brien and Jonathan Opie (1999).

23. Ryle 1954.

24. Fauconnier and Turner 2002.

25. Fauconnier 1997, Coulson and Matlock 2001, Coulson 1996, Fauconnier and Turner 2002.

26. See P. M. Churchland 2001.

27. See, for example, Rosch 1973 and 1978, and the discussions in Lakoff 1987 and Nosofsy and Palmeri 1997.

28. See again P. M. Churchland 2001.

29. Nor indeed are these the only areas that play a role in spatial knowledge. To do justice to the matter, one should also discuss the superior colliculus (Groh and Sparks 1996), the cerebellum, the basal ganglia, the red nucleus, and the spinal cord for starters. (See especially Jeannerod 1997, Goodale and Milner 1995, and Gross and Graziano 1995.)

30. See Jeannerod 1997.

31. Damasio 1999, Grush 2000.

32. Pouget and Sejnowski 1997a, 1997b.

33. See Andersen, Essick, and Siegel 1985; Andersen et al. 1990; Andersen 1995b; Mazzoni and Andersen 1995; Wise et al. 1997.

34. See Matin, Stevens, and Picoult 1983. In this experiment, run on himself and his colleagues, Stevens immobilized the eye muscles via a procedure known as a retro-bulbar block. When a light is flashed in the visual periphery (e.g., to the right), one

intends to move the eyes to the right to look at it. Because the extraocular muscles are paralyzed, however, no eye movement can happen. This mismatch between intent and performance produces the vivid visual *experience* of the whole world making an abrupt jump to the right, as though the eyes really had moved, but since the world still looks the same, the world must have moved along with them. In fact, of course, nothing moved, neither eyes nor world. One simply *intended* the eyes to move. This is a wonderful example of feedback from the motor command trumping visual motion.

35. Goodale and Milner (1995) use a visual illusion in which a disc visually appears to be larger than it is, but the grasp aperture in *reaching* for the disc is set to the correct size.

36. The units in each hemisphere were organized into maps, with one axis representing sensitivity to horizontal retinal field position (vertical position was not considered) and the other representing sensitivity to eye position. The maps were constructed to have neuronal gradients, in which the right hemisphere had more neurons responsive to the left retinal field and eye positions, and vice versa for the left hemisphere. Parietal cortex is known to have these sorts of gradients for retinal position; eye-position gradients are observed in other areas, but it is not known whether they exist in parietal cortex.

37. Pouget and Sejnowski's theory is based on linear combinations of continuous functions. It may be suggested that such a model can (in principle) be approximated to an arbitrary degree of accuracy by a Turing machine. On the assumption that this is true, nothing is revealed about which model most accurately captures what the brain is really doing. The behavior of the solar system can also be approximated to an arbitrary degree of accuracy by a Turing machine, but insisting that planetary motion actually involves symbol manipulation according to syntactically specified rules is unrewarding. That Turing equivalence is irrelevant here is further illustrated by the fact that Pouget and Sejnowski's model could also be implemented by analog very-large-scale integrated circuits (VLSI), which is about as nonsymbolic as you can get.

38. Kant's "transcendental unity of apperception" is turning out to be the fundamental integration of diverse sensory and motor coordinate systems, exquisitely configured *physically* to represent space. More positively for Kantians, space as a "form of intuition," as Kant characterized it in the *Critique of Pure Reason*, might turn out to have a neurophysiological basis.

39. For a discussion of the computational power of neural nets, see Siegelmann and Sontag 1995 and Bell 1999.

40. See the essays in Gentner, Holyoak, and Kokinov 2001.

41. See Aloimonos 1993; Churchland, Ramachandran, and Sejnowski 1994; Clark 1999; O'Regan 1992.

8　How Do Brains Learn?

1. Sugiura, Patel, and Corriveau 2001.

2. Nieuwenhuys 1985, Finlay and Darlington 1995.

3. Panksepp and Panksepp 2001b, p. 73.

4. One major change may be in what are considered the units of selection. For example, Gilbert et al. (1996) propose that it is really the *morphological field* whose alterations mediate evolution, not simply the gene.

5. On the evolution of the human brain, see Finlay and Darlington 1995, Quartz and Sejnowski 1997, Finlay, Darlington, and Nicastro 2001.

6. See Kolb and Gibb 2001, Elbert, Heim, and Rockstroh 2001.

7. See P. S. Churchland and Sejnowski 1992.

8. Corriveau, in conversation.

9. Real 1991.

10. See their review paper (Montague and Dayan 1998).

11. Berns, McClure, Pagnoni, and Montague 2001.

12. See discussions of this research by Fuster (1973, 1995) and by Goldman-Rakic (1988).

13. See the detailed review of the amnesic patient H. M. in Corkin 2002. Larry Squire has also studied a number of patients of this type in San Diego (see Squire and Kandel 1999).

14. Eichenbaum 1998, Bunsey and Eichenbaum 1996.

15. Transitivity looks like this: If Tom is taller than Sally and Sally is taller than Bill, then Tom is taller than Bill.

16. Wilson and McNaughten 1994, Gais et al. 2000, Stickgold et al. 2000.

17. Gould et al. 1999.

18. See Sutton and Barto 1998.

9　Religion and the Brain

1. Without going into too much detail, this qualifier is meant to avoid discussing whether God is omnipotent even though he cannot square the circle or make $\pi = 5$ or make time go backwards or lift a heavier rock than he can lift, and so forth.

2. A lesser god might be envisioned, that is, one whose power is limited (perhaps quite severely), who knows some things but not everything (or perhaps not even very much), who tends to be good but not without flaw. This would be rather like Zeus, for example, who is quite likable overall, but is only a little more worthy of worship and entreaty than certain humans. In the interests of space, I have not discussed this sort of deity.

3. See *Webster's New Collegiate Dictionary*.

4. Dawkins, *The Blind Watchmaker* (1985); Mayr, *What Evolution Is* (2001).

5. See Ridely 2000.

6. See Williams 1996 and Lewis Wolpert 1991.

7. Joyce and Orgel 1993.

8. Hume's *Dialogues Concerning Natural Religion*.

9. For example, Herbert Jaspers reported on six patients with syphillitic demeita. They described feeling a presence nearby, often feeling that a person was walking behind and propelling them forward. The tendency is to think the presence it out of sight, behind the subject, just out of view. The neurologist Lhermitte refers to this phenomenon as "the feeling of presence." See also Critchely 1979.

10. Persinger 1987.

11. Mike Valpy, Science: neurotheology, *Toronto Globe and Mail*, 25 August 2001, p. F7.

12. As Dave Molfese pointed out, it may be a bit problematic to suppose that a benevolent God uses harmful seizures to make himself known.

13. Ramachandran and Blakeslee 1998, Boyer 2001.

14. For a very different point of view on faith, see MacKay 1974.

15. These figures are taken from *World Christian Encyclopedia*, vol. 2 (2001), edited by D. B. Barrett, G. T. Kurian, and T. M. Johnson. Chinese folk religions are described as a mixture of Confucianism, Taoism, Buddhism, and animism.

16. See a most insightful paper by Robert McCauley, forthcoming.

17. For an interesting speculation concerning the basis for human sacrifices, see Ehrenreich 1997. For a discussion of the role of evolution in religion, see Boyer 2001.

18. Davies 1992.

19. Loftus 1979, Loftus and Hoffman 1989.

20. See Austin 1998.

21. There are informal accounts where someone claimed to have been floating, but when queried, failed to describe highly salient objects on the top of cupboards.

22. On the topic of inexactness, see Anagnostopoulos 1994.

23. In one case of inflexible application of zero-tolerance legislation, disciplinary proceedings were begun against a Canadian doctor who married a woman who had been his patient and had ceased to be his patient fully seven years before he began dating her. The zero-tolerance rule forbids any sexual interaction between a doctor and patient. Canadian Supreme Court Chief Justice Kenneth MacDonald, who threw out the case, was Aristotlian in his comments: "The legislation lacks balance and is incapable of giving proper justice to different situations. Neither the public nor the affected parties benefit from this unbending type of legislation."

24. Hamilton 1964; E. O. Wilson 1975, 1998. See also Sober and Wilson 1998 for an extended discussion.

25. Sober and Wilson 1998, Casebeer 2001, Mark Johnson 1993, Solomon 1995.

26. In *The Critique of Judgment*, Kant's treatise on aesthetics, first published in 1790.

27. *Webster's New Collegiate Dictionary*.

28. In a broadcasted interview many years ago.

References

Abbott, L., and T. J. Sejnowski, eds. 1999. *Neural Codes and Distributed Representations*. Cambridge: MIT Press.

Albright, C. R., and J. B. Ashbrook. 2001. *Where God Lives in the Human Brain*. Naperville, Ill.: Sourcebook.

Allen, R., and A. S. Reber. 1998. Unconscious intelligence. In W. Bechtel and G. Graham, eds., *A Companion to Cognitive Science*, pp. 314–323. Oxford: Blackwell.

Allman, J. M. 1999. *Evolving Brains*. New York: Scientific American Library.

Aloimonos, Y. 1993. *Active Perception*. Hillsdale, N.J.: Lawrence Erlbaum & Associates.

Anagnostopoulos, G. 1994. *Aristotle on the Goals and Exactness of Ethics*. Berkeley: University of California Press.

Andersen R. 1995a. Encoding of intention and spatial location in the posterior parietal cortex. *Cerebral Cortex* 5: 457–469.

Andersen, R. 1995b. Coordinate transformations and motor planning in posterior parietal cortex. In M. Gazzaniga, ed., *The Cognitive Neurosciences*, pp. 519–532. Cambridge: MIT Press.

Andersen, R., C. Asanuma, G. Essick, and R. Siegel. 1990. Corticocortical connections of anatomically and physiologically defined subdivisions within the inferior parietal lobule. *Journal of Comparative Neurology* 296: 65–113.

Andersen, R., G. Essick, and R. Siegel. 1985. Encoding of spatial location by posterior parietal neurons. *Science* 230: 456–458.

Anderson, S. W., A. Bechara, H. Damasio, D. Tranel, and A. R. Damasio. 1999. Impairment of social and moral behavior related to early damage in human prefrontal cortex. *Nature Neuroscience* 2: 1032–1037.

Aristotle. 1955. *The Nichomachean Ethics*. Translated by J. A. K. Thompson. Harmondsworth: Penguin Books.

Aristotle. 1941. *Physica*. In *The Basic Works of Aristotle*, edited by R. McKeon. New York: Random House.

Armstrong, D. 1981. *The Nature of the Mind*. Ithaca: Cornell University Press.

Arthur, W. 1997. *The Origin of Animal Body Plans: A Study in Evolutionary Developmental Biology*. New York: Cambridge University Press.

Austin, J. H. 1998. *Zen and the Brain*. Cambridge: MIT Press.

Baars, B. J. 1989. *A Cognitive Theory of Consciousness*. Cambridge: Cambridge University Press.

Baars, B. J. 2002. The conscious access hypothesis: origins and recent evidence. *Trends in Cognitive Sciences* 6: 47–52.

Bachevalier, J. 2001. Neural basis of memory development: insight from neuropsychological studies in primates. In C. A. Nelson and M. Luciana, eds., *The Handbook of Developmental Cognitive Neuroscience*. Cambridge: MIT Press.

Ballantine, H. T., Jr., A. J. Bouckoms, and E. K. Thomas. 1987. Treatment of psychiatric illness by stereotactic cingulotomy. *Biological Psychiatry* 22: 807–819.

Bar, M., and I. Biederman. 1999. Localizing the cortical region mediating visual awareness of object identity. *Proceedings of the National Academy of Sciences, USA* 96: 1790–1793.

Barondes, S. H. 1993. *Molecules and Mental Illness*. New York: Scientific American Library.

Barrett, D. B., G. T. Kurian, and T. M. Johnson 2001. *World Christian Encyclopedia: A Comparative Survey of Churches and Religions in the Modern World*. 2nd ed. Oxford: Oxford University Press.

Bartoshuck, L. M., and G. K. Beauchamp. 1994. Chemical senses. *Annual Review of Psychology* 45: 419–449.

Bates, E. 1990. Language about me and you: pronominal reference and the emerging concept of self. In D. Cicchetti and M. Beeghly, eds., *The Self in Transition*, pp. 165–182. Chicago: University of Chicago Press.

Bates, E., I. Bretherton, and L. Snyder. 1988. *From First Words to Grammar: Individual Differences and Dissociable Mechanisms*. New York: Cambridge University Press.

Bauman, M. L., and T. L. Kemper. 1995. Neuroanatomical observations of the brain in autism. In J. Panksepp, ed., *Advances in Biological Psychiatry*, pp. 1–26. New York: JAI Press.

Beauregard, M., J. Lévesque, and P. Bourgouin. 2001. Neural correlates of conscious self-regulation of emotion. *Journal of Neuroscience* 21: 1–6.

Bechara, A., A. R. Damasio, H. Damasio, and S. W. Anderson. 1994. Insensitivity to future consequences following damage to human prefrontal cortex. *Cognition* 50: 7–15.

Bechara, A., H. Damasio, D. Tranel, and A. R. Damasio. 1997. Deciding advantageously before knowing the advantageous strategy. *Science* 275: 1293–1294.

Bechtel, W. 2001. Representations: from neural systems to cognitive systems. In W. Bechtel et al., eds., *Philosophy and the Neurosciences*. Oxford: Blackwells.

Bechtel, W., and G. Graham, eds. 1998. *A companion to cognitive science*. Malden, Mass.: Blackwells.

Bechtel, W., P. Mandik, J. Mundale, and R. S. Stufflebeam, eds. 2001. *Philosophy and the Neurosciences: A Reader*. Oxford: Oxford University Press.

Bechtel, W., and R. C. Richardson. 1993. *Discovering Complexity*. Princeton: Princeton University Press.

Beer, R. D. 2000. Dynamical approaches to cognitive science. *Trends in Cognitive Sciences* 4: 91–99.

Beer, R. D. In press. The dynamics of active categorical perception in an evolved model agent. *Behavioral and Brain Sciences*.

Bell, A. 1999. Levels and loops: the future of artificial intelligence and neuroscience. *Philosophical Transactions of the Royal Society of London*, B 354: 2013–2020.

Bermúdez, J. L., A. Marcel, and N. Eilan, eds. 1995. *The Body and the Self*. Cambridge: MIT Press.

Berns, G. S., S. M. McClure, G. Pagnoni, and P. R. Montague. 2001. Predictability modulates human brain response to reward. *Journal of Neuroscience* 21: 2793–2798.

Black, I. 2000. *The Dying of Enoch Wallace: Life, Death and the Changing Brain*. New York: McGraw-Hill.

Blake, R. and N. K. Logothetis. 2002. Visual competition. *Nature Reviews* 3: 13–23.

Blakemore, S.-J., and J. Decety. 2001. From the perception of action to the understanding of intention. *Nature Reviews:Neuroscience* 2: 561–567.

Bogen, J. 1985. Split-brain syndromes. In J. A. M. Frederiks, ed., *Handbook of Clinical Neurology*. Vol. 1 (45): *Clinical Neuropsychology*, pp. 99–105. London: Elsevier.

Bogen, J. 1995. On the neurophysiology of consciousness. I: An overview. *Consciousness and Cognition* 4: 52–62.

Bogen, J., and P. J. Vogel. 1965. Cerebral commissurotomy in man. *Bulletin of the Los Angeles Neurological Society* 27: 169–172.

Bornstein, R. F. 1992. Subliminal mere exposure effects. In R. F. Bornstein and T. S. Pittman, eds., *Perception without Awareness: Cognitive, Clinical, and Social Perspectives*, pp. 191–210. New York: Guilford.

Bourgeois, J.-P. 2001. Synaptogenesis in the neocortex of the newborn: the ultimate frontier of individuation? In C. A. Nelson and M. Luciana, eds., *Handbook of Developmental Cognitive Neuroscience*. Cambridge: MIT Press.

Bowdle, T. A., A. Horita, and E. D. Kharasch, eds. 1994. *The Pharmacologic Basis of Anesthesiology*. New York: Churchill Livingstone.

Boyer, Pascal. 2001. *Religion Explained*. New York: Basic Books.

Brazier, M. A. B. 1984. *A History of Neurophysiology in the 17th and 18th Centuries: From Concept to Experiment*. New York: Raven Press.

Brecht, B. 1939. *Galileo*. Edited by E. Bentley. Translated by C. Laughton. New York: Grove Press, 1966.

Brothers, L. 1997. *Friday's Footprint: How Society Shapes the Human Mind*. New York: Oxford University Press.

Brown, T. H., A. H. Ganong, E. W. Kariss, and C. L. Keenan. 1990. Hebbian synapses: biophysical mechanisms and algorithms. *Annual Review of Neuroscience* 13: 475–511.

Bruce, C., R. Desimone, and C. G. Gross. 1981. Visual properties of neurons in a polysensory area in superior temporal sulcus of the macaque. *Journal of Neurophysiology* 46: 369–384.

Bullock, T. H., R. Orkand, and A. Grinnell. 1977. *Introduction to Nervous Systems*. San Francisco: Freeman.

Bunsey, M., and H. Eichenbaum. 1996. Conservation of hippocampal memory function in rats and humans. *Nature* 379: 255–257.

Butterworth, G. 1995. An ecological perspective on the origins of self. In J. L. Bermúdez, A. Marcel, and N. Eilan, eds., *The Body and the Self*. Cambridge: MIT Press.

Call, J. 2001. Chimpanzee social cognition. *Trends in Cognitive Science* 5: 388–393.

Callender, C. 2001. *Introducing Time*. Crow's Nest, New South Wales, Australia: Allen and Unwin.

Callender, C., and N. Huggett, eds. 2001. *Physics Meets Philosophy at the Planck Scale: Contemporary Theories in Quantum Gravity*. Cambridge: Cambridge University Press.

Campbell, C. A. 1957. Has the self "free will"? In his *On Selfhood and Godhood*, pp. 158–179. London: Allen and Unwin. New Jersey: Humanities Press.

Campbell, N. A. 1996. *Biology*. 4th ed. Menlo Park, Calif.: Benjamin/Cummings Publishing Co.

Campbell, R., and B. Hunter, eds. 2000. *Moral Epistemology Naturalized*. Calgary, Canada: University of Calgary Press.

Canup, R. M., and K. Righter, eds. 2000. *Origin of the Earth and the Moon*. Tuscon: University of Arizona Press.

Carey, S. 2001. Bridging the gap between cognition and developmental neuroscience: the example of number representation. In C. A. Nelson and M. Luciana, eds., *The Handbook of Developmental Cognitive Neuroscience*. Cambridge: MIT Press.

Casebeer, William. 2001. Natural ethical facts: evolution, connectionism, and moral cognition. Ph.D. dissertation, University of California at San Diego.

Chalmers, D. J. 1996. *The Conscious Mind: In Search of a Fundamental Theory*. New York: Oxford University Press.

Cheng, P. 1999. Causal reasoning. In R. A. Wilson and F. C. Keil, eds., *The MIT Encyclopedia of Cognitive Sciences*, pp. 106–107. Cambridge: MIT Press.

Chomsky, N. 1966. *Cartesian Linguistics*. New York: Harper & Row.

Churchland, P. M. 1979. *Scientific Realism and the Plasticity of Mind*. Cambridge: Cambridge University Press.

Churchland, P. M. 1987. How parapsychology could become a science. *Inquiry* 30: 227–239. Reprinted in P. M. Churchland and P. S. Churchland 1998.

Churchland, P. M. 1988. *Matter and Consciousness*. 2nd ed. Cambridge: MIT Press.

Churchland, P. M. 1993. Evaluating our self-conception. *Mind and Language* 8: 211–222.

Churchland, P. M. 1995. *The Engine of Reason, the Seat of the Soul*. Cambridge: MIT Press.

Churchland, P. M. 1996a. The rediscovery of light. *Journal of Philosophy* 93: 211–228.

Churchland, P. M. 1996b. Folk psychology. In S. Guttenplan, ed., *Companion to the Mind*. Oxford: Blackwells.

Churchland, P. M. 2001. Neurosemantics: on the mapping of minds and the portrayal of world. In K. E. White, ed., *The Emergence of the Mind: Proceedings of the International Symposium*, pp. 117–147. Milan: Montedison and Fondazione Carlo Erba.

Churchland, P. M. 2002. Catching consciousness in a neural net. In A. Brook and D. Ross, eds., *Dennett's Legacy*, pp. 64–82. Cambridge: Cambridge University Press.

Churchland, P. M. In press. Outer space and inner space: the new epistemology. *Proceedings and Addresses of the American Philosophical Association.*

Churchland, P. M., and P. S. Churchland. 1990. Could a machine think? Recent arguments and new prospect. *Scientific American* 262 (1): 32–37. Reprinted in H. Geirsson and M. Losonsky, eds., *Readings in Language and Mind*, pp. 273–281. Cambridge, Mass.: Blackwells, 1996.

Churchland, P. M., and P. S. Churchland. 1991. Intertheoretic reduction: a neuroscientist's field guide. *Seminars in the Neurosciences* 2: 249–256.

Churchland, P. M., and P. S. Churchland. 1997. Recent work on consciousness: philosophical, theoretical, and empirical. *Seminars in Neurology* 17: 101–108. Reprinted in P. M. Churchland and P. S. Churchland 1998.

Churchland, P. M., and P. S. Churchland. 1998. *On the Contrary*. Cambridge: MIT Press.

Churchland, P. M., and P. S. Churchland. 2000. Foreword. In John von Neumann, *The Computer and the Brain*, 2nd ed. New Haven: Yale University Press.

Churchland, P. S. 1983. Consciousness: the transmutation of a concept. *Pacific Philosophical Quarterly* 64: 80–95.

Churchland, P. S. 1986. *Neurophilosophy: Towards a Unified Understanding of the Mind-Brain*. Cambridge: MIT Press.

Churchland, P. S. 1996a. Toward a neurobiology of the mind. In R. R. Llinás and P. S. Churchland, eds., *The Mind-Brain Continuum*, pp. 281–303. Cambridge: MIT Press.

Churchland, P. S. 1996b. Feeling reasons. In A. R. Damasio, H. Damasio, and Y. Christen, eds., *Decision-Making and the Brain*, pp. 181–199. Berlin: Springer-Verlag.

Churchland, P. S. 1996c. The hornswoggle problem. *Journal of Consciousness Studies* 3 (5–6): 402–408.

Churchland, P. S. 1997. Can neurobiology teach us anything about consciousness? In N. Block, O. Flanagan, and G. Güzeldere, eds., *The Nature of Consciousness: Philosophical Debates*, pp. 127–140. Cambridge: MIT Press.

Churchland, P. S. 1998. What should we expect from a theory of consciousness? In H. H. Jasper, L. Descarries, V. F. Castellucci, and S. Rossignol, eds., *Consciousness: At the Frontiers of Neuroscience*. Philadelphia: Lippincott-Raven.

Churchland, P. S. 2002. Self-representation in nervous systems. *Science* 296: 308–310.

Churchland, P. S., V. S. Ramachandran, and T. J. Sejnowski. 1994. A critique of pure vision. In C. Koch and J. L. Davis, eds., *Large-Scale Neuronal Theories of the Brain*, pp. 23–60. Cambridge: MIT Press.

Churchland, P. S., and T. J. Sejnowski. 1988. Perspectives in cognitive neuroscience. *Science* 242: 741–745.

Churchland, P. S., and T. J. Sejnowski. 1992. *The Computational Brain.* Cambridge: MIT Press.

Clark, A. 1993. *Being There: Putting Brain, Body, and World Together Again.* Cambridge: MIT Press.

Clark, A. 1999. An embodied cognitive science? *Trends in Cognitive Sciences* 3: 345–350.

Cooper, J. R., F. E. Bloom, and R. H. Roth. 1996. *The Biochemical Basis of Neuropharmacology.* 7th ed. Oxford: Oxford University Press.

Corballis, M. 1988. Review of *Neurophilosophy* by P. S. Churchland. *Biology and Philosophy* 3: 393–402.

Corkin, S. 2002. What's new with the amnesic patient H.M.? *Nature Reviews: Neuroscience* 3: 153–160.

Coulson, S. 1996. The Menendez Brothers Virus: Analogical Mapping in Blended Spaces. In Adele Goldberg, ed., *Conceptual Structure, Discourse, and Language*, pp. 67–81. Palo Alto, Calif.: CSLI.

Coulson, S., and T. Matlock. 2001. Metaphor and the space structuring model. *Metaphor and Symbol* 16: 295–316.

Crick, F. 1994. *The Astonishing Hypothesis.* New York: Scribners.

Crick, F., and C. Koch. 1998. Consciousness and neuroscience. *Cerebral Cortex* 8: 97–107. Reprinted in Bechtel, Mandik, Mundale, and Stufflebeam 2001.

Crick, F., and C. Koch. 2000. The unconscious homunculus. In T. Metzinger, ed., *Neural Correlates of Consciousness*, pp. 103–110. Cambridge: MIT Press.

Crick, F., and C. Koch. In press. What Are the Neural Correlates of Consciousness? In J. L. van Hemmen and T. J. Sejnowski, eds., *Problems in Systems Neuroscience.* Oxford: Oxford University Press.

Critchley, M. 1979. *The Divine Banquet of the Brain.* New York: Raven.

Crowther, J. G. 1969. *A Short History of Science.* London: Methuen.

Cummins, R. 1996. *Representation, Targets, and Attitudes.* Cambridge: MIT Press.

Cytowic, R. E. 1996. *The neurological side of neuropsychology.* Cambridge: MIT Press.

Damasio, A. R. 1994. *Descartes' Error.* New York: Grossett/Putnam.

Damasio, A. R. 1999. *The Feeling of What Happens.* New York: Harcourt Brace.

Damasio, A. R. In press. *Looking for Spinoza: Joy, Sorrow, and the Human Brain.* New York: Harcourt.

Damasio, A. R., D. Tranel, and H. Damasio. 1991. Somatic markers and the guidance of behavior. In H. Levin, H. Eisenberg, and A. Benton, eds., *Frontal Lobe Function and Dysfunction*. New York: Oxford University Press.

Damasio, A. R., and G. Van Hoesen. 1983. Emotional disturbances associated with focal lesions of the limbic frontal lobe. In K. Heilman and P. Satz, eds., *Neuropsychology of Human Emotion*, pp. 268–299. New York: Guilford.

Darwin, C. 1859. *The Origin of Species*. Cambridge: Harvard University Press, 1964.

Davies, P. C. W. 1992. *The Mind of God: The Scientific Basis for a Rational World*. New York: Simon and Schuster.

Dawkins, R. 1985. *The Blind Watchmaker*. New York: Norton.

Dayan, P., and L. F. Abbott. 2001. *Theoretical Neuroscience: Computational and Mathematical Modeling of Neural Systems*. Cambridge: MIT Press.

Deacon, T. W. 1997. *The Symbolic Species: The Co-evolution of Language and the Brain*. New York: Norton.

Dehaene, S., and L. Naccache. 2001. Towards a cognitive neuroscience of consciousness: basic evidence and a workspace framework. *Cognition* 79: 1–37.

Dehaene, S., L. Naccache, L. Cohen, D. L. Bihan, J.-F. Mangin, J.-B. Poline, and D. Riviere. 2001. Cerebral mechanisms of word masking and unconscious repetition priming. *Nature Neuroscience* 4: 752–758.

Dennett, D. C. 1978. *Brainstorms: Philosophical Essays on Mind and Psychology*. Cambridge: MIT Press.

Dennett, D. C. 1984. *Elbow Room: The Varieties of Free Will Worth Wanting*. Cambridge: MIT Press.

Dennett, D. C. 1991. *Consciousness Explained*. Boston: Little Brown.

Dennett, D. C. 1992. The self as a center of narrative gravity. In F. Kessel, P. Cole, and D. Johnson, eds., *Self and Consciousness: Multiple Perspectives*, pp. 103–115. Hillsdale, N.J.: Lawrence Erlbaum & Associates.

Dennett, D. C. 1996. *Kinds of Minds: Towards an Understanding of Consciousness*. New York: Basic Books.

Dennett, D. C. 1998. *Brainchildren: Essays on Designing Minds*. Cambridge: MIT Press.

Dennett, D. C. 2001a. The Zombic Hunch: Extinction of an Intuition? In A. O'Hear, ed., *Philosophy at the New Millennium*, Royal Institute of Philosophy, suppl. 48, pp. 27–43. Cambridge: Cambridge University Press.

Dennett, D. C. 2001b. Are we explaining consciousness yet? *Cognition* 79: 221–237.

Descartes, R. 1637. *Discourse on Method*. In *The Philosophical Works of Descartes*, 2 vols., translated by E. S. Haldane and G. T. R. Ross. Cambridge: Cambridge University Press, 1911–1912.

De Sousa, R. 1990. *The Rationality of Emotion*. Cambridge: MIT Press.

Detlefsen, M. 1999. Gödel's incompleteness theorem. In R. Audi, ed., *The Cambridge Dictionary of Philosophy*, 2nd ed. Cambridge: Cambridge University Press.

De Waal, F. 1996. *Good Natured*. Cambridge: Harvard University Press.

De Waal, F. 2001. Pointing primates: sharing knowledge—without language. *Chronicle of Higher Education*, January 19, 2001, B7–9.

Doetsch, G. S. 2000. Patterns in the brain: neuronal population coding in the somatosensory system. *Physiology and Behavior* 69: 187–201.

Donald, M. 2001. *A mind so rare: the evolution of human consciousness*. New York: Norton.

Duclaux, R., and D. R. Kensahlo. 1980. Response characteristics of cutaneous warm fibres in the monkey. *Journal of Neurophysiology* 43: 1–15.

Eccles, J. C. 1953. *The Neurophysiological Basis of Mind*. New York: Oxford University Press.

Eccles, J. C. 1994. *How the Self Controls Its Brain*. Berlin: Springer-Verlag.

Edelman, G. M., and G. Tononi. 2000. Reentry and the dynamic core: neural correlates of conscious experience. In T. Metzinger, ed., *Neural Correlates of Consciousness*, pp. 139–151. Cambridge: MIT Press.

Edelman, S. 2002. Constraining the neural representation of the visual world. *Trends in Cognitive Sciences* 6: 125–131.

Ehrenreich, B. 1997. *Blood Rites: Origins and History of the Passions of War*. New York: Henry Holt and Co.

Eichenbaum, H. 1996. Is the rodent hippocampus just for "place"? *Current Opinion in Neurobiology* 6: 187–195.

Eichenbaum, H. 1998. Is the rodent hippocampus just for "place"? In L. R. Squire and S. M. Kosslyn, eds., *Findings and Current Opinion in Cognitive Science*, pp. 105–113. Cambridge: MIT Press.

Eichenbaum, H., and N. Cohen. 2001. *From Conditioning to Conscious Recollection*. New York: Oxford University Press.

Elbert, T., S. Heim, and B. Rockstroh. 2001. Neural plasticity and development. In C. A. Nelson and M. Luciana, eds., *The Handbook of Developmental Cognitive Neuroscience*, pp. 191–202. Cambridge: MIT Press.

Elman, J. L. 1995. Language as a dynamical system. In R. Port, and T. Van Gelder, eds., *Mind as Motion: Explorations in the Dynamics of Cognition*, pp. 195–226. Cambridge: MIT Press.

Elman, J., E. Bates, M. Johnson, A. Karmiloff-Smith, D. Parisi, and K. Plunkett. 1996. *Rethinking Innateness: A Connectionist Perspective on Development*. Cambridge: MIT Press.

Farber, I. 2000. Domain integration: a theory of progress in the life sciences. Doctoral dissertation, University of California at San Diego. http://reductio.com/ilya/.

Farber, I., and P. S. Churchland. 1994. Consciousness and the neurosciences: philosophical and theoretical issues. In M. Gazzaniga, ed., *The Cognitive Neurosciences*, pp. 1295–1306. Cambridge: MIT Press.

Farber, I., W. Peterman, and P. S. Churchland. 2001. The view from here: the nonsymbolic structure of spatial representation. In J. Branquinho, ed., *The Future of Cognitive Science*, pp. 55–76. Oxford: Oxford University Press.

Fauconnier, G. 1997. *Mappings in Thought and Language*. Cambridge: Cambridge University Press.

Fauconnier, G., and M. Turner. 2002. *The Way We Think: Conceptual Blending and the Mind's Hidden Complexities*. New York: Basic Books.

Ffytche, D. H., R. J. Howard, M. J. Brammer, A. David, P. Woodruff, and S. Williams. 1998. The anatomy of conscious vision: an MRI study of visual hallucinations. *Nature Neuroscience* 1: 738–742.

Finger, S. 1994. *Origins of Neuroscience: A History of Explorations into Brain Function*. New York: Oxford University Press.

Finlay, B. L., and R. B. Darlington. 1995. Linked regularities in the development and evolution of mammalian brains. *Science* 286: 1578–1584.

Finlay, B. L., R. B. Darlington, and N. Nicastro. 2001. Developmental structure in brain evolution. *Behavioral and Brain Sciences* 24 (2): 263–278, 298–304.

Fiset, P., T. Paus, T. Daloze, G. Plourde, P. Meuret, V. Bonhomme, N. Hajj-Ali, S. B. Blackman, and A. C. Evans. 1999. Brain mechanisms of propofol-induced loss of consciousness in humans: a positron emission tomographic study. *Journal of Neuroscience* 19: 5506–5513.

Flanagan, O. 1992. *Consciousness Reconsidered*. Cambridge: MIT Press.

Flanagan, O. 1996. *Self Expressions: Mind, Morals, and the Meaning of Life*. New York: Oxford University Press.

Fodor, J. A. 1974. Special sciences, or the disunity of science as a working hypothesis. *Synthese* 28: 97–115.

Fodor, J. A. 1975. *The Language of Thought*. New York: Crowell.

Fodor, J. A. 1983. *The Modularity of Mind*. Cambridge: MIT Press.

Fodor, J. A. 1987. *Psychosemantics*. Cambridge: MIT Press.

Fodor, J. A. 1990. *A Theory of Content*. Cambridge: MIT Press.

Fodor, J. A. 1994. *The Elm and the Expert*. Cambridge: MIT Press.

Fodor, J. A. 2000. *The Mind Doesn't Work That Way: The Scope and Limits of Computational Psychology*. Cambridge: MIT Press.

Fodor, J. A., and E. LePore. 1992. *Holism: A Shopper's Guide*. Oxford: Blackwells.

Franks, N. P., and W. R. Lieb. 1994. Molecular and cellular mechanisms of general anaesthesia. *Nature*. 367: 607–614.

Frith, C. D. 1992. *The Cognitive Neuropsychology of Schizophrenia*. Hillsdale, N.J.: Lawrence Erlbaum & Associates.

Frith, C. D., R. Perry, and E. Lumer. 1999.The neural correlates of conscious experience: an experimental framework. *Trends in Cognitive Sciences* 3: 105–114.

Frith, U. 1999. Autism. In R. A. Wilson, and F. Keil, eds. *The MIT Encyclopedia of the Cognitive Sciences*, pp. 58–60. Cambridge: MIT Press.

Fuster, J. M. 1973. Unit activity in prefrontal cortex during delayed-response performance: neural correlates of transient memory. *Journal of Neurophysiology* 36: 61–78.

Fuster, J. M. 1995. *Memory in the Cerebral Cortex*. Cambridge: MIT Press.

Gais, S., W. Plihal, U. Wagner, and J. Born. 2000. Early sleep triggers memory for early visual discrimination skills. *Nature Neuroscience* 3: 1335–1339.

Gallese, V., and A. Goldman. 1998. Mirror neurons and the simulation theory of mind-reading. *Trends in Cognitive Sciences* 2: 493–501.

Garcia, J., W. G. Hankins, and K. W. Rusiniak. 1974. Behavioral regulation of the milieu internal in man and rat. *Science*. 185: 824–831.

Gärdenfors, P. 2000. *Conceptual Spaces: The Geometry of Thought*. Cambridge: MIT Press.

Gardner, E. L., and J. H. Lowinson. 1993. Drug craving and positive/negative hedonic brain states activated by addicting drugs. *Seminars in the Neurosciences* 5: 359–368.

Gazzaniga, M. S., and LeDoux, J. E. 1978. *The Integrated Mind*. New York: Plenum Press.

Gentner, D. , K. J. Holyoak, and B. N. Kokinov. 2001. *The Analogical Mind*. Cambridge: MIT Press.

Gerhardt, J., and M. Kirschner 1997. *Cells, Embryos, and Evolution*. Oxford: Black-wells.

Geschwind, N. 1965. Disconnexion syndromes in animals and man. *Brain* 88: 237–294.

Gibson, R. F., Jr. 1982. *The Philosophy of W. V. Quine*. Tampa: University Presses of Florida.

Glymour, C. 1997. *Thinking Things Through*. Cambridge: MIT Press.

Glymour, C. 2001. *The Mind's Arrows: Bayes Nets and Graphical Causal Models in Psychology*. Cambridge: MIT Press.

Glymour, C., and G. F. Cooper, eds. 1999. *Computation, Causation, and Discovery*. Cambridge: MIT Press.

Goldman-Rakic, P. S. 1988. Topography of cognition: parallel distributed networks in primate association cortex. *Annual Review of Neuroscience* 11: 137–156.

Goldstein, E. B. 1999. *Sensation and Perception*. 5th ed. New York: Brooks/Cole Publishing Co.

Goodale, M. A., and A. D. Milner 1995. *The Visual Brain in Action*. Oxford: Oxford University Press.

Gopnik, A., A. N. Meltzoff, and P. K. Kuhl. 1999. *The Scientist in the Crib*. New York: Morrow.

Gould E., A. Beylin, P. Tanapat, A. Reeves, and T. J. Shors. 1999. Learning enhances adult neurogenesis in the hippocampal formation. *Nature Neuroscience* 2: 260–265.

Grady, M. 2001. *Search for life*. Washington, D.C.: Natural History Museum/Smithsonian Institution Press.

Grafman, J., and Y. Christen, eds. 1999. *Neuronal plasticity: building a bridge from the laboratory to the clinic*. Berlin: Springer.

Griffiths, P. E. 1997. *What Emotions Really Are*. Chicago: University of Chicago Press.

Groh, J., and D. Sparks 1996. Saccades to somatosensory targets. 3: Eye-position-dependent somatosensory activity in the primate superior colliculus. *Journal of Neurophysiology* 75: 439–453.

Gross, C. G. 1999. *Brain, Vision, Memory: Tales in the History of Neuroscience*. Cambridge: MIT Press.

Gross, C. G., and M. S. A. Graziano. 1995. Multiple representations of space in the brain. *Neuroscientist* 1: 43–50.

Grush, R. 1997. The architecture of representation. *Philosophical Psychology* 10: 5–23. Reprinted in Bechtel, Mandik, Mundale, and Stufflebeam 2001.

Grush, R. 2000. Self, world, and space: the meaning and mechanisms of ego- and allo-centric spatial representation. *Brain and Mind* 1: 59–92.

Grush, R., and P. S. Churchland. 1995. Gaps in Penrose's toilings. *Journal of Consciousness Studies* 2: 10–29. Reprinted in P. M. Churchland and P. S. Churchland 1998.

Hacker, P. 1987. Languages, minds, and brains. In C. Blakemore and S. Greenfield, eds., *Mindwaves*. Oxford: Blackwells.

Hacking, I. 2001. *An Introduction to Probability and Inductive Logic*. Cambridge: Cambridge University Press.

Haeckel, E. 1874. *Anthropogenie, oder Entwicklungsgeschicte des Menschen*. Leipzig: Engleman.

Hamilton, W. 1964. The genetical evolution of social behavior. *Journal of Theoretical Biology* 7: 1–52.

Hammer, M. 1993. An identified neuron mediates the unconditioned stimulus in associative olfactory learning in honeybees. *Nature* 366: 59–63.

Harvey, W. 1847. *The Works of William Harvey*. Translated from the Latin by R. Willis. London: Sydenham Society.

Haug, M., and R. E. Whalen, eds. 1999. *Animal Models of Human Emotions and Cognition*. Washington, D.C.: American Psychological Association.

Hebb, D. O. 1949. *The Organization of Behavior: A Neuropsychological Theory*. New York: Wiley.

Heeger, D. J., and D. Rees. 2002. What does fMRI tell us about neuronal activity? *Nature Reviews: Neuroscience* 3: 142–151.

Heimer, L. 1983. *The Human Brain and Spinal Cord*. New York: Springer-Verlag.

Heinrich, B. 1999. *Mind of the Raven*. New York: Harper-Collins.

Heinrich, B. 2000. Testing insight in ravens. In C. Heyes and L. Huber, ed., *The Evolution of Cognition*, pp. 289–306. Cambridge: MIT Press.

Henderson, J. M. 1993. Visual attention and saccadic eye movements. In G. d'Ydewalle, and J. Van Rensbergen, eds., *Perception and Cognition*, pp. 37–50. New York: North-Holland.

Heyes, C. 2001. Causes and consequences of imitation. *Trends in Cognitive Sciences* 5: 253–261.

Hobart, R. E. 1934. Free will as involving determinism and inconceivable without it. *Mind* 43: 1–27.

Hobson, J. A. 1993. Understanding persons: the role of affect. In S. Baron-Cohen, H. Tager-Flusberg, and D. J. Cohen, eds., *Understanding Other Minds: Perspectives From Autism*, pp. 204–227. Oxford: Oxford University Press.

Hobson, J. A. 1999. *Consciousness*. New York: Scientific American Library.

Hobson, J. A. 2001. *The Dream Drugstore: Chemically Altered States of Consciousness*. Cambridge: MIT Press.

Hoffman, D. 1998. *Visual Intelligence*. New York: Norton.

Hooker, C. A. 1995. *Reason, Regulation, and Realism: Towards a Regulatory Systems Theory of Reason and Evolutionary Biology*. New York: State University of New York Press.

Hubel, D. H. 1988. *Eye, Brain, and Vision*. New York: Freeman.

Hubel, D. H., and T. N. Wiesel. 1959. Receptive fields of single neurons in the cat's striate cortex. *Journal of Physiology* 148: 574–591.

Hubel, D. H., and T. N. Wiesel. 1977. Functional architecture of macaque monkey visual cortex. *Proceedings of the Royal Society of London*, B 198: 1–59.

Huber, L. 2000. Psychophylogenesis: innovations and limitations in the evolution of cognition. In C. Heyes and L. Huber, eds., *The Evolution of Cognition*, pp. 23–41. Cambridge: MIT Press.

Hume, David. 1739. *A Treatise of Human Nature*. Edited by L. A. Selby-Bigge, 1888 and 1896. Oxford: Oxford University Press.

Hume, David. 1779. *Dialogues Concerning Natural Religion*. Edited by Norman Kemp Smith, 1962. Oxford: Oxford University Press.

Hutchins, E. 1995. *Cognition in the Wild*. Cambridge: MIT Press.

Huttenlocher, P. R., and A. S. Dabholkar 1997. Regional differences in synaptogenesis in human cerebral cortex. *Journal of Comparative Neurology* 387: 167–178.

Jacob, F. 1999. *Of Flies, Mice, and Men*. Cambridge: Harvard University Press.

James, W. 1890. Chapter 10 of *The Principles of Psychology*. Edited by Frederick Burkhardt and Fredson Bowers, 1981. Cambridge: Harvard University Press.

Jeannerod, Marc. 1997. *The Cognitive Neuroscience of Action*. Oxford: Blackwells.

Jeannerod, Marc. 2001. Neural simulation of action: a unifying mechanism for motor cognition. *NeuroImage* 14: S103–S109.

Jeannerod, Marc, and Victor Frak. 1999. Mental imaging of motor activity in humans. *Current Opinion in Neurobiology* 9: 735–739.

Jennings, C. 2001. Analyzing functional imaging studies. *Nature neuroscience* 4: 333.

Johnson, G. 1995. *Fire in the Mind: Science, Faith, and the Search for Order*. New York: Knopf.

Johnson, M. 1993. *Moral Imagination: Implications of Cognitive Science for Ethics*. Chicago: University of Chicago Press.

Johnson, M. H. 1995. The development of visual attention: a cognitive neuroscience perspective. In M. Gazzaniga, ed., *The Cognitive Neurosciences*, pp. 735–747. Cambridge: MIT Press.

Johnson, M. H. 1997. *Developmental Cognitive Neuroscience: An Introduction*. Malden, Mass.: Blackwells.

Joyce, G. F., and L. E. Orgel. 1993. Prospects for understanding the origin of the RNA world. In R. F. Gersteland, T. Cech, and J. F. Atkins, eds., *The RNA World*. New York: Cold Spring Harbor Laboratory Press.

Jung, C. G. 1959. *The Archetypes and the Collective Unconscious*. Translated by R. F. C. Hull. New York: Pantheon Books.

Kagan, J. 1981. *The Second Year: The Emergence of Self-Awareness*. Cambridge: Harvard University Press.

Kagan, J. 1994. *Galen's Prophecy: Temperament in Human Nature*. New York: Basic Books.

Kandel, E. R., J. H. Schwartz, T. M. Jessell, eds. 2000. *Principles of Neural Science*. 4th ed. New York: McGraw-Hill.

Kane, R. 1996. *The Significance of Free Will*. New York: Oxford University Press.

Kant, I. 1797. Fragments of a moral catechism. In his *Metaphysical Principles of Virtue*, translated by James Ellington, pp. 148–153. New York: Bobbs-Merrill, 1964.

Kant, Immanuel. 1790. *The Critique of Judgment*. Edited and translated by J. C. Meredith. Oxford: Clarendon Press, 1952.

Kanwisher, N. 2001. Neural events and perceptual awareness. *Cognition* 79: 89–113.

Katz, P., ed. 1999. *Beyond Neurotransmission*. New York: Oxford University Press.

Kelly, K. T. 1996. *The Logic of Reliable Inquiry*. New York: Oxford University Press.

Kenny, A. 1992. *The Metaphysics of Mind*. Oxford: Oxford University Press.

Kitcher, P. W. 1996. From neurophilosophy to neurocomputation: searching for the cognitive forest. In R. M. McCauley, ed., *The Churchlands and Their Critics*, pp. 48–85. Cambridge, Mass.: Blackwell.

Klüver, H., and P. C. Bucy. 1937. "Psychic blindness" and other symptoms following bilateral temporal lobectomy in rhesus monkeys. *American Journal of Physiology* 119: 352–353.

Klüver, H., and P. C. Bucy. 1938. An analysis of certain effects of bilateral temporal lobectomy in the rhesus monkey, with special reference to "psychic blindness." *Journal of Psychology* 5: 33–54.

Kolb, B., and R. Gibb. 2001. Early brain injury, plasticity, and behavior. In C. A. Nelson and M. Luciana, eds., *The Handbook of Developmental Cognitive Neuroscience*, pp. 175–190. Cambridge: MIT Press.

Kolb, B., and I. Q. Whishaw. 1990. *Fundamentals of Human Neuropsychology*. New York: W. H. Freeman.

Kosslyn, S. M., G. Ganis, and W. L. Thompson. 2001. Neural foundations of imagery. *Nature Reviews: Neuroscience* 2: 635–642.

Kravitz, H., D. Goldenberg, and C. A. Neyhus. 1978. Tactile exploration by normal human infants. *Developmental Medicine and Child Neurology* 20: 720–726.

Kreiman, G., I. Fried, and C. Koch. 2002. Single-neuron correlates of subjective vision in the human medial temporal lobe. *Proceedings of the National Academy of Science* 99: 8378–8383.

Kuffler S. W. 1953. Discharge patterns and functional organization of mammalian retina. *Journal of Neurophysiology* 16: 37–68.

Lakoff, G. 1987. *Women, Fire, and Dangerous Things*. Chicago: Chicago University Press.

Lakoff, G., and M. Johnson. 1999. *Philosophy in the Flesh*. New York: Basics Books.

Land, M. F., and D. N. Lee. 1994. Where we look when we steer. *Nature* 369: 742–744.

Lawrence, P. A. 1992. *The Making of a Fly: The Genetics of Animal Design*. Cambridge, Mass.: Blackwells Science.

Le Doux, J. 1996. *The Emotional Brain*. New York: Simon and Schuster.

Le Doux, J. 2002. *Synaptic Self*. New York: Viking Press.

Lehky, S. R., and T. J. Sejnowski. 1999. Seeing white: qualia in the context of decoding population codes. *Neural Computation* 11: 1261–1280.

Leibniz, G. W. 1989. *G. W. Leibniz: Philosophical Essays*. Translated by R. Ariew and D. Garber. Indianapolis: Hackett Publishing.

Leopold, D. A., and N. K. Logothetis. 1999. Multistable phenomena: changing views in perception. *Trends in Cognitive Sciences* 3: 154–264.

Leslie, A. M., and S. Keeble. 1987. Do sixth-month-old infants perceive causality? *Cognition* 25: 265–288.

Levitan, I. B., and L. K. Kaczmarek. 1991. *The Neuron: Cell and Molecular Biology.* Oxford: Oxford University Press.

Libet, B. 1985. Unconscious cerebral initiative and the role of conscious will in voluntary action. *Behavioral and Brain Sciences* 8: 529–566.

Llinás, R. R. 2001. *I of the Vortex.* Cambridge: MIT Press.

Llinás, R. R., and D. Pare. 1996. The brain as a closed system modulated by the sense(s). In Llinás and P. S. Churchland 1996.

Llinás, R., and P. S. Churchland. 1996. *The Mind-Brain Continuum: Sensory Processes.* Cambridge: MIT Press.

Loftus, E. F. 1979. *Eyewitness Testimony.* Cambridge: Harvard University Press.

Loftus, E. F. 1997. Creating false memories. *Scientific American* 277 (3): 71–75.

Loftus, E. F., and H. G. Hoffman. 1989. Misinformation and memory: the creation of new memories. *Journal of Experimental Psychology: General* 118: 100–104.

Loftus, E. F., and K. Ketcham. 1994. *The Myth of Repressed Memory.* New York: St. Martin's.

Logothetis, N. K., and J. Schall. 1989. Neuronal correlates of subjective visual perception. *Science* 245: 761–763.

Logothetis, N. K., H. Guggenberger, S. Peled, and J. Pauls. 1999. Functional imaging of the monkey brain. *Nature Neuroscience.* 2: 555–562.

Lotto, R. B., and D. Purves. 2002. A rationale for the structure of color space. *Trends in neurosciences* 25: 84–88.

Lotze, M., P. Montoya, M. Erb, E. Hulsmann, H. Flor, U. Klose, N. Birbaumer, and W. Grodd. 1999. Activation of cortical and cerebellar motor areas during executed and imagined hand movements: an fMRI study. *Journal of Cognitive Neuroscience* 11: 491–501.

Lumer, E. D., G. M. Edelman, and G. Tononi. 1997. Neural dynamics in the model of the thalamocortical system. 1: Layers, loops, and the emergence of fast synchronous rhythms. *Cerebral Cortex* 7: 228–236.

Lumer, E. D., K. J. Friston, and G. Rees. 1998. Neural correlates of perceptual rivalry in the human brain. *Science* 280: 1930–1934.

Lumer, E. D., and G. Rees. 1999. Covariation of activity in visual prefrontal cortex associated with subjective visual perception. *Proceedings of the National Academy of Sciences, USA* 96: 1669–1673.

Lycan, W. 1997. Consciousness as internal monitoring. In N. Block, O. Flanagan, and G. Güzeldere, eds., *The Nature of Consciousness*, pp. 755–771. Cambridge: MIT Press.

Lyons, J. W. 1985. *Fire*. New York: Scientific American Library.

MacKay, D. M. 1974. *The Clockwork Image: A Christian Perspective on Science*. Downers Grove, Ill.: Intervarsity Press.

MacLean, P. D. 1949. Psychosomatic disease and the "visceral" brain: recent developments bearing on the Papez theory of emotion. *Psychosomatic Medicine* 11: 338–353.

MacLean, P. D. 1952. Some psychiatric implications of physiological studies on frontotemporal portion of limbic system visceral brain. *Electrophysiological and Clinical Neurophysiology* 4: 407–418.

Maddy, P. 1992. *Realism in Mathematics*. Oxford: Clarendon Press.

Maddy, P. 1997. *Naturalism in Mathematics*. Oxford: Clarendon Press.

Makeig, S. , T.-P. Jung, A. J. Bell, D. Ghahremani, and T. J. Sejnowski. 1997. Blind separation of auditory event-related brain responses into independent components. *Proceedings of the National Academy of Sciences, USA* 94: 10979–10984.

Malcolm, N. 1971. *Problems of Mind*. Ithaca: Cornell University Press.

Marcel, A. J. 1983. Conscious and unconscious perception: experiments on visual masking and word recognition. *Cognitive Psychology* 15: 197–237.

Marshall, B. J., and J. R. Warren. 1984. Unidentified curved bacilli in the stomach of patients with gastritis and peptic ulceration. *Lancet* 1 (8390): 1311–1315.

Maudlin, T. 1994. *Quantum Non-locality and Relativity*. Oxford: Blackwells.

May, L., M. Friedman, A. Clark, eds. 1996. *Mind and Morals*. Cambridge: MIT Press.

Mayr, E. 2001. *What Evolution Is*. New York: Basic Books.

Mazzioni, P., and R. Andersen. 1995. Gaze coding in posterior parietal cortex. In M. Arbib, ed., *The Handbook of Brain Theory and Neural Networks*, pp. 432–426. Cambridge: MIT Press.

McCauley, R. N., ed. 1996. *The Churchlands and Their Critics*. Oxford: Blackwells.

McCauley, R. N. 2000. The naturalness of religion and the unnaturalness of science. In F. Keil and R. Wilson, eds., *Explanation and Cognition*. Cambridge: MIT Press.

McConkie, G. W., and K. Rayner. 1975. The span of the effective stimulus during a fixation in reading. *Perception and Psychophysics* 17: 578–586.

McGinn, C. 1994. Can we solve the mind-body problem? In R. Warner and T. Szubka, eds., *The Mind-Body Problem: A Guide to the Current Debate*, pp. 349–366. Oxford: Blackwells.

McHugh, T. J., K. I. Blum, J. Z. Tsien, S. Tonegawa, and M. A. Wilson. 1996. Impaired hippocampal representation of space in CA1-specific NMDAR1 knockout mice. *Cell* 87: 1339–1349.

McIntosh, A. R., M. N. Rajah, and N. J. Lobaugh. 1999. Interactions of prefrontal cortex in relation to awareness in sensory learning. *Science* 284: 1531–1533.

Medawar, P. 1984. *The Limits of Science*. Oxford: Oxford University Press.

Meltzoff, A. N. 1995. Understanding the intentions of others: re-enactment of intended acts by 18-month-old children. *Developmental Psychology* 31: 838–850.

Meltzoff, A. N., and A. Gopnik. 1993. The role of imitation in understanding persons and developing a theory of mind. In S. Baron-Cohen, H. Tager-Flusberg, and D. J. Cohen, eds., *Understanding Other Minds*, pp. 335–366. Oxford: Oxford University Press.

Meltzoff, A. N., and M. K. Moore. 1977. Imitation of facial and manual gestures by human neonates. *Science* 198: 75–78.

Meltzoff, A. N., and M. K. Moore 1983. Newborn infants imitate adult facial gestures. *Child Development* 54: 702–709.

Menand, L. 2001. *The Metaphysical Club*. New York: Farrar, Straus & Giroux.

Meno, D. K., A. M. Owen, E. J. Williams, P. S. Minhas, C. M. C. Allen, S. J. Boniface, J. D. Pickard, I. V. Kendall, S. P. M. J. Downer, J. C. Clark, T. A. Carpenter, and N. Antoun. 1998. Cortical processing in persistent vegetative state. *Lancet* 352: 800.

Menon, R. S., and S.-G. Kim. 1999. Spatial and temporal limits in cognitive neuro-imaging with fMRI. *Trends in Cognitive Sciences* 3: 207–216.

Metzinger, T. 2000. The subjectivity of subjective experience: A representationalist analysis of the first-person perspective. In T. Metzinger, ed., *Neural Correlates of Consciousness*, pp. 285–306. Cambridge: MIT Press.

Metzinger, T. 2003. *Being No One: The Self-Model Theory of Subjectivity*. Cambridge: MIT Press.

Millar, S. 1994. *Understanding and Representing Space: Theory and Evidence from Studies with Blind and Sighted Children*. Oxford: Oxford University Press.

Millikan, R. 1984. *Language, Thought, and Other Biological Categories*. Cambridge: MIT Press.

Mithen, S. 1996. *The Prehistory of the Mind*. London: Thames and Hudson.

Montague, P. R., and P. Dayan. 1998. Neurobiological modeling. In W. Bechtel and G. Graham, eds., *A Companion to Cognitive Science*, pp. 526–541. Oxford: Blackwells.

Montague, P. R., P. Dayan, and T. J. Sejnowski. 1993. Foraging in an uncertain environment using predictive Hebbian learning. In J. D. Cowan, G. Tesauro, and J.

Alspector, eds., *Advances in Neural Information Processing Systems, 6*. San Mateo, Calif.: Morgan Kaufman Publishers.

Montague, P. R., and S. R. Quartz. 1999. Computational approaches to neural reward and development. *Mental Retardation and Developmental Disabilities Research Reviews* 5: 1–14.

Moser, P. K., and J. D. Trout, eds. 1995. *Contemporary Materialism: A Reader*. London: Routledge.

Mountcastle, V. B. 1957. Modality and topographic properties of single neurons of cat's somatic sensory cortex. *Journal of Neurophysiology* 20: 408–434.

Murray, D. S. 1988. *A History of Western Psychology*. 2nd ed. Englewood Cliffs, N.J.: Prentice-Hall.

Nagel, T. 1994. Consciousness and objective reality. In R. Warner and T. Szubka, eds., *The Mind-Body Problem: A Guide to the Current Debate*, pp. 63–68. Oxford: Blackwells.

Necker, L. A. 1832. Observations on some remarkable phenomena seen in Switzerland: an optical phenomenon which occurs on viewing of a crystal or geometrical solid. *Philosophical Magazine* 3: 329–337.

Nelson, C. A., and M. Luciana, eds. 2001. *The Handbook of Developmental Cognitive Neuroscience*. Cambridge: MIT Press.

Nieder, A., and H. Wagner. 1999. Perception and neuronal coding of subjective contours in the owl. *Nature Neuroscience* 2: 660–663.

Nieuwenhuys, R. 1985. *Chemoarchitecture of the Brain*. New York: Springer-Verlag.

Nieuwenhuys, R., J. Voogd, and C. van Huijzen. 1981. *The Human Central Nervous System: A Synopsis and Atlas*. New York: Springer-Verlag.

Northcutt, R. G. 1977. Nervous system (vertebrate). In *McGraw-Hill Encyclopedia of Science and Technology*, vol. 9, pp. 90–96.

Nosofsky, R. M., and T. J. Palmeri. 1997. An exemplar-based random walk model of speeded classification. *Psychological Review* 104: 266–300.

O'Brien, G., and J. Opie. 1999. A connectionist theory of phenomenal experience. *Behavioral and Brain Sciences* 22: 127–148.

O'Keefe, J., and J. Dostrovsky. 1971. The hippocampus as a spatial map. Preliminary evidence from unit activity in the freely moving rat. *Experimental Brain Research* 34: 171–175.

O'Regan, J. K. 1992. Solving the "real" mysteries of visual perception: the world as an outside memory. *Canadian Journal of Psychology* 46: 461–488.

Orgel, L. E. 1999. The origin of life on Earth. In *Revolutions in Science*, pp. 18–25. New York: Scientific American.

Osherson, D., ed. 1990. *Invitation to Cognitive Science*. Vols. 1–3. Cambridge: MIT Press.

Oxford Dictionary of Physics. 1996. Oxford: Oxford University Press.

Packard, M., and L. Teather. 1998a. Amygdala modulation of multiple memory systems: hippocampus and caudate-putamen. *Neurobiology of Learning and Memory* 69: 163–203.

Packard, M., and L. Teather. 1998b. Double dissociation of hippocampal and dorsal-striatal memory systems by post-training intra-cerebral injections of 2-amino-phospho-pentanoic acid. *Behavioral Neuroscience* 111: 543–551.

Paine, T. 1794. *The Age of Reason: Being an Investigation of True and Fabulous Theology*. New York: Putnam's Sons, 1896.

Palmer, S. E. 1999. *Vision Science: Photons to Phenomenology*. Cambridge: MIT Press.

Panksepp, Jaak. 1998. *Affective Neuroscience*. New York: Oxford University Press.

Panksepp, Jaak, and Jules B. Panksepp. 2000. The seven sins of evolutionary psychology. *Evolution and Cognition* 6: 108–131.

Panksepp, Jaak, and Jules B. Panksepp. 2001a. A synopsis of "The seven sins of evolutionary psychology." *Evolution and Cognition* 7: 2–5.

Panksepp, Jaak, and Jules B. Panksepp. 2001b. A continuing critique of evolutionary psychology. *Evolution and Cognition* 7: 56–80.

Papez, J. W. 1937. A proposed mechanism of emotion. *Archives of Neurology and Psychiatry* 38: 725–744.

Parvizi, J., and A. R. Damasio. 2001. Consciousness and the brainstem. *Cognition* 79: 135–159.

Pascual-Leone, A., and V. Walsh. 2001. *Science* 292: 510–512.

Patel, A. D., and E. Balaban. 2001. Human pitch perception is reflected in the timing of stimulus-related cortical activity. *Nature Neuroscience* 4: 839–844.

Pearl, J. 1988. *Probabilistic Reasoning in Intelligent Systems: Networks of Plausible Inference*. San Mateao: Morgan Kaufman.

Penrose, R. 1994. *Shadows of the Mind*. Oxford: Oxford University Press.

Penrose, R., and S. Hameroff. 1995. What "gaps"? Reply to Grush and Churchland. *Journal of Consciousness Studies* 2: 99–112.

Perry, J. 2001. *Knowledge, Possibility, and Consciousness.* Cambridge: MIT Press.

Persinger, Michael A. 1987. *Neuropsychological Bases of God Beliefs.* New York: Praeger.

Peterhans, E., and R. von der Heydt. 1991. Subjective contours—bridging the gap between psychophysics and physiology. *Trends in Neurosciences* 14: 112–119.

Pinker, S. 1997. *How the Mind Works.* New York: Norton.

Plato. 1997. *Euthyphro.* Trans by G. M. A. Grube. In J. M. Cooper, and D. S. Hutchinson, eds., *Plato: Complete Works*, pp. 1–16. Indianapolis: Hackett Publishing Co.

Plotkin, H. C., and F. J. Odling-Smee. 1981. A multiple-level model of evolution and its implications for sociobiology. *Behavioral and Brain Sciences* 4: 225–268.

Poeck, K. 1969. Pathophysiology of emotional disorders associated with brain damage. In P. J. Vinken and G. W. Bruyn, eds., *Handbook of Clinical Neurology*, vol. 3. Amsterdam: North-Holland Publishing Co.

Polonsky, A., R. Blake, J. Braun, and D. Heeger. 2000. Neuronal activity in human primary visual cortex correlates with perception during binocular rivalry. *Nature Neuroscience* 3: 1153–1159.

Popper, K. R. 1959. *The Logic of Scientific Discovery.* New York: Harper & Row.

Posner, M. I. 1995. Attention in cognitive neuroscience: an overview. In M. Gazzaniga, ed., *The Cognitive Neurosciences*, pp. 615–624. Cambridge: MIT Press.

Posner, M. I., and M. E. Raichle. 1994. *Images of Mind.* New York: Scientific American Library.

Pouget, A., and T. J. Sejnowski. 1997a. Spatial transformations in the parietal cortex using basis functions. *Journal of Cognitive Neuroscience* 9 (2): 222–237.

Pouget, A., and T. J. Sejnowski. 1997b. Lesion in a basis function model of parietal cortex: comparison with hemineglect. In P. Thier and H.-O. Karnath, eds., *Parietal Contributions to Orientation in 3D Space*, pp. 521–538. Heidelberg: Springer-Verlag.

Povinell, D. 2000. *Folk Physics for Apes: The Chimpanzee Theory of How the World Works.* Oxford: Oxford University Press.

Premack, D. 1988. "Does the chimpanzee have a theory of mind" revisited. In R. W. Byrne and A. Whiten, eds., *Machiavellian Intelligence, Social Expertise, and the Evolution of Intellect in Monkeys, Apes, and Humans*, pp. 160–179. Oxford: Oxford University Press.

Puccetti, R. 1981. The case for mental duality: evidence from split-brain data and other considerations. *Behavioral and Brain Sciences* 4: 93–123.

Purpura, K. P., and N. D. Schiff. 1997. The thalamic intralaminar nuclei: a role in visual awareness. *Neuroscientist* 3: 314–321.

Purves, D., G. J. Augustine, D. Fitzpatrick, L. C. Katz, A.-S. LaMantia, J. O. McNamara, and S. M. Williams. 2001. *Neuroscience.* 2nd ed. Sunderland, Mass.: Sinauer Associates.

Putnam, H. 1967. Psychological predicates. In W. H. Capitan and D. D. Merrill, eds., *Art, Mind, and Religion*, pp. 37–48. Pittsburgh: University of Pittsburgh Press.

Putnam, H. 1994. The best of all possible brains? Review of *Shadows of the Mind*, by R. Penrose. *New York Times Book Review*, November.

Pylyshyn, Z. 1984. *Computation and Cognition.* Cambridge: MIT Press.

Quartz, S. R. 1999. The constructivist brain. *Trends in Cognitive Sciences* 3 (2): 48–57.

Quartz, S. R. In press. Toward a developmental evolutionary psychology: genes, development, and the evolution of the human cognitive architecture. In S. J. Scher and F. Rauscher, eds., *Evolutionary Psychology: Alternative Approaches.* Boston: Kluwer Press.

Quartz, S. R., and T. J. Sejnowski. 1997. The neural basis of cognitive development: a constructivist manifesto. *Behavioral and Brain Sciences* 3: 48–57.

Quartz, S. R., and T. J. Sejnowski. 2002. *Liars, Lovers, and Heroes: What the New Brain Science Reveals about How We Become Who We Are.* New York: Harper-Collins.

Quine, W. V. O. 1960. *Word and Object.* Cambridge: MIT Press.

Quine, W. V. O. 1969. Epistemology naturalized. In his *Ontological Relativity and Other Essays*, pp. 69–90. New York: Columbia University Press.

Raine, A., J. R. Meloy, S. Bihrle, J. Stoddard, L. LaCasse, and M. S. Buchsbaum. 1998. Reduced prefrontal and increased subcortical brain functioning assessed using positron emission tomography in predatory and affective murderers. *Behavioral Sciences and the Law* 16: 319–332.

Raine, A., M. S. Buchsbaum, and L. LaCasse. 1997. Brain abnormalities in murderers indicated by positron emission tomography. *Biological Psychiatry* 42: 495–508.

Ramachandran, V. S., and S. Blakeslee. 1998. *Phantoms in the Brain: Probing the Mysteries of the Human Mind.* New York: Morrow.

Real, Leslie. 1991. Animal choice behavior and the evolution of cognitive architecture. *Science* 253: 980–986.

Rennie, J. ed. 1999. *Revolutions in Science.* New York: Scientific American.

Ridley, M. 1999. *Genome: The Autobiography of a Species in 23 Chapters.* New York: Harper Collins.

Rizzolatti, G., L. Fogassi, and V. Gallese. 2001. Neurophysiological mechanisms underlying the understanding and imitation of action. *Nature Reviews: Neuroscience* 2: 661–670.

Robbins, T. W., and B. J. Everitt. 1995. Arousal systems and attention. In M. Gazzaniga, ed., *The Cognitive Neurosciences*, pp. 703–720. Cambridge: MIT Press.

Rock, I. 1975. *An Introduction to Perception*. New York: Macmillan.

Rodman, H. 1999. Temporal cortex. In G. Adelman and B. H. Smith, eds., *Encyclopedia of Neuroscience*, pp. 2022–2025. New York: Elsevier.

Rolls, E. T. 1989. Parallel distributed processing in the brain: implications of the functional architecture of neuronal networks in the hippocampus. In R. G. M. Morris, ed., *Parallel Distributed Processing: Implications for Psychology and Neuroscience*, pp. 286–308. Oxford: Oxford University Press.

Rorty, A. O. 1986. *Essays on Descartes' Meditations*. Berkeley: University of California Press.

Rorty, R., ed. 1967. *The Linguistic Turn: Recent Essays in Philosophical Method*. Chicago: University of Chicago Press.

Rosch, E. (Eleanor Heider). 1973. Natural categories. *Cognitive Psychology* 4: 328–350.

Rosch, E. 1978. Principles of categorization. In E. Rosch and B. Lloyd, eds., *Cognition and Categorization*, pp. 27–48. Hillsdale, N.J.: Lawrence Erlbaum & Associates.

Rosenthal, D. M. 1997. A theory of consciousness. In N. Block, O. Flanagan, and G. Güzeldere, eds., *The Nature of Consciousness*, pp. 729–754. Cambridge: MIT Press.

Rumford, T. 1798. Heat is a form of motion: an experiment in boring cannon. *Philosophical Transactions* 88.

Ruse, M. 1991. Evolutionary ethics and the search for predecessors: Kant, Hume, and all the way back to Aristotle? *Society for Philosophy and Politics* 8: 59–85.

Russell, B. 1935. *Religion and Science*. London: Oxford University Press.

Ryle, G. 1954. *Dilemmas*. Cambridge: Cambridge University Press.

Sakata, H., and M. Taira. 1994. Parietal control of hand action. *Current Opinion in Neurobiology* 4: 847–856. Reprinted in Squire and Kosslyn 1998.

Savage-Rumbaugh, S., and R. Lewin. 1994. *Kanzi: The Ape at the Brink of the Human Mind*. New York: John Wiley and Sons.

Saver, J. L., and A. R. Damasio. 1991. Preserved access and processing of social knowledge in a patient with acquired sociopathy due to ventromedial frontal damage. *Neuropsychologia* 29: 1241–1249.

Schaal, S. 1999. Is imitation learning the route to humanoid robots? *Trends in Cognitive Sciences* 3: 233–242.

Schacter, D. L. 1996. *Searching for Memory: The Brain, the Mind, and the Past*. New York: Basic Books.

Schleiden, M. J. 1838. Beiträge zur Phytogenesis. *Arch. Anat. Physiol. Wiss. Med.*, 137–176.

Schlick, M. 1939. When is a man responsible? In his *Problems of Ethics*, pp. 143–156. New York: Prentice-Hall.

Schore, A. N. 1994. *Affect Regulation and the Origin of the Self*. Hillsdale, N.J.: Lawrence Erlbaum & Associates.

Schulkin, J. 2000. *Roots of Social Sensibility and Neural Function*. Cambridge: MIT Press.

Schultz, W., P. Dayan, and P. R. Montague. 1997. A neural substrate of prediction and reward. *Science* 275: 1593–1599.

Schwann, T. 1839. Mikroskopische Untersuchungen über die Übereinstimmung in der Structur und dem Wachsthum der Thiere und Pflanzen. Berlin: G. E. Reimer, Sandersche Buchh.

Searle, J. 1992. *The Rediscovery of the Mind*. Cambridge: MIT Press.

Sekuler, R., and R. Blake. 1994. *Perception*. 3rd ed. New York: McGraw-Hill.

Sellars, W. 1956. Empiricism and the philosophy of mind. In H. Fiegl and and M. Scriven, eds., *The Foundations of Science and the Concepts of Psychology and Psychoanalysis*, Minnesota Studies in the Philosophy of Science, no. 1, pp. 253–329. Minneapolis: University of Minnesota Press. Reprinted in W. Sellars, *Science, Perception, and Reality*. New York: Routledge and Kegan Paul, 1963.

Semendeferi, K., A. Lu, N. Schenker, and H. Damasio. 2002. Humans and great apes share a large frontal cortex. *Nature Neuroscience* 5: 272–276.

Sharp, F. R., M. Tomitaka, M. Bernaudin, and S. Tomitaka 2001. Psychosis: pathological activation of limbic thalamocortical circuits by psychomimetics and schizophrenia? *Trends in Neurosciences* 6: 330–334.

Sheinberg, N. L., and N. K. Logothetis. 1997. The role of temporal cortical areas in perceptual organization. *Proceedings of the National Academy of Sciences, USA* 94: 3408–3414.

Shepherd, G. M. 1979. *The Synaptic Organization of the Brain*. 2nd ed. Oxford: Oxford University Press.

Siegelmann, H. T., and E. D. Sontag. 1995. On the computational power of neural nets. *Journal of Computer and System Sciences* 50: 132–150.

Singer, W. 2000. Phenomenal awareness and consciousness from a neurobiological perspective. In T. Metzinger, ed., *Neural Correlates of Consciousness*, pp. 121–137. Cambridge: MIT Press.

Skyrms, B. 1966. *Choice and Chance· An Introduction to Inductive Logic*. Belmont, Calif.: Dickenson.

Smullyan, R. 1992. *Gödel's Incompleteness Theorems*. Oxford: Oxford University Press.

Sober, E., and D. Wilson. 1998. *Unto Others: The Evolution and Psychology of Unselfish Behavior*. Cambridge: Harvard University Press.

Solomon, R. 1995. Living well: the virtues and the good life. In his *Handbook for Ethics*. New York: Harcourt Brace and Jovanovich.

Sperry, R. W. 1974. Lateral specialization in the surgically separated hemispheres. In F. O. Schmitt and F. G. Worden, eds., *The Neurosciences: Third Study Program*, pp. 5–19. Cambridge: MIT Press.

Spirtes, P., C. Glymour, and R. Scheines. 2000. *Causation, Prediction, and Search*. 2nd, rev. ed. Cambridge: MIT Press.

Squire, L. R., and P. Alvarez. 1995. Retrograde amnesia and memory consolidation: a neurobiological perspective. *Current Opinion in Neurobiology* 5: 169–177. Reprinted in L. R. Squire and S. M. Kosslyn, eds., *Findings and Current Opinion in Cognitive Neuroscience*, pp. 75–83. Cambridge: MIT Press, 1998.

Squire, L. R., and B. H. Knowlton. 1995. Memory, hippocampus, and brain systems. In M. S. Gazzaniga, ed., *The Cognitive Neurosciences*. Cambridge: MIT Press.

Squire, L. R., and E. R. Kandel. 1999. *Memory: From Mind to Molecules*. New York: Scientific American Library.

Squire, L. R., and S. M. Kosslyn, eds. 1998. *Findings and Current Opinion in Cognitive Neuroscience*. Cambridge: MIT Press.

Squire, L. R., and S. M. Zola. 1996. Ischemic brain damage and memory impairment: a commentary. *Hippocampus* 6: 546–552.

Squire, L. R., and S. Zola-Morgan. 1991. The medial temporal lobe memory system. *Science* 253: 1380–1386.

Stapp, H. P. 1999. Attention, intention, and will in quantum physics. In B. Libet, A. Freeman, and K. Sutherland, eds., *The Volitional Brain: Towards a Neuroscience of Free Will*, pp. 143–164. New York: Academic Press.

Stephens, G. L., and G. Graham. 2000. *When Self-Consciousness Breaks: Alien Voices and Inserted Thoughts*. Cambridge: MIT Press.

Stevens, J. K., R. C. Emerson, G. L. Gerstein, T. Kallos, G. R. Neufeld, C. W. Nichols, and A. C. Rosenquist. 1976. Paralysis of the awake human: visual perception. *Vision Research* 16: 93–98.

Stickgold, R., A. James, and J. A. Hobson. 2000. Visual discrimination learning requires sleep after training. *Nature Neuroscience* 3: 1237–1238.

Stiles, J. 2001. Spatial cognitive development. In C. A. Nelson and M. Luciana, eds., *The Handbook of Developmental Cognitive Neuroscience*, pp. 399–414. Cambridge: MIT Press.

Sugiura, N., R. G. Patel, and R. A. Corriveau. 2001. NMDA receptors regulate a group of transiently expressed genes in the developing brain. *Journal of Biological Chemistry* 276: 14257–14263.

Suri, R. E. 2001. Anticipatory responses of dopamine neurons and cortical neurons reproduced by internal model. *Experimental Brain Research* 140: 234–240.

Sutton, R. S., and A. G. Barto. 1998. *Reinforcement Learning: An Introduction.* Cambridge: MIT Press.

Swinburne, R. 1994. Body and soul. In R. Warner and T. Szubka, eds., *The Mind-Body Problem: A Guide to the Current Debate*, pp. 311–316. Oxford: Blackwells.

Taylor, R. 1992. *Metaphysics.* 4th ed. Englewood Cliffs, N.J.: Prentice-Hall.

Thagard, P. 1998a. Ulcers and bacteria. I: Discovery and acceptance. *Studies in History and Philosophy of Science. Part C: Studies in History and Philosophy of Biological and Biomedical Sciences* 29: 107–136.

Thagard, P. 1998b. Ulcers and bacteria. II: Instruments, experiments, and social interactions. *Studies in History and Philosophy of Science. Part C: Studies in History and Philosophy of Biological and Biomedical Sciences* 29: 317–342.

Thagard, P. 1999. *How Scientists Explain Disease.* Princeton: Princeton University Press.

Thelen, E. 1995. Time-scale dynamics and the development of an embodied cognition. In R. Port and T. van Gelder. *Mind as Motion: Explorations in the Dynamics of Cognition*, pp. 69–100. Cambridge: MIT Press.

Tomasello, M. 1992. *First verbs: a case study of early grammatical development.* Cambridge: Cambridge University Press.

Tomasello, M. 1999. The cultural ecology of children's interactions with objects and artifacts. In E. Winograd, R. Fivush, and W. Hirst, eds., *Ecological Approaches to Cognition: Essays in Honor of Ulrich Neisser.* Hillsdale, N.J.: Lawrence Erlbaum & Associates.

Tomasello, M. 2000. *The Cultures and Origins of Human Cognition.* Cambridge: Harvard University Press.

Tomasello, M., and J. Call. 1997. *Primate Cognition*. New York: Oxford University Press.

Tononi, G., G. M. Edelman, and O. Sporns. 1998. Complexity and coherency: integrating information in the brain. *Trends in Cognitive Sciences* 12: 474–484.

Tootell, R. B. H., J. B. Reppas, A. M. Dale, R. B. Look, and M. I. Sereno. 1995. Visual motion aftereffect in human cortical area MT revealed by functional magnetic resonance imaging. *Nature* 375: 139.

Torres, E. B. 2001. Theoretical framework for the study of sensory-motor integration. Ph.D. dissertation, University of California at San Diego.

Torres, E., and D. Zipser. 1999. Constraint satisfaction and error correction in multi-joint arm reaching movements. *Annual Society for Neuroscience Meeting Abstracts*, abstract no. 760.9.

Tsien, J. Z., P. T. Huerta, and S. Tonegawa. 1996. The essential role of hippocampal CA1 NMDA receptor-dependent synaptic plasticiy in spatial memory. *Cell* 87: 1327–1338.

Turrigiano, G. 1999. Homeostatic plasticity in neuronal networks: the more things change, the more they stay the same. *Trends in Neurosciences* 22: 221–227.

Van Inwagen, P. 1975. The incompatibility of free will and determinism. *Philosophical Studies* 27: 185–199. Reprinted in G. Watson, ed., *Free Will*, pp. 46–58. Oxford: Oxford University Press, 1982.

Vendler, Z. 1994. The ineffable soul. In R. Warner and T. Szubka, eds., *The Mind-Body Problem: A Guide to the Current Debate*, pp. 317–328. Oxford: Blackwells.

Vogt, B. A., D. M. Finch, and C. R. Olson. 1992. Functional heterogeneity in the cingulate cortex: the anterior executive and the posterior evaluative regions. *Cerebral Cortex* 2: 435–443.

Von Neumann, J. 2000. *The Computer and the Brain*. 2nd ed. Foreword by P. M. Churchland and P. S. Churchland. New Haven: Yale University Press.

Walsh, V., and A. Cowey. 2000. Transcranial magnetic stimulation and cognitive neuroscience. *Nature Reviews: Neuroscience* 1: 73–80.

Walter, H. 2000. *Neurophilosophy of Free Will: From Libertarian Illusions to a Concept of Natural Autonomy*. Cambridge: MIT Press.

Wann, J., and M. Land. 2000. Steering with or without the flow: is retrieval of heading necessary? *Trends in Cognitive Sciences* 4: 319–324.

Warner, R. 1994. In defense of a dualism. In R. Warner and T. Szubka, eds., *The Mind-Body Problem: A Guide to the Current Debate*, pp. 343–354. Oxford: Blackwells.

Webster's New Collegiate Dictionary. 1981. Toronto: Allen and Son.

Wegner, D. M. 2002. *The Illusion of Conscious Will*. Cambridge: MIT Press.

Weiskrantz, L. 1997. *Consciousness Lost and Found: A Neuropsychological Exploration*. Oxford: Oxford University Press.

Wellman, H. M., A. K. Hickling, and C. A. Schult. 1997. Young children's psychological, physical, and biological explanations. In H. M. Wellman and K. Inagaki, eds., *The Emergence of Core Domains of Thought: Children's Reasoning about Physical, Psychological and Biological Phenomena*, pp. 7–25. San Francisco: Jossey-Bass.

Wertheim, A. H., B. S. Mesland, and W. Bles. 2001. Cognitive suppression of tilt sensations during linear self-motion in the dark. *Perception* 30: 733–741.

Willatts, P. 1984. The stage-IV infant's solution to problems requiring the use of supports. *Infant Behavior and Development* 7: 125–134.

Willatts, P. 1989. Development of problem-solving in infancy. In A. Slater and G. Bremmer, eds., *Infant Development*, pp. 143–182. Hillsdale, N.J.: Lawrence Erlbaum & Associates.

Williams, G. C. 1996. *Plan and Purpose in Nature*. London: Weidenfeld and Nicolson.

Wilson, E. O. 1975. *Sociobiology: The New Synthesis*. Cambridge: Harvard University Press.

Wilson, E. O. 1998. *Consilience: The Unity of Knowledge*. New York: Knopf.

Wilson, M. A., and B. L. McNaughton. 1994. Reactivation of hippocampal ensemble memories during sleep. *Science* 265: 676–679.

Wilson, R. A., and F. Keil, eds. 1999. *The MIT Encyclopedia of the Cognitive Sciences*. Cambridge: MIT Press.

Wittgenstein, L. 1958. *Philosophical Investigations*. Translated by G. E. M. Anscombe. Oxford: Blackwells.

Wolpert, D. M., Z. Ghahramani, and M. I. Jordan. 1995. An internal model for sensorimotor integration. *Science* 269: 1880–1882.

Wolpert, L. 1991. *The Triumph of the Embryo*. Oxford: Oxford University Press.

Wundt, W. 1862. *Beiträge zur Theorie der Sinneswahrnehmung* (Contributions to the theory of sense-perception). The introduction, entitled "On the methods of psychology," is translated in T. Shipley, ed., *Classics in Psychology*. New York: Philosophical Library, 1961.

Yarbus, A. L. 1967. *Eye Movements and Vision*. Translated by L. A. Riggs. New York: Plenum.

Yates, J. 1985. The content of consciousness is a model of the world. *Psychological Review* 92: 249–284.

Young, R. M. 1970. *Mind, Brain, and Adaptation in the Nineteenth Century*. New York: Oxford University Press.

Zajonc, R. 1980. Feeling and thinking: preferences need no inferences. *American Psychologist* 35: 151–175.

Zhang, K., I. Ginzburg, B. L. McNaughten, and T. J. Sejnowski. 1998. Interpreting neuronal population activity by reconstruction: unified framework with application to hippocampal place cells. *Journal of Neurophysiology* 79: 1017–1044.

Zigmond, M. J., F. E. Bloom, S. C. Landis, J. L. Roberts, L. R. Squire. 1999. *Fundamental Neuroscience*. San Diego: Academic Press.

Zipser, D., B. Kehoe, G. Littlewort, and J. Fuster. 1993. A spiking network model of short-term active memory. *Journal of Neuroscience* 13: 3406–3420.

Websites

BioMedNet Magazine: http://news.bmn.com/magazine

Encyclopedia of Life Sciences: http://www.els.net

The MIT Encyclopedia of the Cognitive Sciences: http://cognet.mit.edu/MITECS

Moon illusion: http://www.uwsp.edu/acad/psych/sh/moon.htm

Index

Bogen, Joseph, 44
Bonobo chimpanzees, 253
  verbal behavior of, 143
Brain(s), chimpanzee, 248
Brain(s), human, 1
  abnormal effects of stress on, 395
  and access, 159
  as active constructor, 271, 279, 368
  of autistics, 116–117
  and awareness vs. nonawareness of
    stimulus, 136, 137
  vs. brains of other primates, 202
  as causal machine, 204–205
  cleverness of whole from stupidity of
    components in, 329
  coherencing functions of, x, 17, 165
  and computers, 284–285, 329
  diagram of
    from medial aspect, 138
    showing interhemispheric connections,
      45
    showing motor areas, 89
    showing position of V1, 151
    showing temporal lobe, 139
    3-D reconstructions of, 60
  emulators in, 80–88
  as evolutionary product, 40, 283
    vs. product of clever engineer, 254
  function of, 31
  hemispheres of, 44–47
  Hippocrates on, 6, 10
  and knowledge, 329
  and mind or mental phenomena, 30, 46,
    47–50, 254, 393
    and soul-brain hypothesis, 47
  and other mammalian brains, 248, 250,
    252
  and other selves, 107
  parallel networks in, 304
  and pragmatists' view of metaphysics, 40
  and representations, 64–65, 271, 273,
    275, 321 (*see also* Representations)
    of external world, 106
  scientific discoveries regarding, 43
  and self, 61–62, 124–125
  self-concept as derived from, 61–62
  somatosensory signals in, 94
  study of, 10–20, 368–369
  and sublime feeling, 401
  ventricles in, 257
Brain(s), monkey, 89, 111, 161, 213
  mirror neurons in, 101, 109
  predictor neurons in, 340
Brain(s), mouse, 248
Brain(s), rat, 215, 217
Brain(s), vertebrate
  evolution of, 246
  major divisions in, 247
Brain-averse approach to representations,
  273–274, 305
Brain damage/lesions, 256
  and avoidance, 342
  and decision-making habits, 230
  and feeling of fear (case of S.M.), 231,
    235
  and neural emulators, 85
  and practical judgment (case of E.V.R.),
    222–227, 235
  and religion, 373 (*see also* Religion)
  and self-representation, 70
  in amnesia patient, 65
  in parietal cortex, 67–68
  and spatial problem solving, 277
  and voluntary movement, 212–213
Brain-friendly approach to
  representations, 273, 274
Brain-mapping techniques, 18, 19
Brainstem, 60, 73, 92, 104
  and attentional functions, 169
  of monkey, 339
  of rat, 93
  and temporal-lobe seizures, 386
Brecht, Bertolt, quoted, 1
British Empiricism
  epistemology of, 244
  theory of inferential vs. noninferential
    judgments of, 123
Brunschwig, Hieronymous, 257
Buddhism, 374, 391
Bulimia, 70

Neuronal structures and representational
  mapping, 275
Neurons, 12–16
  back-projecting vs. forward-projecting,
    148–149
  coding in, 285–290
  computations performed by, 26
  vs. computer chips, 285
  connectivity modifications in, 330–334
  coordination through, 71
  discovery of, 10, 12
  examination of, 255–256
  imaging techniques for, 18–20
  integrate-and-fire model of, 258
  long-axon, 160
  mirror, 101, 108, 109
  networks of (*see* Neural networks)
  place, 277
  place coding in, 289, 290, 291
  projective fields of, 288
  receptive fields of, 287–288
  reinforcement learning in vum neuron,
    336–337
  schematic diagram of, 194
  similarity of, throughout animal
    kingdom, 252, 254
  tuning of, 138, 287–288
  vector coding in, 289, 290, 290–291
  vector/parameter space of, 292
  weight configurations of, 300, 302
Neurophilosophy, 2–5
  advent of, vii
  integration of, with cognitive science and
    philosophy, 2
  questions for, 369
Neurophilosophical explanation of
    consciousness, naysaying arguments
    against, 173–174, 198
  argument from ignorance, 174–176
  consciousness as subatomic effect, 195–
    197
  limitations of science, 174, 197
  problem is excessively difficult, 178–180
  scientific fact vs. phenomenal experience,
    180–193
  zombies as logical possibility, 176–178

Neurophysiology and declarative
  memory, 358–361
Neuroscience, viii–ix
  antireductionist view of, 25–27
  and brain, 1
  and brain-averse approach, 273–274
  and brain studying itself, 368
  and causation, 50, 53
  cognitive, 53, 123
  and cognitive science, 2, 27, 30
  and decision making, 236
  discovery in, 2
  and humans as knowers, 366
  as nascent, 4
  and philosophers/philosophy, vii, viii, x,
    32
  progress in, 169–170
  and quantum indeterminacy, 233–234
  and religion, 373 (*see also* Religion)
Neurosemantics, 302–305
Neurotransmitters, 14, 286
  and attention, 158
  in decision making, 214
  and microtubules, 195
Newborn humans
  body representation of, 100–101
  causal knowledge of, 106–107
Newton, Sir Isaac, 12, 25, 38, 131, 172,
  243
Nicomachean Ethics (Aristotle), 211
Nicotine, 111
NMDA (N-methyl-D-aspartate), 326,
  346, 348, 357
NMDA receptors, 345, 349, 358
N-methyl-D-aspartate (NMDA), 326,
  346, 348, 357
Nonconscious cognition, 48–50, 51, 52
  in sensorimotor problem, 77
Nonconscious processing in experience of
  self, 118–119
Nonconscious representation, 158–159
Nondeclarative memory, 354
Nonexistence, demonstration of, 172
Norepinephrine (NE), 103
  in decision making, 214
Nucleus accumbens, 74, 341